NAVIGATIONAL SURGERY OF THE FACIAL SKELETON

A. Schramm, N.-C. Gellrich,
R. Schmelzeisen

Navigational Surgery of the Facial Skeleton

With 129 Figures

Springer

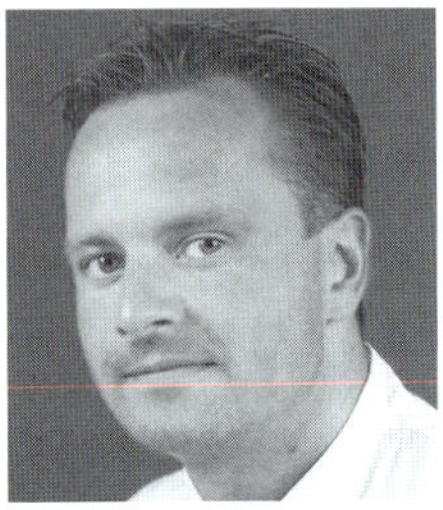

Alexander Schramm, MD DDS
Professor and Vicechairman
Dept. of Oral and Maxillofacial Surgery
Medical School Hannover
Carl-Neuberg-Straße 1
30625 Hannover, Germany

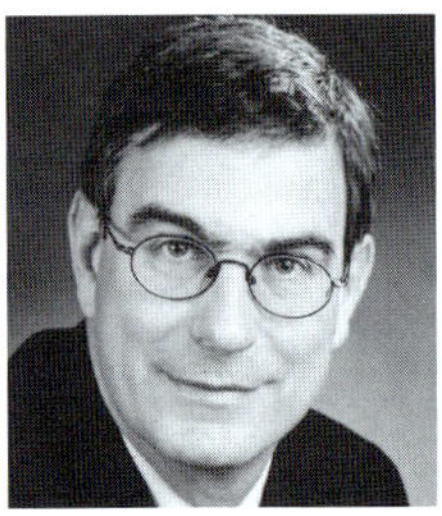

Nils-Claudius Gellrich, MD DDS
Professor and Chairman
Dept. of Oral and Maxillofacial Surgery
Medical School Hannover
Carl-Neuberg-Straße 1
30625 Hannover, Germany

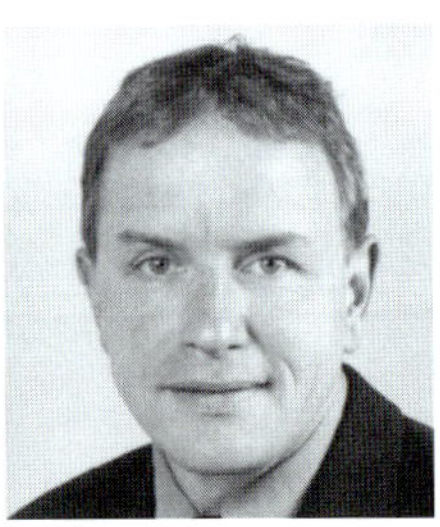

Rainer Schmelzeisen, MD DDS
Professor and Chairman
Dept. of Oral and Maxillofacial Surgery
University Hospital Freiburg
Hugstetterstraße 55
79106 Freiburg i. Br., Germany

Library of Congress
Control Number 2006935422
ISBN-10 3-540-22357-6
Springer Berlin Heidelberg New York
ISBN-13 978-3-540-22357-3
Springer Berlin Heidelberg New York

Springer is a part of Springer Science+Business Media

springer.com

Editor: Gabriele Schröder, Heidelberg, Germany
Desk Editor: Martina Himberger, Heidelberg, Germany
Cover design: Frido Steinen-Broo, EStudio Calamar, Spain
Production: LE-TeX Jelonek, Schmidt & Vöckler GbR, Leipzig, Germany
Reproduction and typesetting: AM-productions GmbH, Wiesloch, Germany

Printed on acid-free paper 27/3100/YL – 5 4 3 2 1 0

Preface

Navigational surgery in the craniomaxillofacial field started to become clinically applicable in the 1990s. Its distribution into daily routine, however, was limited due to the fact that all navigation systems narrowly addressed neurosurgical needs, which are basically to find a 3D structure within a 3D volume. However, in the field of craniomaxillofacial surgery these neurosurgery-oriented navigation systems had to be adapted and the software changed, especially with respect to preoperative planning, including virtual model building and following the pre-op plan during surgery. This changed the workflow in the field of navigational surgery in the craniomaxillofacial field so greatly that a separate imaging analysis platform for pre- and postoperative assessment and quality control became more and more demanding.

The authors have promoted the idea of pre- and postoperative planning and the interface of these imaging analysis achievements with intraoperative navigation. This has led, over recent years, to a very beneficial implementation of modern technology into the area of patient care. We implemented this technique into our daily routines in our departments and we even promoted the idea of preoperative planning in teaching of our residents and students, so that every voxel-based data set is now assessed on an imaging analysis platform. Furthermore, we found it useful that pre- and postoperative image fusion of voxel-based datasets led to a unique type of quality control with respect to surgically achieved results.

We hope that through this book we can share the ideas we had and achievements we made during the last ten years. We hope that the next generation of surgeons will have the chance to include these achievements in their daily practical work.

Alexander Schramm, Nils-Claudius Gellrich
and Rainer Schmelzeisen

Acknowledgement

The authors wish to thank all our colleagues and coworkers who participated and contributed to the treatment of our patients. (Dr. Barth, Dr. Bormann, Dr. Rücker, Dr. Brachvogel, Prof. Eckardt, Dr. Dini, Dr. Eulzer, Dr. Wenzel, Dr. Glaum, Dr. Mölle, Dr. Tavassol, Dr. Sinikovic, Dr. Kokemüller, Dr. Grotzer, Dr. Schrader, Dr. Sendic, Dr. Starke, Dr. Schumann, Dr. Becker, Dr. Stöver, Dr. Majdani, Dr. Leinung, Dr. Götz, Dr. Donnerstag, Dr. Keberle, Prof. Piepenbrock, Prof. Haubitz, Prof. Galanski, Prof. Krauss, Prof. Schwestka-Polly, Prof. Stiesch-Scholz, Prof. Lenarz, the OR teams and the in- and outpatient teams from the Medical School Hannover, Germany; Dr. Schön, Dr. Zizelmann, Dr. Hohlweg-Majert, Dr. Stricker, Dr. Sakkas, Dr. Gutwald, Dr. Schwarz, Dr. Fakler, Dr. Swaid, Dr. Cufi, Dr. Held, Dr. Schimming, Dr. Schupp, Dr. Spreer, Dr. Galli, Dr. Schneider, Dr. Randelzhofer, Mr. Gläser, Dr. Nilius, Dr. Spetzger, Dr. Hubbe, Dr. Buitrago-Télles, Dr. Aschendorf, Dr. Henne, Dr. Schendera, Dr. Opferkuch, Dr. Berlis, Dr. Vougioukas, Dr. Bloss, Dr. Hustedt, Prof. Tatagiba, Prof. Lagréze, Prof. Mittelviefhaus, Prof. Langer, Prof. Maier, Prof. Schipper, Prof. Zentner, Prof Laszig, Prof. Schumacher, Prof. Strub, Prof. Jonas, Prof. Otten, Prof. Krekeler, Prof. Düker, Prof. Frommhold, the OR teams and the in- and outpatient teams from the University Hospital Freiburg, Germany; Dr. Rohner, Dr. Kunz, Prof. Hammer and Prof. Prein from the University Hospital Basel, Switzerland; Dr. Caversaccio, Prof. Nolte, Dr. Hallermann, Mrs. DeMomi, Mr. Chapuis, Mr. Bläuer, Mr. Langlotz and Mr. Papas from the University Hospital Bern, Switzerland; Prof. Eufinger and Mr. Wehmöller from Cranio Construct, Bochum, Germany; Mrs. Thoma, Mrs. Engelhard, Mr. Bühner and Mr. Moctezuma from Stryker-Leibinger, Freiburg, Germany; Mr. Fischer and Mr. Stockmann from IVS Solutions AG, Chemnitz, Germany).

Our special thanks go to Ms. Schröder and Ms. Himberger from Springer Verlag, Heidelberg, Germany and Ms. Strohbach and Mr. Telger for their excellent support throughout the publication process.

Contents

1 Introduction 1

2 Historical Evolution of Computer-assisted Surgery
Frame-based Stereotaxy 3
Frameless Stereotaxy 4

3 Evolution of the Clinical Use of Navigation Systems in the Head and Neck 7

4 Intraoperative Navigation 9

5 Registration Process
Invasive Registration 12
Noninvasive Registration 15
Anatomical Landmarks 15
Adhesive Skin Markers 16
Headset 17
Surface Matching 18
Dental Arch Splints 18
Vacuum-formed Maxillary Splint 18
Maxillary Silicone Impression Splint 21
Vestibular Silicone Impression Splint 21
Invasive Head Registration 22
Noninvasive Head Registration 24

6 Imaging Procedures 25

7 Preoperative Planning and Simulation
Stereolithographic Method 27
Computer-assisted Planning 28
Fusion of Image Data Sets 32
Feature-based Fusion 33
Image-based Fusion 33
Monomodal Image Fusion 34

8 Preoperative Preparations
Definition of the Reference Points 39
Intraoperative Setup 42
Registration 43

9 Intraoperative Accuracy 47

10 Patient-friendly Navigation 51

11 Computer-assisted Therapy
Minimally Invasive Surgeries and Biopsies 53
Optic Nerve Decompression 66
Recommendations for the Treatment of Traumatic Optic Nerve Injury 67

Resections and Reconstructions 72
Lateral Skull Base
and Temporomandibular Joint 73
Anterior Skull Base 86
Midface 86
Intraoperative Radiotherapy 104
Secondary Reconstructions
after Tumor Resections 105

Traumatological Procedures 114
Primary Orbital and Midfacial Reconstructions . . 114
Secondary Orbital
and Midfacial Reconstructions 126
Reconstruction with CAD-CAM Implants 135
Procedures for Midfacial Correction 142
Implant Insertions 154

References 161

Introduction

Surgical procedures in the head and neck region require a detailed knowledge of head and neck anatomy. Particularly in the skull, structures of major functional and aesthetic importance are spaced close together within a relatively confined area. Anatomical changes due to tumor growth, trauma-related defects or displacements, and craniofacial deformities and dysgnathias present special challenges for the surgeon. Besides the clinical examination, which is still of fundamental importance, imaging procedures are used in the preoperative assessment of anatomical changes. Imaging studies enable us to analyze the pathological condition and plan the operation accordingly. Two-dimensional techniques such as conventional radiography are seriously limited due to the presence of superimposed structures. Computed tomography (CT) was the first imaging modality to provide a three-dimensional (3D) representation of the clinical situation. Recent developments in 3D shadowing software can produce high-contrast simulated 3D models of the skull that are particularly useful in traumatology. Once an image data set has been acquired, it can be digitally processed without further radiation exposure to provide detailed views of the bones and soft tissues. Magnetic resonance imaging (MRI) may offer similar advantages, depending on the nature of the investigation.

These examination techniques also have major importance as postoperative studies. They provide an objective, detailed basis for evaluating the results of operative procedures, planning adjuvant therapies, and conducting follow-ups. There is still a need, however, to avoid negative postoperative surprises caused by faulty intraoperative judgments, and this problem has sparked a desire among surgeons for improved methods of intraoperative visualization. Recent developments in 3D sectional imaging technology such as volume tomography and C-arm techniques from traumatology may provide simpler and more practical options for intraoperative use. These new developments involve less radiation exposure and are considerably more cost-effective than conventional CT. The intraoperative use of CT or MRI is associated with high staffing and equipment costs. These modalities hamper the clinical course and may interfere with certain operating room procedures, precluding several interventions. Intraoperative CT also subjects the patient to extra radiation exposure, making it inappropriate for routine operative use.

Intraoperative navigation is free of these disadvantages. It enables the surgeon to correlate the anatomy of the operative site with the data set acquired before the operation. This makes it possible to locate anatomical and pathological structures without having to rely on subjective assessments and interpretations of image data sets. When we supplement preoperative analysis with the ability to plan surgical access routes and mark tumor boundaries and surgical clearance margins, we have a new treatment modality known as computer-assisted surgery. Unlike robotic techniques, the operation is conducted without the use of manipulators or of semi- or fully automatic cutting, burring, or drilling instruments.

Historical Evolution of Computer-assisted Surgery

Contents

Frame-based Stereotaxy 3
Frameless Stereotaxy 4

Frame-based Stereotaxy

Stereotaxy was first used by Dittmar in 1873 to obtain tissue samples from the medulla oblongata. Horsley and Clarke (1908) developed a method for localizing intracranial structures by using a head frame combined with a stereotactic atlas. In 1947, Spiegel was the first surgeon to use a head frame for orientation and instrument guidance in a human patient (Spiegel et al. 1947). Stereotactic procedures were planned and carried out with the aid of frames that were rigidly secured to the patient's head. For this purpose the frame had to maintain a constant position during image data acquisition and during the operation itself. Thus it remained attached to the patient's head throughout the preoperative period. Instruments were mounted on the frame to guide the surgeon during the operative procedure.

This method is based on the use of a stereotactic atlas in which every internal structure is correlated with a particular external reference mark in a coordinate system. Any of a variety of stereotactic frames can be used to define the external coordinate system for targeting intracranial structures. The stereotactic atlas is used to assign coordinates to an external structure. CT- or MRI-guided stereotactic surgery began with modified conventional stereotactic instruments (Leksell and Jernberg 1980; Goerss et al. 1982) and evolved through the development of new, specialized instrumentation (Perry et al. 1980; Patil 1982; Apuzzo and Sabshin 1983). With modern imaging techniques, it became possible to make a precise morphological analysis of each individual patient. Stereotactic atlases became less important because they could provide only an approximate representation of individual anatomy and pathology. With the development of CT, new methods were needed to define and correlate the stereotactic coordinates based on the CT data acquired from the patient (Leksell and Jernberg 1980).

The disadvantages of stereotaxy are that the instantaneous position of the surgical instrument cannot be reliably determined (Anon et al. 1997) and the complicated frame assembly may restrict access to the operative field (Bale et al. 1997). The screws driven into the skull increase the invasiveness of the procedure. Artifacts also make the frame incompatible with CT scanning, despite the development of alternative devices made of carbon and plastics (Brown 1979; Goerss et al. 1982). Because of these problems and the practical inconvenience of the frame, stereotaxy has been unable to achieve maximum clinical efficiency in neurosurgery (Smith et al. 1994). Carini et al. (1992) suggested the idea of fixing the frame noninvasively to the maxillary dental arch. An additional aid to orientation is definitely needed in cases where it is necessary to target deep subcortical tumors and in regions where it is difficult to define the boundaries between the tumor and surrounding edematous brain (Kelly 1986).

Frameless Stereotaxy

Computer-assisted surgery has its origin in frameless stereotaxy, first introduced to neurosurgery in 1987 (Watanabe et al. 1987). This technique, called "neuronavigation," enabled the selective intraoperative localization of anatomical structures based on CT or MRI data sets acquired before the operation (Zamorano et al. 1992). The navigation instrument consists of an articulated mechanical arm linked to a computer workstation. Detectors in the joints of the arm measure the angular deflections, making it possible to calculate the position of the pointer tip, which is designed as a tracking sensor. Generally the arms have six degrees of freedom. One problem with tracking arms is that they are cumbersome to use due to the spring mountings and the overall weight of the assembly. The first commercially available system to be used clinically was the Viewing Wand System (ISG Technologies, Toronto, Ontario, Canada) (Guthrie and Adler 1992; Maciunas et al. 1992a; Olivier et al. 1994; Golfinos et al. 1995). The Viewing Wand was widely utilized (Anon et al. 1994; Dyer et al. 1995; Golfinos et al. 1995; Nabavi et al. 1995; Carney et al. 1996; Carrau et al. 1996; Sipos et al. 1996; Tronnier et al. 1996; Freysinger et al. 1997a; Gunkel et al. 1997a; Marmulla et al. 1997a, 1998; Thumfart and Gunkel 1997; Arginteanu et al. 1998; Hassfeld et al. 1998a; Hilbert et al. 1998a). However, the mechanical coupling shortens the radius of action and limits the applications of this system, and more innovative systems had to be developed.

Ultrasound-based and electromagnetic navigation systems were the first systems to eliminate the need for mechanical coupling by applying the principle of satellite tracking. In electromagnetic systems, a low-frequency magnetic field is superimposed over the operative site. The position of a tracking probe is determined by analyzing the effect of its ferromagnetic parts on the magnetic field. Kato et al. (1991), Manwaring et al. (1994), Wagner et al. (1995, 1996), and Metson et al. (1998) presented magnetic field-based systems that had a reported accuracy of 2–4 mm (Fried et al. 1997). The problem with these systems is the variable stability of the magnetic field. Several metallic objects (e.g., surgical instruments) as well as electromagnetic radiation can distort the magnetic field and compromise the accuracy of the localization. There is no effective way to eliminate interference from extraneous electromagnetic fields and moving metallic objects in the operating suite (Cutting 1992).

In ultrasound-based systems, the position of the pointer is determined by measuring the time it takes for a transducer-emitted tone to reach the microphone-bearing frame, whose geometry has been precisely calibrated (Reinhardt and Zweifel 1990; Reinhardt et al. 1991, 1996; Barnet et al. 1993; Koivukangas et al. 1993; Horstmann and Reinhardt 1994a; Kalfas et al. 1995; Barnett 1996). However, the frame geometry varies with temperature, and a temperature gradient may exist between the transmitter and the microphone. Echoes and air currents may also produce unwanted effects. Thus, the disadvantages of ultrasound-based systems relate to a lack of intraoperative accuracy (Mösges 1998).

An optical instrument-based navigation system was first introduced by Heilbrunn et al. in 1992, and other systems followed (Reinhardt et al. 1993; Buchholz et al. 1994; Henderson et al. 1994; Smith et al. 1994; League 1995; Westermann et al. 1995). Instrument tracking in optical systems is based on the detection of light-emitting diodes (LEDs) by infrared cameras (Fig. 1). Passive systems were also developed in which the active light sources are replaced by reflectors on the surgical instruments. The cameras illuminate the reflectors with infrared flashes so that the instruments can be tracked. The advantage of passive systems is that instruments can be tracked without electrical wires or batteries (Fig. 2). As for their disadvantages, natural and artificial light sources may interfere with tracking, and sterile draping of the reflectors cannot be achieved (Engelhardt 2000). Owing to their high technical precision (Bucholz et al. 1993) and their insensitivity to ambient operating room conditions, navigation systems based on the use of infrared light have become commercially popular (Hassfeld 2000; Hassfeld and Mühling 2001).

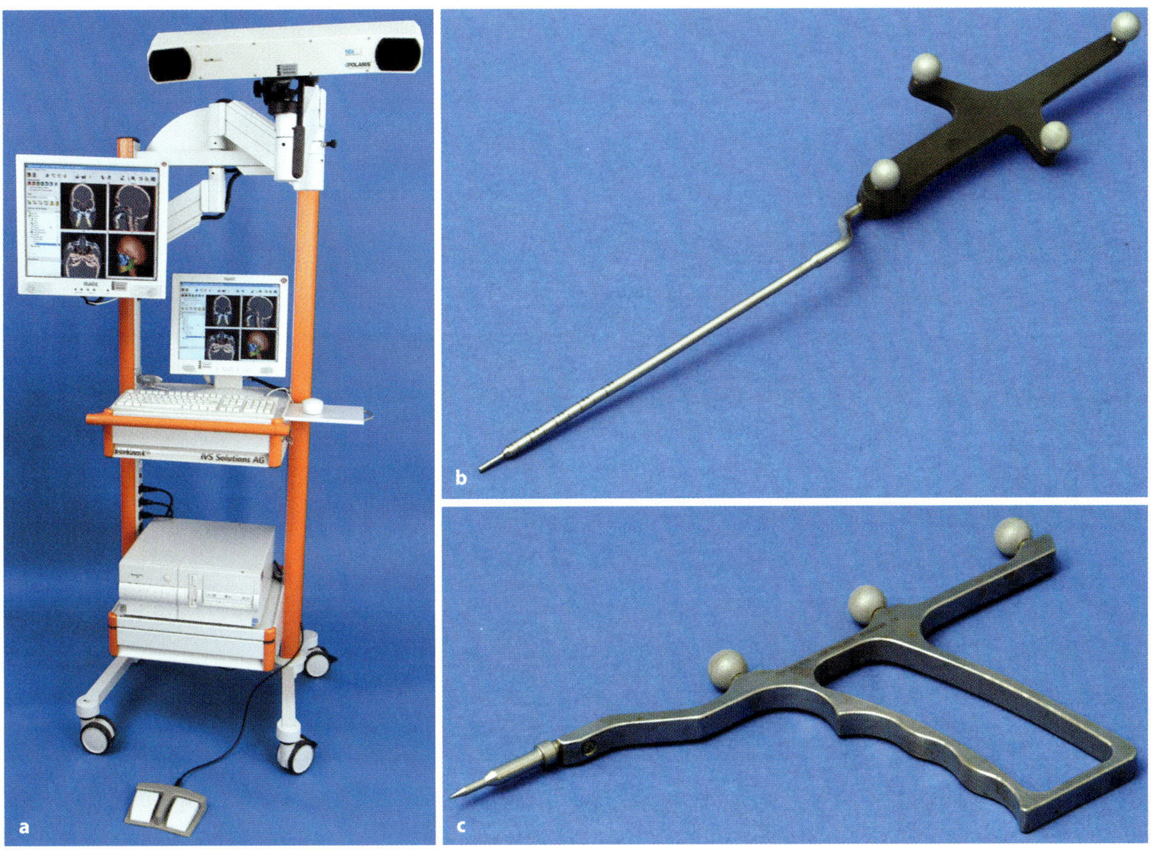

Fig. 1. Passive optical navigation system. **a** The infrared cameras are combined with infrared emitters and detect the infrared light reflected from the instruments (IVS Solutions, Chemnitz, Germany). **b, c** The instruments used in passive optical navigation systems are fitted with infrared light reflectors

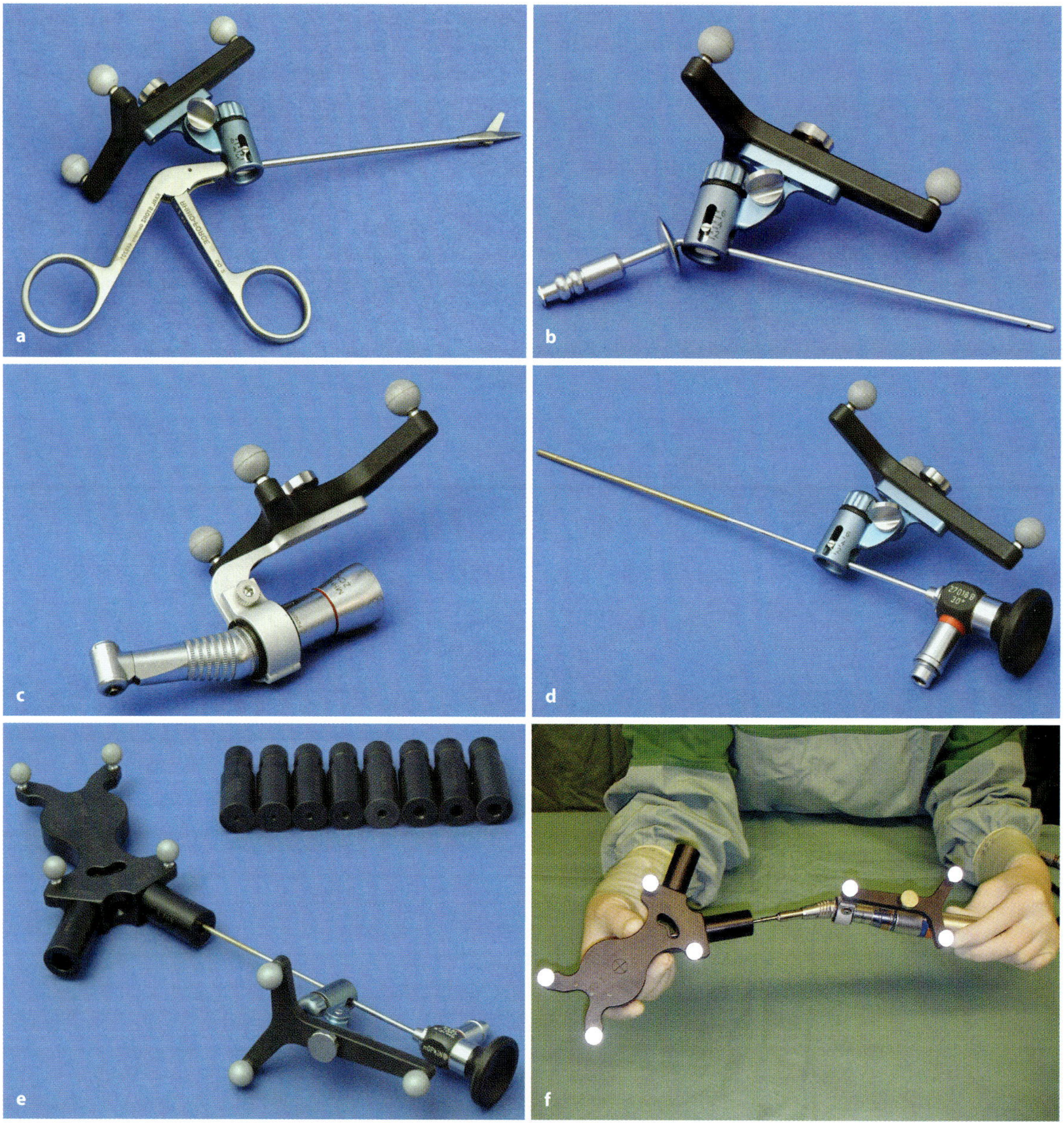

Fig. 2. Universal adapters make it possible to use any nonflexible surgical instrument such as a biopsy forceps (a), suction probe (b), elbow piece (c), or endoscope (d). The instruments can be calibrated before or after surgery. e, f Calibration of an operating endoscope. Sleeves of various diameters are used for precision guidance of the instruments during the calibration process

Evolution of the Clinical Use of Navigation Systems in the Head and Neck

Navigation systems were first used in neurosurgery for the detailed visualization of brain anatomy based on the use of modern neuroimaging procedures (CT, MRI). During the 1990s, initial reports were published on the successful use of intraoperative navigation for improved orientation in pediatric neurosurgery (Drake et al. 1991), the resection of brain tumors (Barnett et al. 1993; Iseki et al. 1994; Spetzger et al. 1996), the drainage of brain abscesses (Laborde et al. 1993), epilepsy surgery (Olivier et al. 1994; Chabrerie et al. 1998), the guidance of biopsy needles and ventricular catheters (Dorward et al. 1997), functional neurosurgical procedures, and in patients with multiple lesions and biopsies (Thumfart et al. 1997; Roessler et al. 1998b; Wirtz and Kunze 1998). Navigation systems also appeared feasible in the brachytherapy of neurosurgical tumors (Mösges et al. 1991), but intraoperative accuracy in all intracranial procedures was significantly limited (1–2 cm) due to the "brain shift" that occurred following craniotomy (Kikinis et al. 1996).

Thus, the paranasal sinuses and skull base, with their close relationship to stationary bony structures, offered an excellent area for the application of frameless stereotaxy (Kavanagh 1994). Foreign-body removal (Klimek et al. 1992a, 1993c), optic nerve decompression (Kurzeja et al. 1994), and endoscopically navigated sinus operations were described (Mösges and Klimek 1993; Ossoff and Reinisch 1994; Gunkel et al. 1995; Roth et al. 1995; Carrau et al. 1996; Hauser et al. 1996; Krückels et al. 1996; Freysinger et al. 1997b; Gunkel et al. 1997c). In 1994, Anon et al. described the use of frameless navigation in previously operated areas, extensive lesions, in the sphenoid bone, and in patients with Onodi cells or other anomalies that could lead to complications. In frontal sinusotomy, Carrau et al. (1994) described the advantages of navigation in preventing dural perforations and frontal lobe injuries. Caversaccio et al. (1997) found that navigation systems could reduce the high risks associated with procedures on the anterior or lateral skull base and arteriovenous malformations with risk of vision loss, deafness, facial nerve paralysis, and intracerebral neurological complications. Various authors have described the use of navigation systems in surgery of the paranasal sinuses and anterior skull base (Freysinger et al. 1997b), intranasal endoscopic or microscopic sinus surgery (Hauser et al. 1997), preoperatively operated areas, patients with massive polyposis or hemorrhage (Klimek et al. 1993a), and in surgical procedures on the orbit, nasopharynx, pituitary gland, and the middle and anterior cranial fossae (Schlöndorff et al. 1989; Klimek and Mösges 1998). Endonasal surgery of the paranasal sinuses involving more than just the maxillary sinus, revision sinus surgery, and the surgical removal of sinonasal and orbital tumors can be performed more easily with the aid of image guidance and computer assistance. It is easier to locate foreign bodies in the orbital region (Klimek et al. 1993b). Navigation also facilitates orientation in procedures on the lateral skull base, especially the transtemporal surgery of acoustic neuroma and the insertion of cochlear implants (Mösges 1993).

The use of a mechanically coupled navigation system in oromaxillofacial surgery was first described in 1994 for the removal of skull base tumors, foreign body extractions, and the transfer of osteotomy lines (Hassfeld et al. 1994). These publications were followed by isolated reports on navigated tumor resections (Wagner et al. 1995; Hoffmann et al. 2004; Westendorff et al. 2004), implant insertions (Ploder et al. 1995), and corrective osteotomies (Marmulla et al. 1997b; Marmulla and Niederdellmann 1998, 1999; Heiland et al. 2004; De Greef et al. 2005; Ewers et al. 2005; Westermark et al. 2005). Surgeons had not yet incorporated this very promising technology into routine oromaxillofacial operations, however. The main reasons for this were a lack of intraoperative accuracy, an inability to plan and simulate surgical procedures with existing computer software, the high technical costs, and the learning curve for mastering the software and hardware components of the navigation systems.

Intraoperative Navigation

Intraoperative navigation is comparable to the navigation systems used in automobiles. While the position of an automobile is determined by satellite receivers that track waves emitted from the vehicle, an optical-based intraoperative navigation system uses infrared cameras to detect the light waves emitted by LEDs mounted on the surgical instruments. Road maps are analogous to the CT or MRI data sets that are acquired from the patient prior to the operation. To calibrate the system, it is necessary to define a starting position so that the virtual patient on the monitor corresponds anatomically to the real patient on the operating table. This is done by using reference points that can be uniquely identified on the patient and can be located in the data set. This process of correlating the patient's images to the patient's actual anatomy is called *registration*. Usually it is based on three non-coplanar reference points that can be uniquely identified in the image data and on the skull of the patient. At the start of the operation, these reference points are sequentially touched with a localizing system, such as an instrument fitted with LEDs, and they are simultaneously digitized in the image data. When registration (spatial correlation) is complete, the computer can calculate the spatial position of the instrument in the 3D model and display it in relation to the preplanned trajectory and the targeted surgical site. It must also be possible to continually update changes in the patient's position ("reregistration"), because movements during the operation cannot be prevented and are even necessary for some maneuvers. This is accomplished with an LED array that is securely attached to the patient. Generally a metal clamp with three steel prongs is mounted on the patient's head for this purpose – a procedure that is done routinely in almost all neurosurgical operations. When the setup is complete, the surgeon can move a tracking instrument during the operation while watching the corresponding movements of the instrument tip on the monitor. Any rigid surgical instrument such as a drill, chisel, or even an endoscope or the focus of an operating microscope can be tracked in this way, providing a means of intraoperative navigation.

Registration Process

Contents

Invasive Registration 12
Noninvasive Registration. 15
Anatomical Landmarks. 15
Adhesive Skin Markers 16
Headset 17
Surface Matching 18
Dental Arch Splints 18
Vacuum-formed Maxillary Splint. 18
Maxillary Silicone Impression Splint 21
Vestibular Silicone Impression Splint. 21
Invasive Head Registration. 22
Noninvasive Head Registration 24

To define the position of the instrument in the patient data set, the computer must be able to convert between the coordinate systems of the patient, instrument, camera, and data set. The basis for these transformations is the "local rigid body" concept, which states that an object must have at least three fixed reference elements that span the coordinate system of the object in question (Zamorano et al. 1993b). Registration, or the process of correlating the physical reference points to those in the data set, is done by carrying out multiple computer transformations. The first transformation, designated T_1 (Fig. 3), calculates the position of the instrument in relation to the camera coordinate system. Because the reference elements are placed on the instrument in a fixed pattern, their position can be used to calculate the position of the instrument tip. Another essential part of surgical navigation is registering intraoperative movements of the operative field. These position changes may result from deliberate or accidental intraoperative changes in the position of the patient or operating table. With an optical system, these movements are registered by LEDs mounted directly or indirectly on the patient's head ("dynamic reference frame," DRF). In the second transformation, designated T_2 (Fig. 3), the position of the DRF is calculated in relation to the camera. The reference elements of the DRF must also be mounted in a fixed position in space. The DRF is securely attached to the patient's head so that the reference points maintain a fixed relationship to the DRF. This means that a fixed quantity is calculated in T_3. In the final step, T_4, the reference points in space are correlated to the corresponding points in the image data set. Once registration has been completed, the initial relationships of the camera, DRF, instrument, and

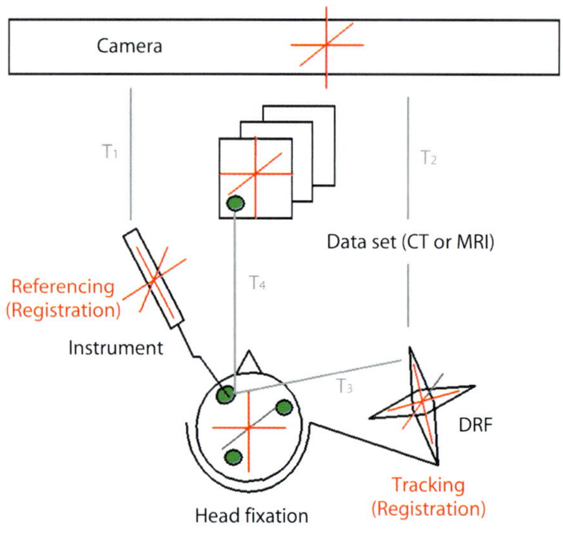

Fig. 3. Transformation process used in correlating the position of the instrument to the image data (registration). The head is fixed in a head frame to which the dynamic reference frame (*DRF*) is attached. The registration points are shown in *green*, and the different coordinate systems are shown in *red*. The four steps in the transformation process are designated as T_1–T_4

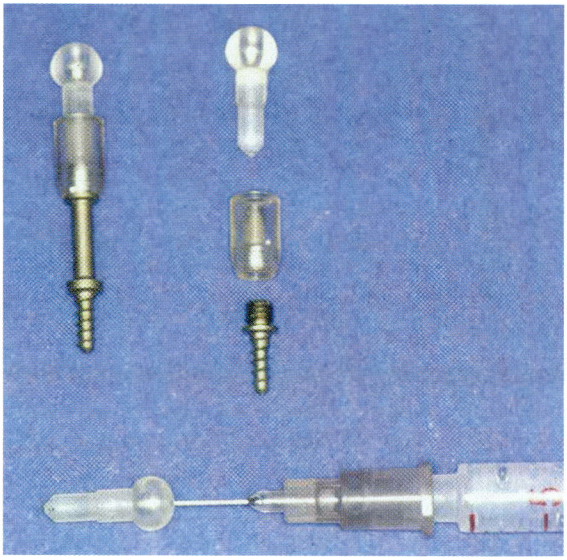

Fig. 4. Screw markers for invasive registration (Cranial Marker Set, Stryker-Leibinger, Freiburg, Germany). The heads of the titanium screws have external threads for mounting the base components. Markers for CT and MRI can be inserted into the base components

data set have been uniquely defined in relation to one another. Then, whenever a position change occurs in any of the elements, its new position can be calculated. Registration of the patient and virtual image (CT or MRI image data set) and the reregistration of intraoperative movements can be done in either of two ways: invasively and noninvasively.

Invasive Registration

Prior to data acquisition, "screw markers" are placed transcutaneously in the patient's head under local anesthesia. This may be done extraorally (e.g., on the calvarium or lateral orbital margin) or intraorally by placing markers in the maxilla, mandible, or both (Schramm et al. 1999a). Commercially available marker systems (Cranial Marker Set, Stryker-Leibinger, Freiburg, Germany) consist of titanium screws (2-mm-diameter) with an additional external thread on the screw head for mounting the base component (Fig. 4). These base components function as holders for applying the CT and MRI markers. Both the base component and markers are made of polymethylmethacrylate (PMMA) plastic. CT markers are fitted with a gold bead for visualization, while MRI markers have a spherical cavity that can be filled with gadolinium contrast agent. Multimodal markers that are compatible with CT and MRI are also available commercially. These systems are suitable for both intra- and extraoral use. Extraoral screws are placed in the facial bones or cranial vault under local anesthesia, and then the base components are screwed into place. The markers are then applied for CT or MRI data acquisition and can be removed afterward. The screws with the base components must remain in place until the start of the operation (Fig. 5).

The disadvantages of invasive registration techniques are the need for operative insertion and the limited time interval between data acquisition and navigated surgical procedure. They may also delay the initiation of operative treatment. Invasive mark-

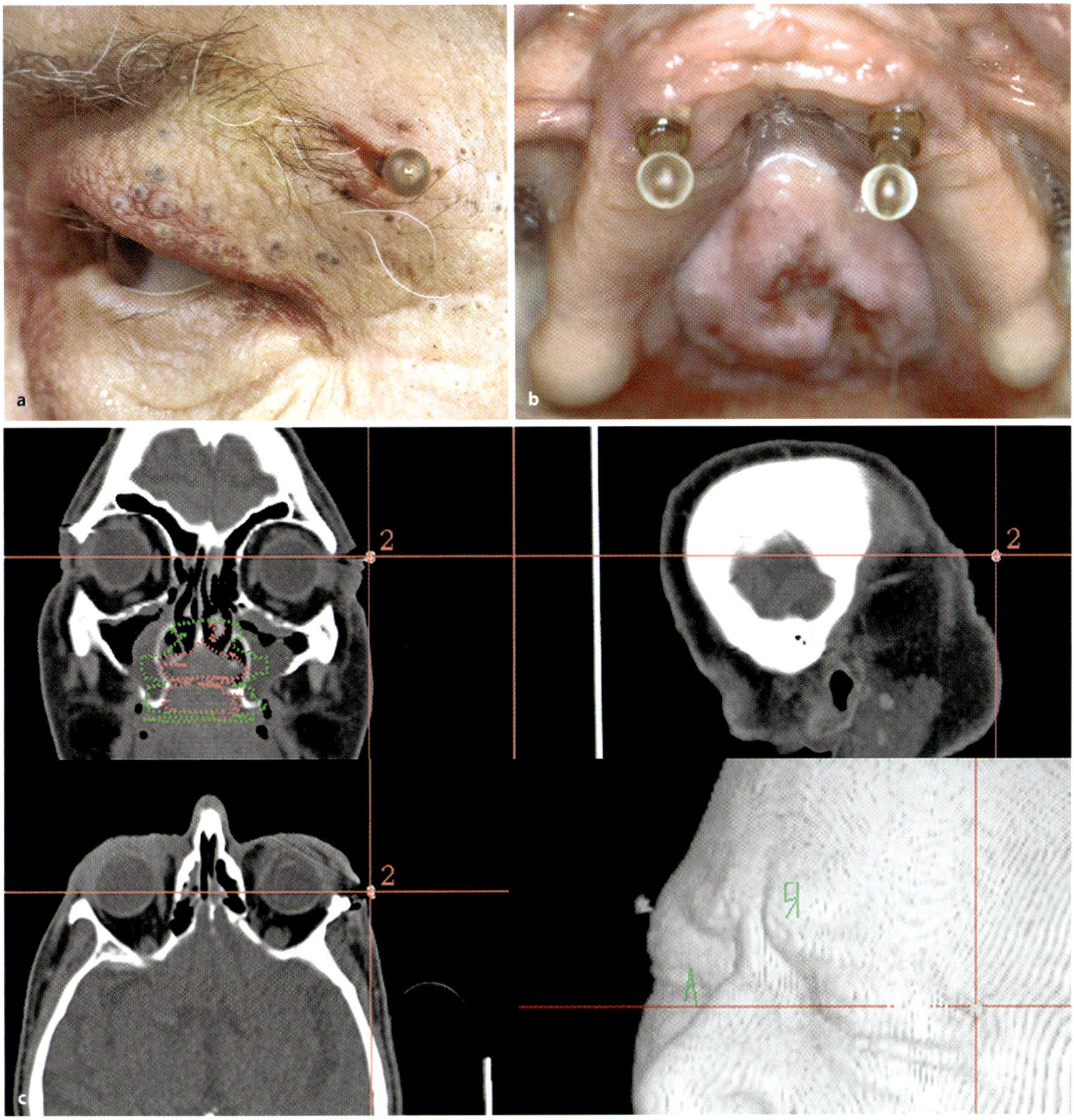

Fig. 5. Clinical application of screw-based invasive registration. Markers placed extraorally (a) or intraorally (b) under local anesthesia are visualized in the CT data set and used as registration points (c)

ers have been used in neurosurgery (Maciunas et al. 1992a,b, 1996; Nabavi et al. 1995; Colchester et al. 1996) but are rarely used in otolaryngological or oro-maxillofacial surgery because of these disadvantages.

In secondary operations, internal fixation material that is already in place, such as titanium screws, may provide acceptable reference points for surgical navigation (Maciunas et al. 1992b; Marmulla et al.

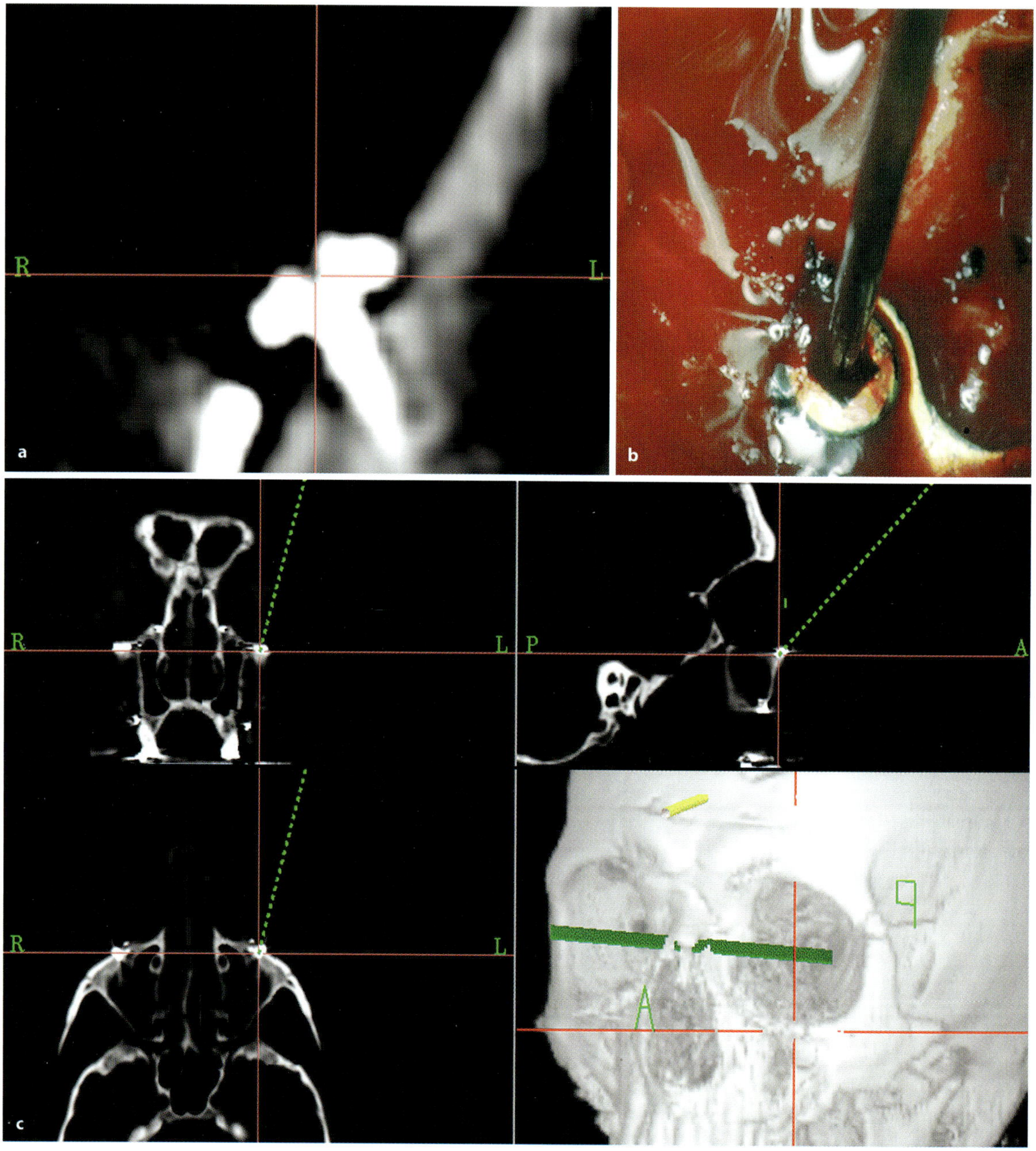

Fig. 6. Use of internal fixation screws as reference markers. The center of the screw head marked in the CT data set (**a**) is touched intraoperatively with the pointer (**b**) and functions as a reference point (**c**). Before acquisition of the data set, internal fixation miniscrews are inserted through a stab incision under local anesthesia (**d**). During the operation these points are touched with the pointer for registration. They can be removed at the end of the operation

Fig. 6. (continued)

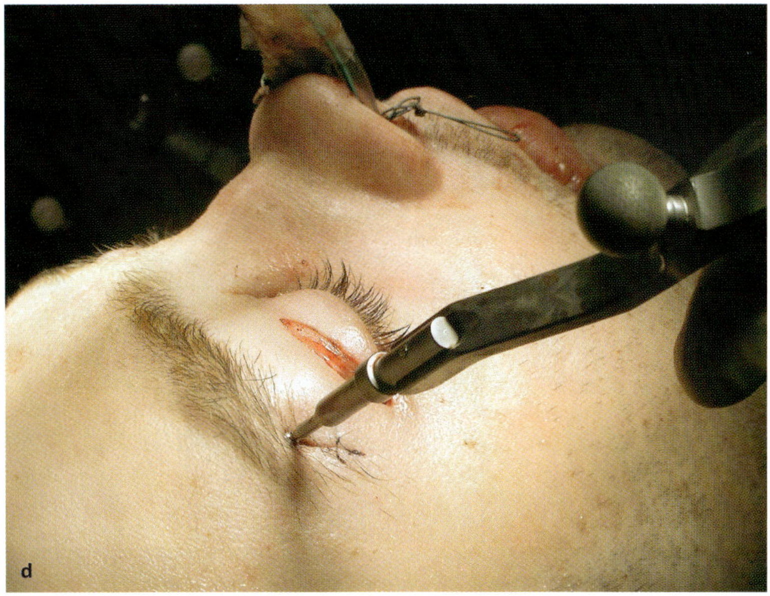

1997a). While this type of registration can be done only in secondary procedures, it is an elegant and reliable method (Fig. 6). Thus, in cases where CT data sets are used exclusively, as in traumatology, internal fixation screws are inserted subcutaneously prior to data acquisition. Generally this is done under local anesthesia, placing the screws in the lateral orbital margins and temporoparietal areas on both sides. Intraoral maxillary placement is another option.

Noninvasive Registration

Noninvasive registration is advantageous because it is technically easier to perform and makes it possible to provide immediate surgical treatment (optic nerve decompression, trauma care) in urgent cases.

Anatomical Landmarks

The development of increasingly powerful computers in the early 1990s led to the use of anatomical landmarks for registration (Boesecke et al. 1990; Hassfeld et al. 1995a; Carney et al. 1996; Desgeorges et al. 1997). The anatomical landmarks are well-defined structures, usually bony prominences, that provide definite reference points for instrument tracking (Golfinos et al. 1995; Vrionis et al. 1997). Edinger et al. (1999) described the use of teeth and filling contours for navigation. For navigating in the nose and paranasal sinuses, Anon et al. (1994) suggested using the nose as a landmark. The tragi and canthi have been used in oromaxillofacial surgery (Horstmann and Reinhardt 1994a; Golfinos et al. 1995; Freysinger et al. 1997b).

Registration is done by correlating soft tissue or bony points on the facial skeleton of the patient to corresponding points in the CT or MRI image data set (Fig. 7). This registration method is time-consuming, difficult to reproduce, and therefore operator-dependent. The correlation process can be particularly difficult and unreliable when MRI data sets are used. Landmark-based registration can achieve an intraoperative positional accuracy of only about 4–6 mm (Horstmann and Reinhardt 1994b; Kondziolka and Lunsford 1996; McDermott and Gutin 1996). Thus, intraoperative navigation in oromaxillofacial surgery based on landmark registration is feasible only when it is used as an adjunct to other registration methods.

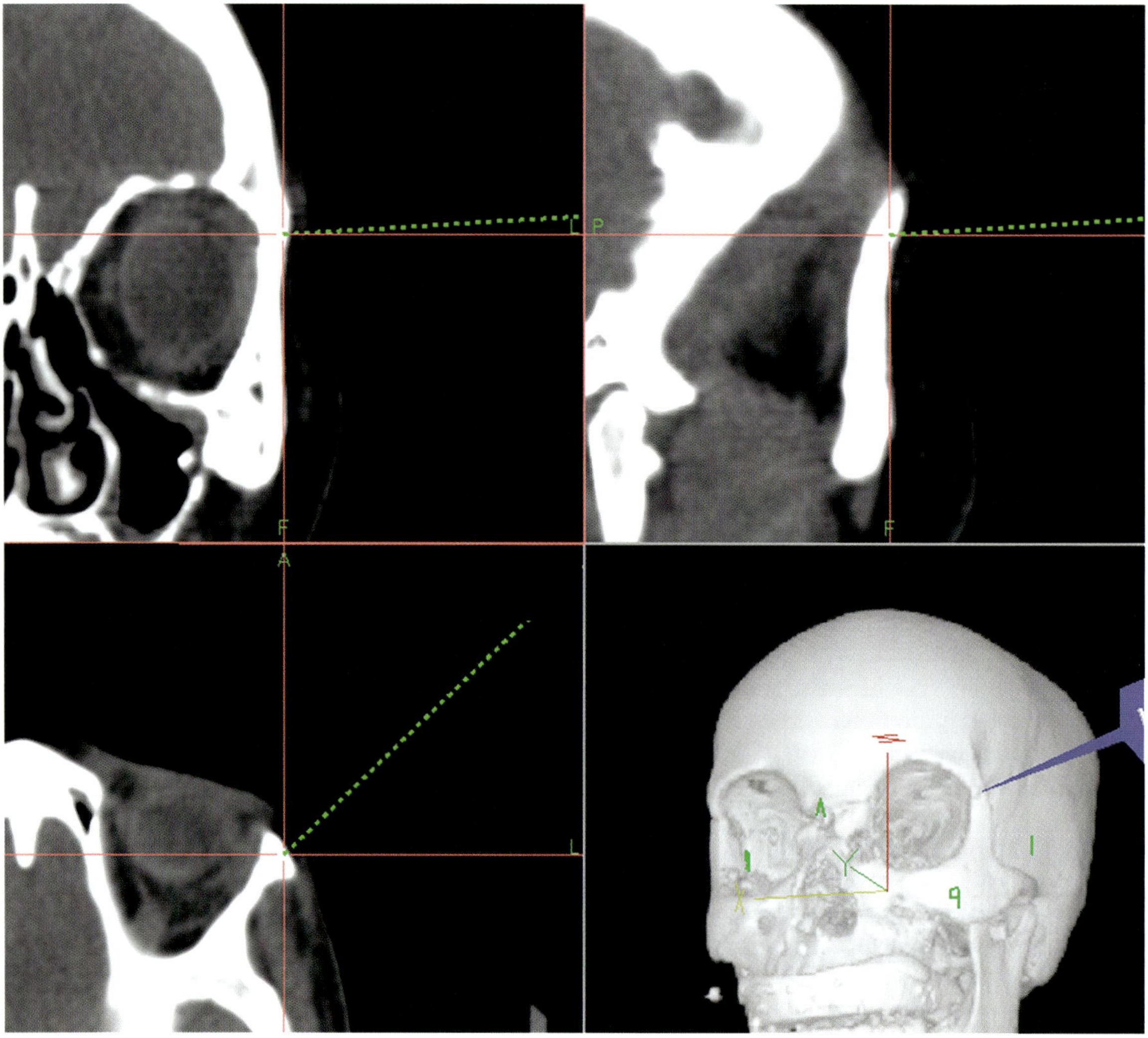

Fig. 7. Landmark-based registration. Here the left frontozygomatic suture is registered as a reference point with the pointer. This landmark may be used as an adjunct to other reference points, such as the registration splint shown here

Adhesive Skin Markers

Adhesive markers are attached to the skin of the patient's head prior to data acquisition (Fig. 8) and are defined as registration points at the start of the operation. This is the most widely used registration method (Roberts et al. 1986; Giller and Purdy 1990; Watanabe et al. 1991; Guthrie and Adler 1992; Laborde et al. 1992, 1993; Takizawa 1993; Sandemann et al. 1994). Cutaneous marker systems are small plastic pads with adhesive on one side and a major diameter of 1–1.5 cm. They are fitted with a central radiopaque marker such as a lead bead (Hassfeld et al. 1995b, 1998b). At least four markers are placed on the patient's skin and remain there until the start of the operation (Klimek et al. 1995; Nabavi et al. 1995; Vinas et al. 1997; Alp et al. 1998). To allow for the risk of premature marker loss, extra markers are usually ap-

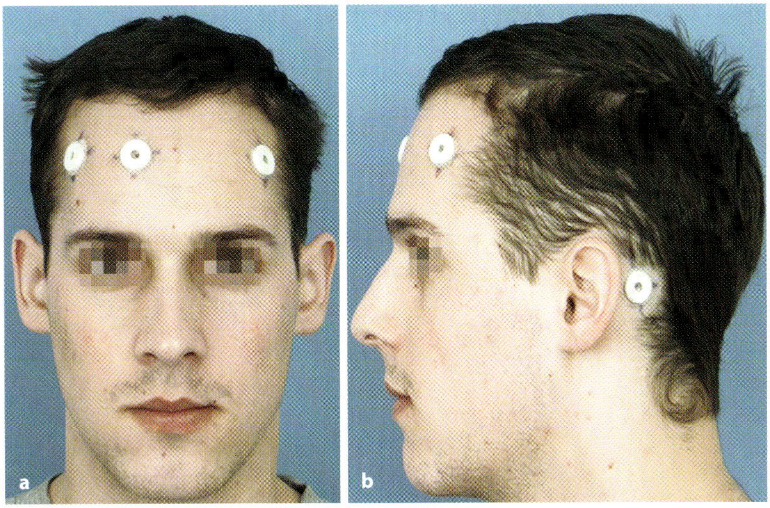

Fig. 8 a, b. Adhesive skin markers. The reference markers are placed on the patient's skin prior to data acquisition and must remain in place until the operation

plied and the skin area is marked with a waterproof skin marker so that a dislodged adhesive marker can be easily reattached (Barnett et al. 1993; Wenzel et al. 1994; Desgeorges et al. 1997; Freysinger et al. 1997b; Roessler et al. 1998a). The adhesive markers are easy to apply and locate during the operation. They are said to provide a positional accuracy of approximately 2 mm, but studies to date are based on phantom models or human preparations that do not take into account movements of the plastic or skin. But even changes in skin tone during data acquisition and during the operation itself may lead to unpredictable errors of correlation.

The clinical application of noninvasive registration methods such as adhesive skin markers or the use of anatomical landmarks has shown an intraoperative accuracy of no better than 2 mm (Anon et al. 1994; Hassfeld et al. 1995a, 1998b; Nabavi et al. 1995; Roth et al. 1995; Desgeorges et al. 1997; Alp et al. 1998; Edinger 1999) and often considerably higher (Horstmann and Reinhardt 1994b; Golfinos et al. 1995; Vinas et al. 1997). In the case of adhesive skin markers, this results from the soft tissue-based attachment of the markers and the consequent inability to predict position changes during application, data set acquisition, and the operation itself (Hauser et al. 1996; Fried et al. 1997). Orientation and registration based on anatomical landmarks may be compromised by poor reproducibility, especially in revisions and operations for recurrent disease, because in many cases the reference structures are no longer present, are inaccessible, or have been displaced from their original position (Klimek and Mösges 1998). This is such a serious drawback that the use of anatomical landmarks is no longer considered appropriate in oromaxillofacial surgery (Hassfeld 2000). Like the newer video- and laser-based registration methods, they are used chiefly in paranasal sinus surgery and neuronavigation.

Headset

In this method the markers are attached to a headset that resembles a dental frame. The headset is placed on designated soft tissue points of the facial skeleton (the bridge of the nose and the external auditory canals). This method is commonly used in endoscopically navigated sinus surgery (Thomas et al. 1990; Takizawa et al. 1993; Howard et al. 1995; Hauser et al. 1997; Klimek and Mösges 1998). Head masks are also used for noninvasive registration (Smith et al. 1994; Walker et al. 2002) and provide a reported positional accuracy of 1.2–2.8 mm (Heermann et al. 2001; Wang et al. 2002). But this registration method has limited reliability due to its soft tissue-based support and, unlike maxillary splints, is poorly tolerated by children (Postec et al. 2002). The headset or cap must remain in place during the operation, which limits their application to endonasal procedures because other approaches would require a different position. The soft tissue support also prevents accurate reregistration, resulting in a low degree of intraoperative accuracy. The use of headsets should thus be limited to endoscopic sinus surgery, although facial neuropathies have been described following the use of a headset for image-guided surgery (Hwang et al. 2002).

Surface Matching

"Surface matching" is a markerless technique in which surfaces on the patient are scanned and correlated with congruent areas in the image data set. The accuracy of this method depends on the algorithm that is used, and scanning skin surfaces is no more accurate than the use of adhesive skin markers, despite several promising reports on laser-based techniques (Raabe et al. 2002; Marmulla et al. 2003, 2004, 2005; Troitzsch et al. 2003; Hoffmann et al. 2005a). Matching bony surfaces yields satisfactory results, but it is necessary to use large, well-curved bony surfaces in order to achieve good accuracy. Thus, surface matching can be used only in operations on the facial skeleton that involve extensive exposure, such as a bicoronal incision (Fig. 9).

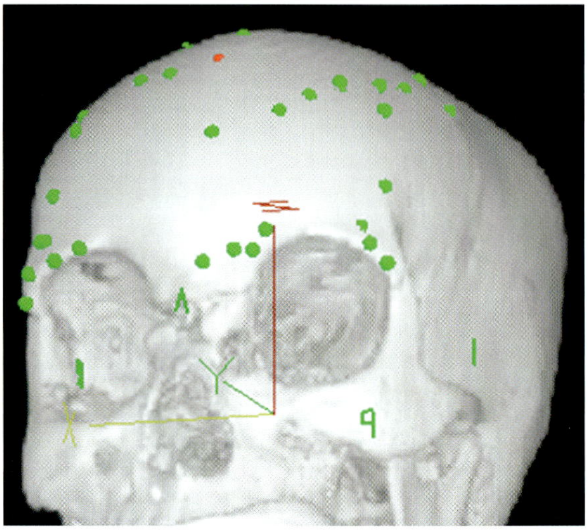

Fig. 9. Surface matching. Registration is done by correlating surface points in the image data set to designated points on the surface of the patient

Dental Arch Splints

This noninvasive registration system encompasses various types of splints (Schramm et al. 2002a).

Vacuum-formed Maxillary Splint

An impression of the maxilla is taken and is used to fabricate a plaster model. After the model has hardened, a plastic plate 1–2 mm thick is "deep-drawn" over the plaster model in a vacuum. The splint is worked to follow the dental equator on the vestibular and palatal surfaces. The base components for attaching the CT markers are polymerized to the base of the splint (Fig. 10). The effect of the geometrical arrangement of the markers on the accuracy of registration is greater than the effect of the number of markers used. It is essential, then, to place the reference markers in an optimum configuration so that they encompass the largest possible volume. The gain in intraoperative accuracy is independent of the registration method used. Thus the base components should be positioned in an XYZ array that provides a maximum separation of the vectors in all three spatial planes. The use of navigation splints for follow-up examinations, which may be done up to several years after the initial examination, requires a splint with long-term durability, like that provided by the vacuum-forming process. This is why vacuum-formed PMMA splints are the standard splints used in all elective treatments, multiple examinations, and staged operative procedures (Fig. 11).

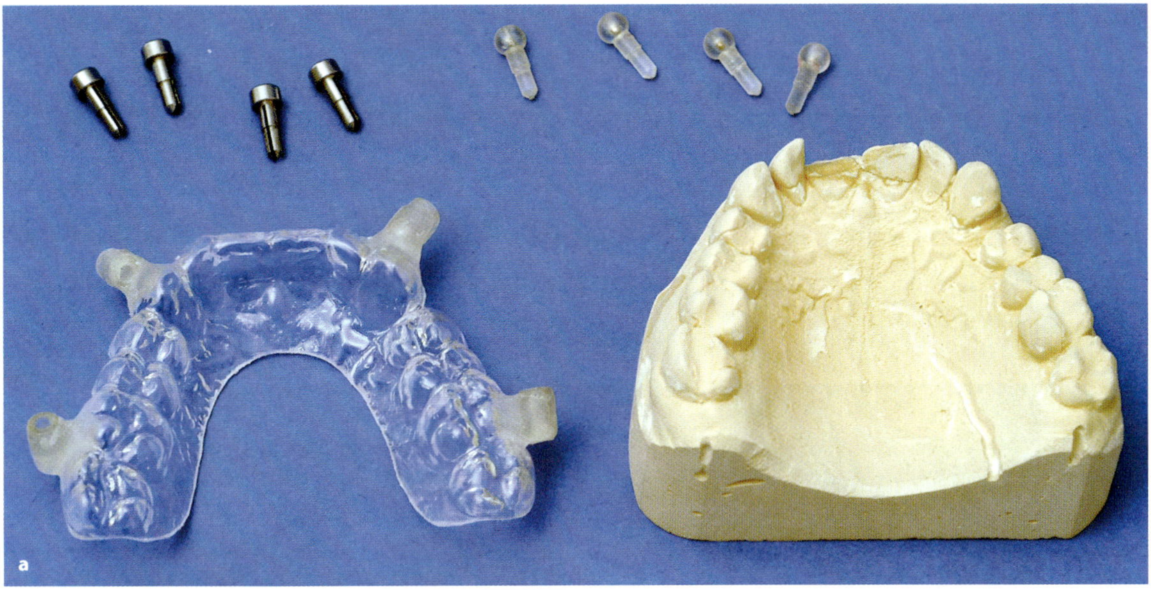

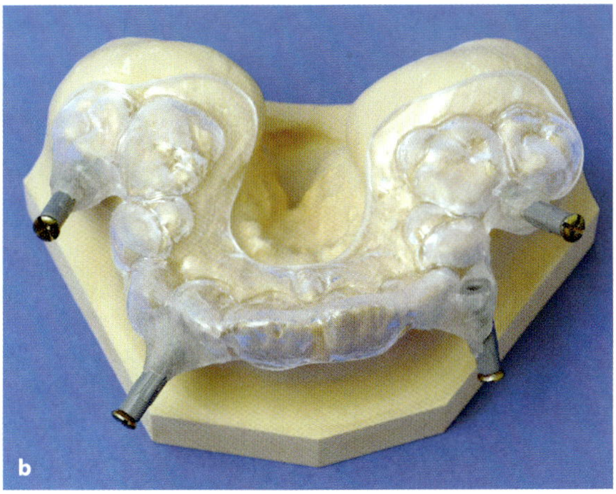

Fig. 10 a, b. Vacuum-formed maxillary splint. A vacuum-formed splint is custom-made in the laboratory and includes four base components that are polymerized to the splint. Gold-bead markers are inserted into the sockets for CT data acquisition. Reference markers made of stainless steel are used during the operation. Another option is to use titanium miniscrews, which are screwed into saw model pins that are polymerized to the splint

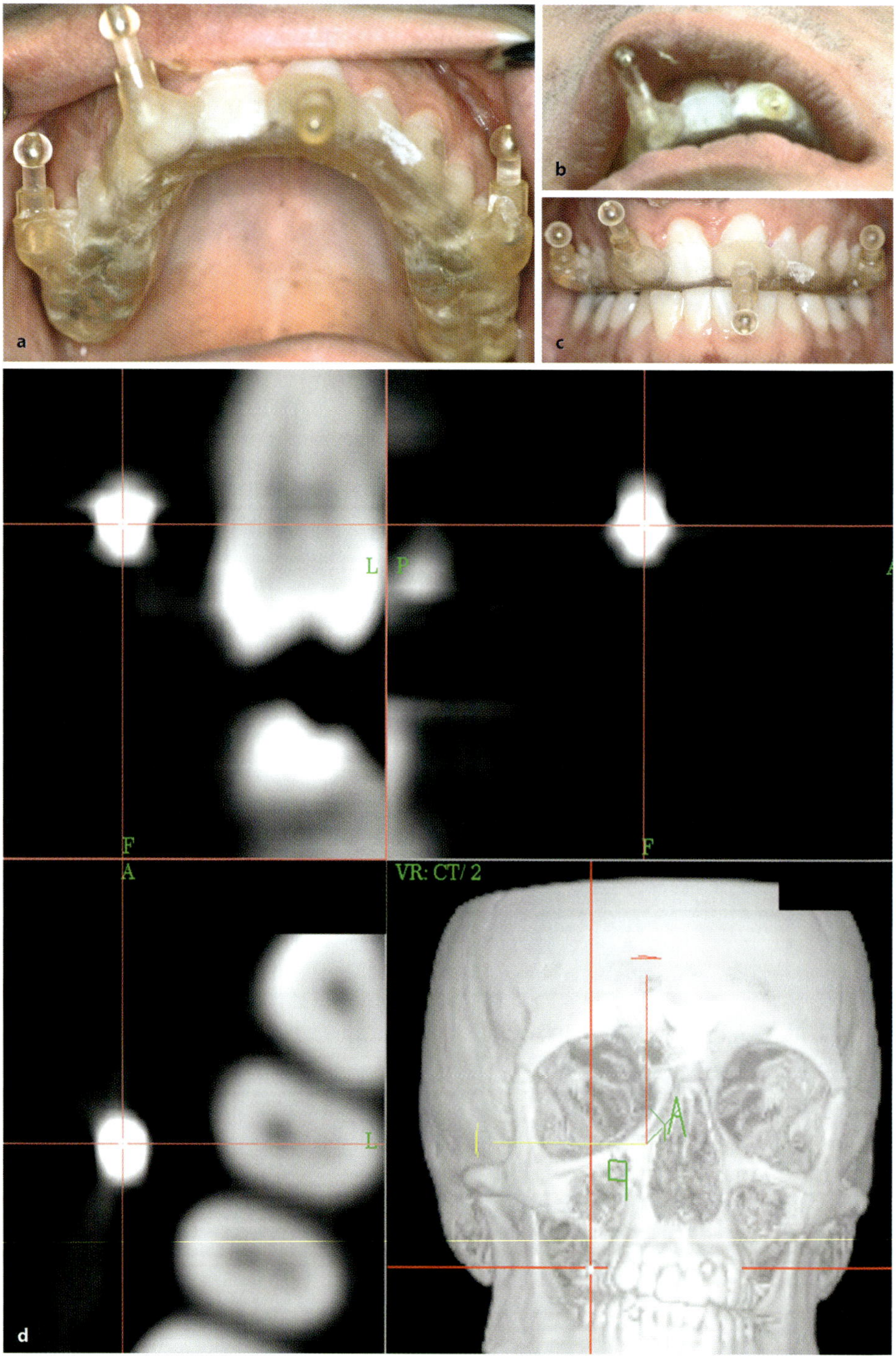

Fig. 11. Noninvasive splint-based registration. The reference markers are attached to a vacuum-formed maxillary splint (a–c). The center of the marker serves as a reference point in the image data set (d)

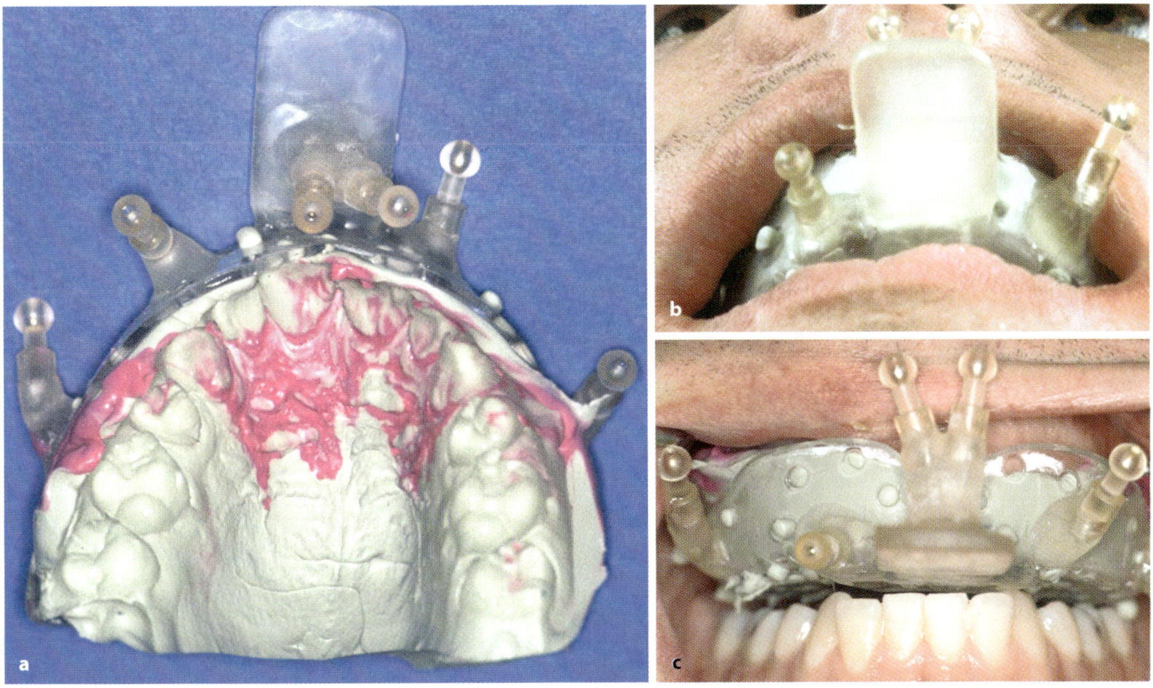

Fig. 12a–c. Maxillary silicone impression splint. The prefabricated, ready-made maxillary splints are fitted to the patient's dental arch with silicone impression material

Maxillary Silicone Impression Splint

The basic shape of the maxillary splint is determined by disposable impression trays, which come in various sizes. The ready-made sockets for receiving the standard navigation markers are attached to the vestibular surfaces of the trays. This prefabricated maxillary splint is lined with silicone impression material and fitted to the patient's jaw. One- and two-phase impression methods can be used (Fig. 12).

After setting for 2–5 minutes, the splint is removed from the mouth and sterilized. The patient watches the splint insertion in a mirror and can then practice positioning the splint without help. With this method, navigation splints can be fabricated in minutes without having to suction saliva or having an absolutely dry dental arch and oral mucosa, allowing for emergency care even in orally intubated patients. It is therefore used mainly in primary posttraumatic reconstructions and optic nerve decompressions.

Vestibular Silicone Impression Splint

The basis for this type of navigation splint is an elliptical, ready-made, perforated oral vestibular plate made of photosetting plastic (Fig. 13). The external dimensions of the plate are based on the sizes of the disposable impression trays. The splint has an individual handle-tab at the front and four integrated base components for attaching the reference markers. As in the maxillary splint, the base components are oriented in the sagittal, coronal, and transverse planes to achieve maximum separation of the marker vectors in space. After the CT or MRI markers are attached, the basic shape of the splint is fitted to the patient's dental arch. Full denture wearers and patients who have a partial denture and few remaining teeth should wear their dentures intraoperatively to maintain their occlusal relationship. Edentulous patients and patients who do not have functional dentures due to trauma can be fitted with a modified

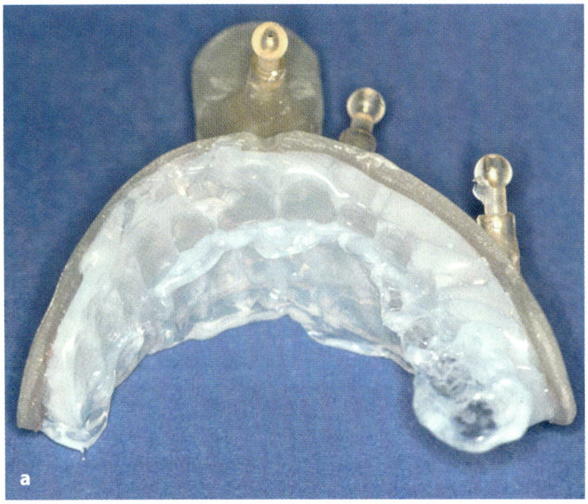

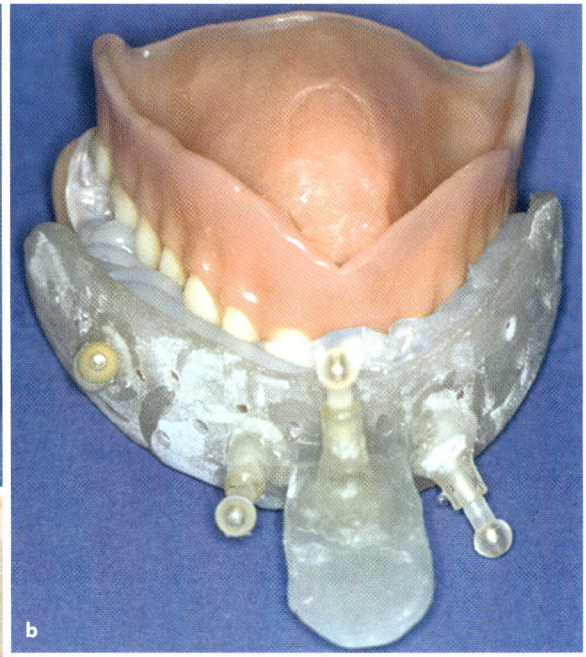

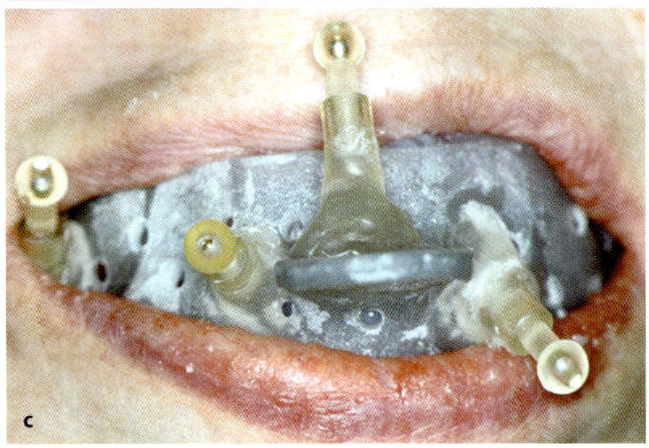

Fig. 13 a–c. Vestibular silicone impression splint. The prefabricated, ready-made vestibular plate is fitted to the maxillary and mandibular dental arches with silicone impression material. This noninvasive registration method is particularly recommended in patients with very limited mouth opening and in full denture wearers

vestibular splint that includes an occlusal stop. The bite plate will aid in fitting the splint along the atrophied alveolar ridges and will help stabilize the silicone impression material. In cases where the splint can be anchored on one side only, extensions should be added to optimize the distribution of the markers. In these cases it is better to use vestibular splints that can be anchored in the upper and lower jaw than vacuum-formed splints or maxillary silicone impression splints.

In partially dentulous patients, the edentulous areas should be partially bridged with an occlusal stop. Edentulous patients who cannot be fitted with a maxillary splint due to limited mouth opening can be fitted with a vestibular splint that does not have an occlusal stop. This type of splint permits the use of an orotracheal tube during general endotracheal anesthesia or the placement of an orogastric feeding tube by the pre- or intraoperative removal of excess impression material from the posterior third (distal free end) of the splint.

Invasive Head Registration

The simplest invasive head tracking device is the Mayfield clamp, which provides acceptable accuracy and is used routinely in neurosurgical operations. This device fixes the position of the patient's head in relation to the operating table. Infrared LEDs or reflectors are attached to the head clamp for registration, making it possible to detect all position changes

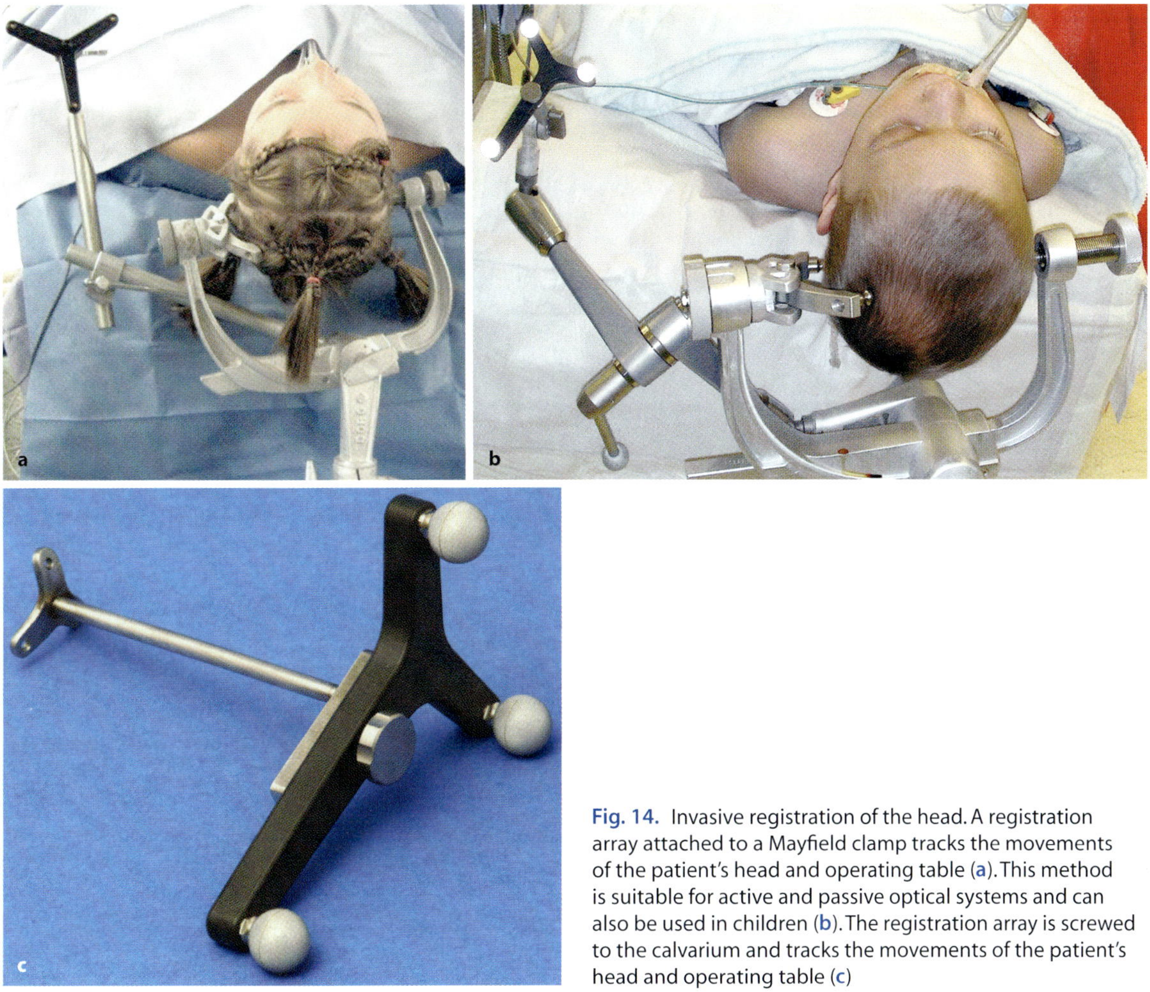

Fig. 14. Invasive registration of the head. A registration array attached to a Mayfield clamp tracks the movements of the patient's head and operating table (a). This method is suitable for active and passive optical systems and can also be used in children (b). The registration array is screwed to the calvarium and tracks the movements of the patient's head and operating table (c)

and register movements of the operating table and clamp during intraoperative navigation (Fig. 14a,b). A potential drawback is unnoticed slippage of the head within the clamp. This prompted the development of holding devices for infrared LEDs (Nolte et al. 1995; Bettega et al. 1996; Schramm et al. 2006) that can be screwed directly or transcutaneously into the bony skull (Fig. 14c). Invasive registration methods require general anesthesia, and this may be cited as a disadvantage in oral implant procedures.

Noninvasive Head Registration

The splint described above can also be used for noninvasive tracking of the patient's head. Because it restricts surgical access, however, its use is limited to operations on the paranasal sinuses. Another noninvasive option is a silicone maxillary splint with an integrated LED array (Caversaccio et al. 1998). Its use has been described in procedures on the skull base and paranasal sinuses (Caversaccio et al. 2002). This method is not compatible with intraoral approaches, which are necessary in the great majority of oromaxillofacial operations. Attaching a registration array (DRF) to a maxillary dental arch splint makes it possible to perform navigation-assisted implant insertions in the mobile lower jaw under local anesthesia (Schramm et al. 2000d; Fig. 15). This registration method is also used in all commercially available implant navigation systems.

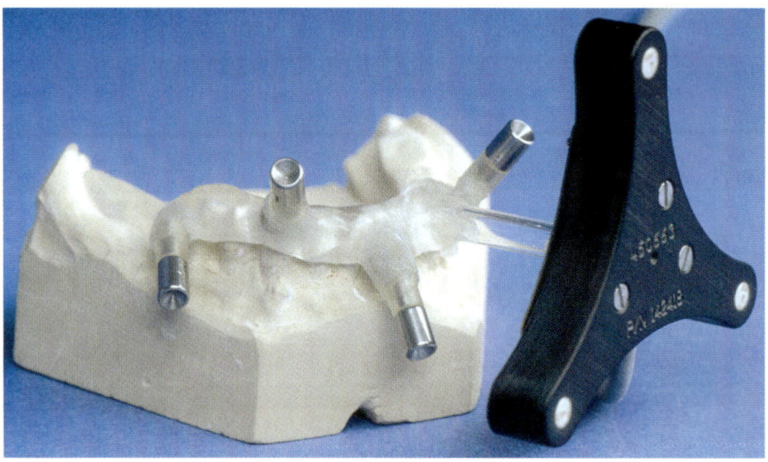

Fig. 15. Noninvasive registration of the jaw. The registration system is attached to a dental arch splint and tracks the movements of the jaw. In this way navigation-assisted implant insertions can be performed under local anesthesia, even on the mobile lower jaw

Imaging Procedures

A sectional imaging study is needed in order to produce a virtual 3D model of the patient. The software programs process data sets that have been acquired by CT, digital volume tomography (DVT), MRI, or a combination of these modalities. The advantages of MRI are better visualization of soft tissue and the ability to acquire images without exposure to ionizing radiation. But since the diagnostic workup is based largely on bony structures, the principal source of image data is spiral CT, which may be supplemented by MRI data sets in selected cases. The advantages of CT include the markedly better delineation of bony structures, better visualization of foreign bodies, relatively short acquisition times, and considerably lower costs. The use of DVT can significantly reduce the radiation exposure associated with CT scanning. DVT should not be used in tumor patients because of its relatively poor soft tissue discrimination, but it is preferred over standard CT scans in implantology, dysgnathic surgery, and especially in traumatology. The disadvantages of MRI-acquired data sets in the head region are poor delineation of bony structures as well as current technical limitations. For example, a phase distortion of up to several millimeters may occur in MRI data sets. Accuracy is also compromised by the use of 3- to 4-mm slice thicknesses (thinner slices are extremely difficult to acquire for technical reasons). Moreover, the relatively long acquisition time increases the risk of motion unsharpness (especially of the eye), making the data difficult to interpret.

The limiting factors in the head region with regard to radiation exposure are the ocular lens and the thyroid gland. The acquisition of axial CT scans can decrease radiation exposure by a factor of 30 compared with coronal CT scans (Hassfeld 2000). The slice thickness used for CT data acquisition is 1 mm. Slice thicknesses of 2 mm or more may introduce errors of up to 2 mm, particularly along the Z-axis. With a slice thickness of 1 mm, a table increment of 1 mm, and a pixel size of 0.5 mm, an effective accuracy of approximately 0.4 mm can be achieved.

Preoperative Planning and Simulation

Contents

Stereolithographic Method 27
Computer-assisted Planning. 28
Fusion of Image Data Sets 32
Feature-based Fusion 33
Image-based Fusion 33
Monomodal Image Fusion 34

Stereolithographic Method

Numerous methods of planning and simulating maxillofacial surgical procedures have been described in the literature – particularly stereolithographic models, which were developed during the 1980s and became increasingly popular during the 1990s (Hemmy et al. 1983; Vannier et al. 1984; Brix et al. 1985; Marsh and Vannier 1985; Gillespie and Isherwood 1986). A real model is sculpted with a cutting drill or fabricated by the stereolithographic method based on the CT data sets (Fleiner et al. 1994; Komori et al. 1994; Bill et al. 1995; Sader et al. 1997; Petzold et al. 1999). The advantage of having a real model is that the altered anatomy is easier to grasp than in a digital model and the surgical procedure can be planned directly on the model. This method has been used in an effort to simulate corrective osteotomies of the calvarium and facial skeleton. It has been applied in the surgical treatment of craniostenosis (Lambrecht and Brix 1990), callus distraction osteogenesis (Takato et al. 1993), the reconstruction of mandibular and midfacial defects (Klimek et al. 1993b), orthognathic and maxillofacial corrective osteotomies (Lindner et al. 1995; Santler 1998), and reconstructive orbital surgery (Perry et al. 1998).

The fabrication of these models is a costly and time-consuming process. For planning cranial reconstructions, stereolithographic models made from spiral CT data sets make more complete use of the available radiological information, although this information is basically limited to osseous structures. Another disadvantage is the appearance of "pseudoforamina," which result from the fact that thin bony lamellae cannot be accurately represented (Holck et

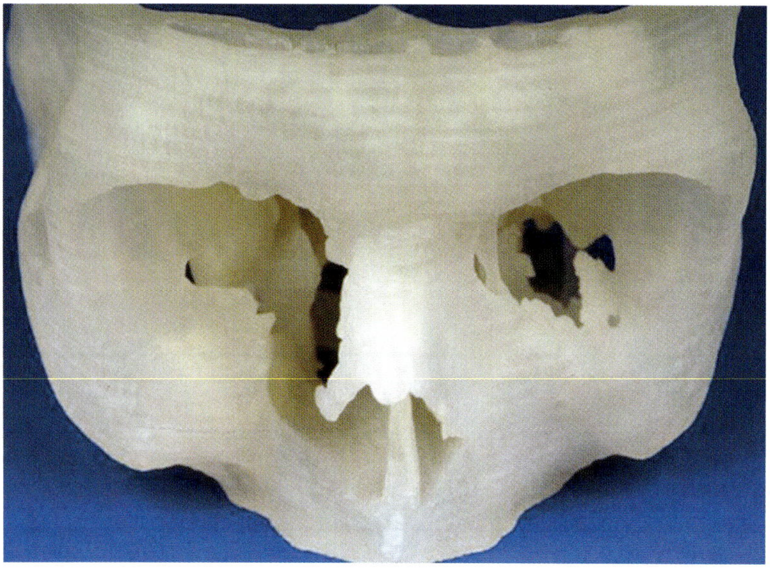

Fig. 16. Stereolithographic model of the naso-orbitoethmoid region. The frequent appearance of pseudoforamina in areas of very thin bone is a serious hindrance to planning, especially in orbital wall reconstructions

al. 1999). This lack of detail makes it impossible to plan certain skull base operations, and consequently this method does not provide a sufficiently accurate basis for planning primary and secondary reconstructions (Fig. 16). The further limitation of stereolithography to only a few corrective simulations has prevented its clinical application on a broad scale.

Computer-assisted Planning

By contrast, computer-assisted virtual planning and surgical simulations (CAP) offer the advantages of exceptionally high detail without information loss and the ability to conduct an almost limitless number and variety of simulations. Computer-assisted planning in virtual patient models (3D models) is based on preoperative sectional images obtained by CT or MRI. The first step is visualization of the image data acquired in the patient, i.e., calculating and displaying a virtual 3D model (Linney et al. 1989). This improves spatial orientation and facilitates diagnostic evaluation. The next step is to analyze the virtual model. This includes determining the extent of a defect by two- and three-dimensional measurements (distances, angles, volumes) performed in arbitrary planes of section. These steps supplement the information supplied by conventional imaging procedures and serve as a foundation. Actual planning in the virtual model begins with a virtual modification of the individual situation (simulation). The goal of preoperative planning is to create a virtual model that corresponds to the desired result of the operation (Schramm et al. 2002b). This is intended to improve the predictability of the operation in terms of the desired outcome, especially in complex reconstructions, and to increase intraoperative safety (Fig. 17).

Planning systems have been developed for the individual preoperative simulation of surgical procedures (Paul et al. 1992; Zamorano et al. 1993a; Hilbert et al. 1998b). Simulation programs have been described for craniofacial surgery (Altobelli et al. 1993; Girod et al. 1995; Vannier et al. 1995; Vannier and Marsh 1996; Bohner et al. 1997; Gladilin et al. 2004; Haegen et al. 2005) and for dysgnathic surgery (Carls et al. 1994). Basic criteria have been formulated for these systems (Klimek et al. 1992b, 1995; Papadopoulos et al. 2002). Besides basic model movements such as rotation and translation, the systems should be able to calculate sections viewed from arbitrary directions, define skin incisions and approaches to the operative site, and provide an interactive environ-

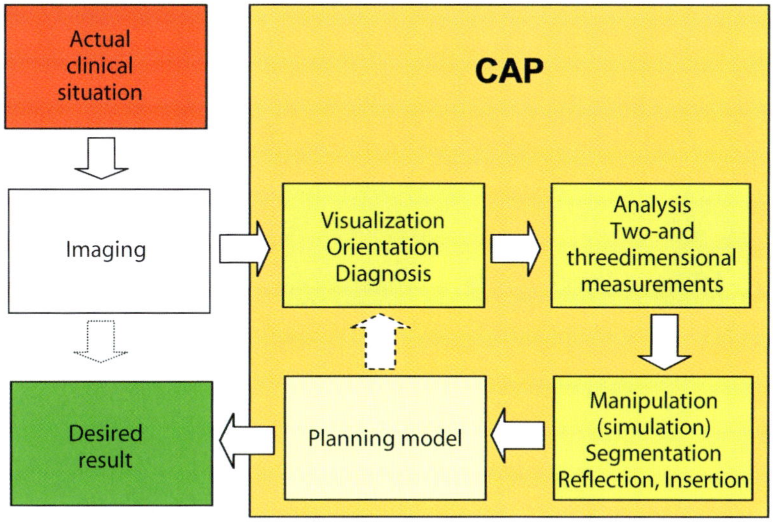

Fig. 17. Flowchart for computer-assisted planning (*CAP*)

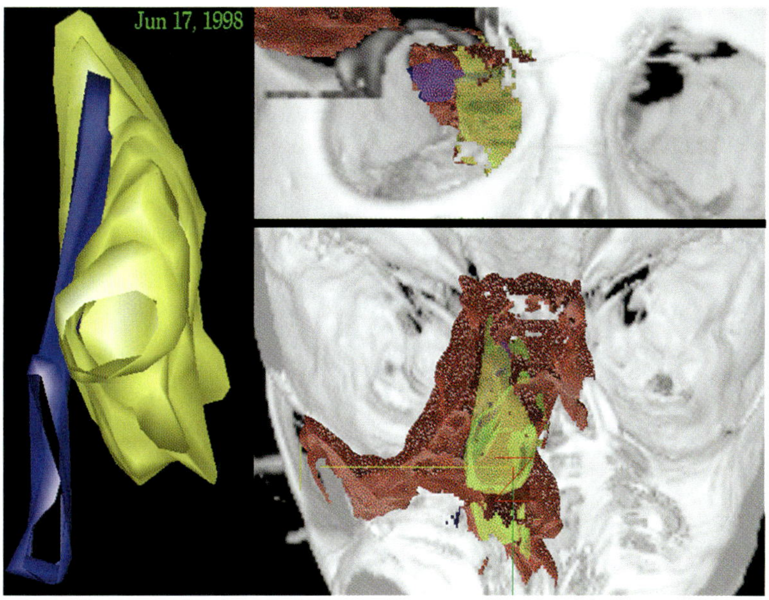

Fig. 18. Three-dimensional (3D) visualization of a large recurrent meningioma (*red*) compressing the optic nerve. The optic nerve (*blue*) and the tumor area to be resected for optic nerve decompression (*yellow*) are displayed separately in the *left window* as a surface-rendered model

ment for simulating the effects of operating instruments (Figs. 18–20). First, however, it must be possible to isolate segments of an arbitrary shape from the skull and position them as desired. Next, it should be possible to carry out these manipulations as realistically as possible. To date, simple software solutions for creating, programming, and implementing a reflection (mirroring) program for preoperative analysis and virtual surgical planning have been integrated into clinical use (Gellrich et al. 1999a; Schramm et al. 1999b; Thoma 1998).

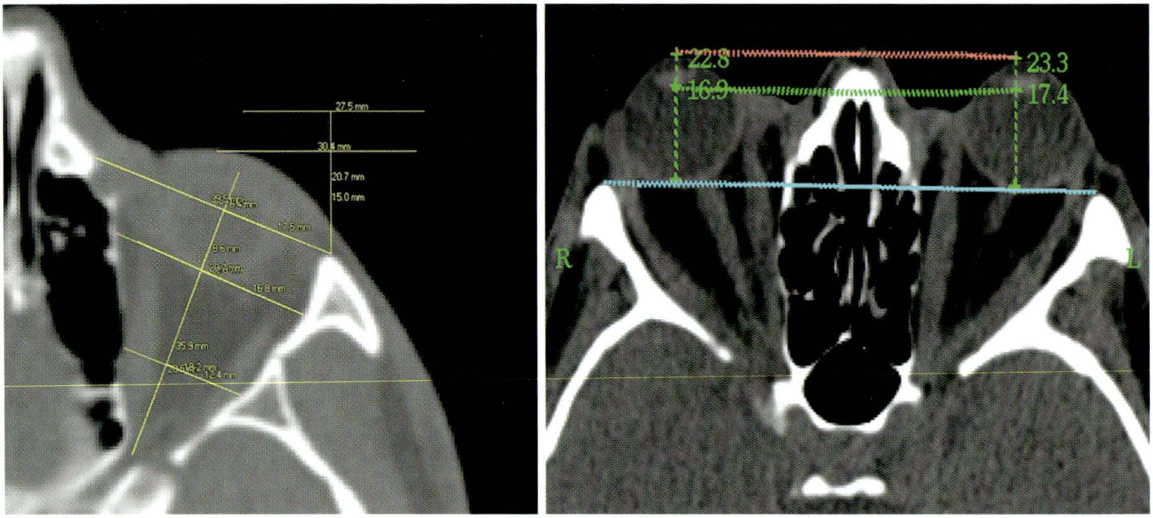

Fig. 19. Computer-based analysis for orbital measurements. The bony orbital dimensions (*left*) and CT-based Hertel measurements (*right*) are shown

Besides enabling the segmentation and mirroring of selected portions of the data set, modern surgical planning systems such as VoXim (IVS-Solutions, Chemnitz) also let the surgeon freely move the segments in relation to one another. This makes it possible to perform virtual bone-based reconstructions and bone-moving operations, and the result of the simulation, or the virtual model, can be used intraoperatively as a virtual template when intraoperative instrument navigation is used (Hohlweg-Majert et al. 2005; Schipper et al. 2005).

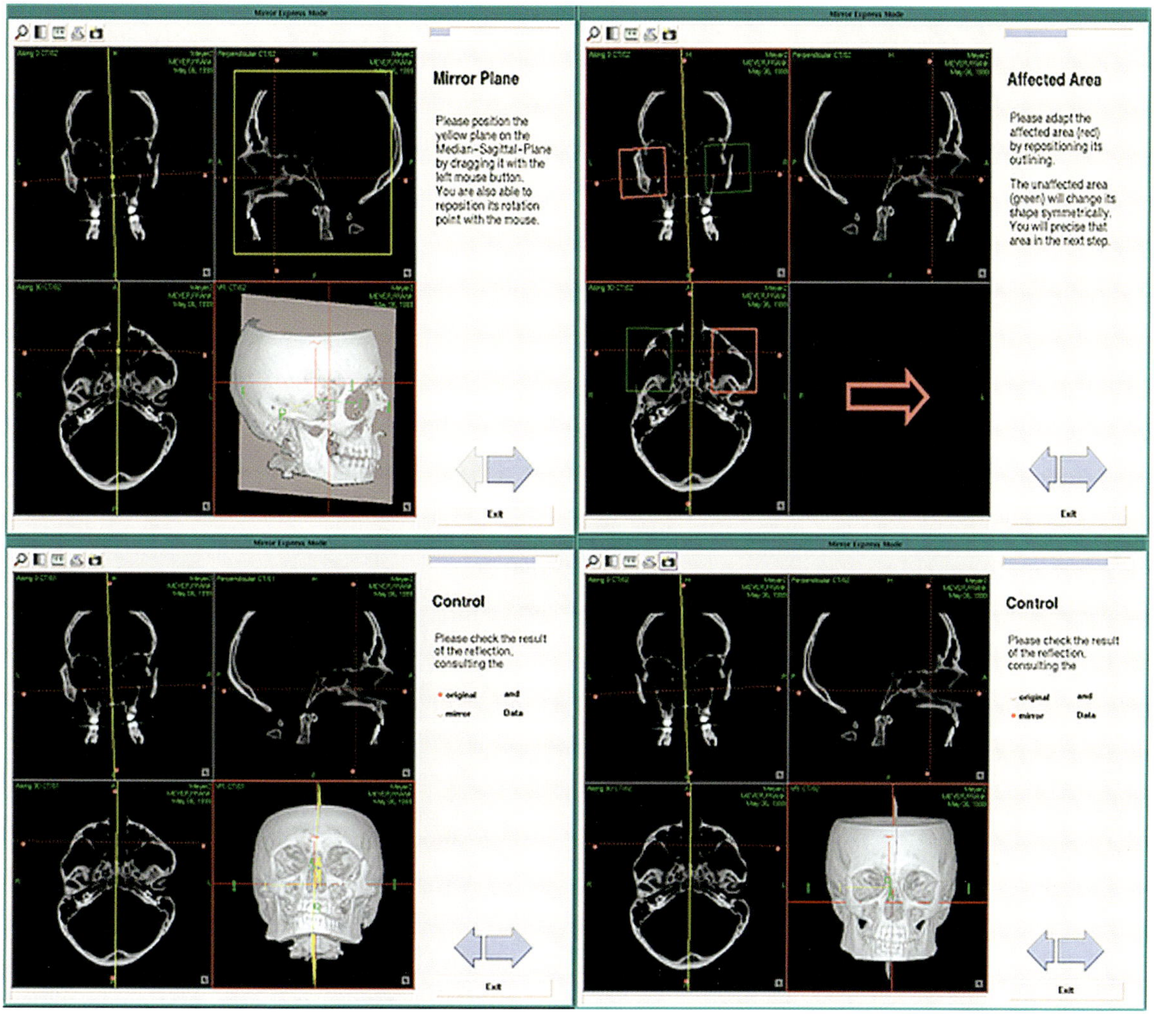

Fig. 20. Computer-assisted simulation for orbital reconstruction. After the plane of symmetry is defined in three dimensions (*upper left*), the surgeon marks the volume of the deformed orbit that is to be replaced (*upper right*). Three-dimensional reflection (mirroring) of the volume data set generates a virtual surgical template for making an idealized reconstruction. By comparing the original (*lower left*) and reflected data set (*lower right*), it is possible to analyze and validate the result of the simulated reconstruction

Fusion of Image Data Sets

Major diagnostic advances have been achieved through the combination of CT and MRI data sets (Hill et al. 1993). A multimodal image display, especially when it includes additional modalities [positron emission tomography (PET), single-photon emission computed tomography (SPECT), magnetic resonance angiography (MRA)], can significantly enhance operative planning (Woods et al. 1993; Hill et al. 1994; Peters et al. 1994; Cohen et al. 1995; Leemüller et al. 1996; Mukherji et al. 1996). The technology of image fusion is still in its early stages, and many groups of authors throughout the world are making rapid advances in this area. In the field of medicine, the fusion of image data is being utilized to improve preoperative planning and diagnosis (Hassfeld 2000). One diagnostic technique involves superimposing the images from different modalities ("multimodal image fusion") in order to combine their specific advantages. Several technical problems

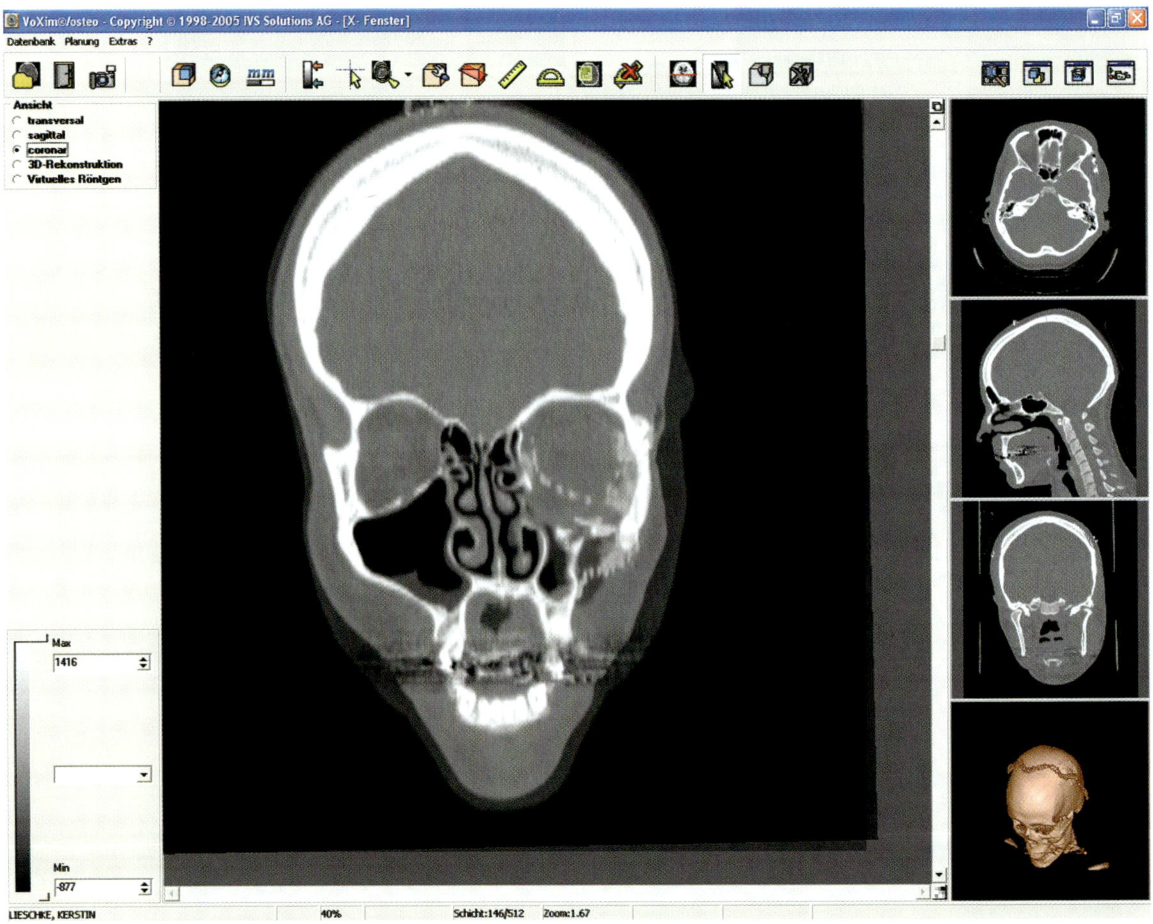

Fig. 21. Image fusion for postoperative evaluation of reconstructive procedures. The result of the reconstruction can be visualized and quantitatively evaluated by a landmark-based overlay of the pre- and postoperative CT data sets from the patient

still need to be resolved in order to achieve the successful fusion of multimodal images. For example, the images usually have different properties with regard to pixel size, threshold values, spatial resolution, and slice thickness. There are inconsistencies in the position and projection of the sensor, including the distance of the sensor from the patient, the inclination angle, and the table increment, as well as differences in patient position and data acquisition times, which may lead to motion artifacts.

These inconsistencies result in images with different information contents that vary in their proportions, orientation, and resolution and cannot be meaningfully correlated and superimposed without preliminary measures. For this reason, we must first transform the images into a "common representation" that has the same proportions before proceeding with the actual image fusion and orientation in a common matrix (Fig. 21). Various techniques can be used for this purpose.

Feature-based Fusion

Techniques of "feature-based fusion" involve the use of characteristic quantities. This means that it is first necessary to define and segment known features in the data sets that are to be fused. These feature may be surface textures or objects, for example.

One feature-based fusion technique is "landmark matching," which is based on the principles of coordinating two different spatial coordinate systems, analogous to the principles of landmark-based registration. The advantages of this technique are rapid computation and high accuracy. Mongioj et al. (1999) and Amdur et al. (1999) superimposed CT and MRI data sets obtained with the use of skin markers and anatomical landmarks, respectively, and documented respective accuracies of 0.9 mm and 1.3–1.4 mm.

Techniques based on the "surface matching" principle employ an algorithm that interpolates and matches previously extracted (segmented) portions of anatomical contours. Parsai et al. (1997) used a surface matching technique to fuse CT and SPECT images from the same patient and reported an accuracy of 3–4 mm. Lattanzi et al. (1997) fused CT and MRI data sets and used a fixation apparatus to place the patient in an ideal position for superimposing the images. "Likelihood registration" is a type of feature-based fusion that is useful in other areas, especially pattern recognition. In this technique image fusion is accomplished with an algorithm based on hypotheses and probabilities on the definition of a surface or an object.

In this type of fusion, as in registration, at least three non-collinear reference points must be identified in each of the two data sets. But in contrast to registration, where the reference points (e.g., markers) must be accessible to a tracking instrument, each uniquely identifiable anatomical reference point can be used for the fusion of two data sets, regardless of its location. These points are located manually, which results in loss of accuracy. But calculating the standard deviation of the points by computer tells us nothing about the overall accuracy of the fusion, only on the segmented region. For example, the result of the fusion may be more accurate for selected points spaced far apart (large segment) with a greater standard deviation than for points spaced close together (small segment) with a smaller standard deviation.

Accordingly, we can increase the accuracy of the fusion by spacing the reference points farther apart and also by identifying additional points. The computer-calculated standard deviation can be used as a good approximation. In doubtful cases, the relevant region can be visually inspected at high magnification to assess the accuracy of the fusion.

Image-based Fusion

These fusion techniques are based on image information, i.e., elements that are already contained in the image such as pixel size, color intensity, wavelength, and threshold values. "Intensity matching" and "voxel-based fusion" are examples of the techniques that are used in medical image processing. The grayscale threshold information of the individual voxels in different modalities (e.g., CT and MRI), initially different, are correlated with an intermediate algorithm and are then superimposed. This computer operation is relatively time-consuming, however. Besides accuracy, speed is an important factor in certain applications (e.g., the fusion of images in real time). Various algorithms with different degrees of accuracy and computation times have been described in the literature (Maes et al. 1997). Because these techniques do not employ characteristic quantities and do not require user interaction, they have a broad range of applications.

The techniques of image fusion described above are also known collectively as "rigid transformation." The fusion of moving images, or nonrigid transformation, affords access to the "fourth dimension" and opens up new possibilities in diagnosis. Another data fusion method, still in the developmental stage, is called "sensor fusion." Involving the use of a recording device equipped with various sensors, this method yields images from different modalities on a single medium.

Monomodal Image Fusion

In monomodal image fusion, images acquired with the same imaging modality are superimposed. To date, relatively few articles on this topic have appeared in the literature. This method of image fusion is particularly well suited for computer-assisted planning and follow-ups in the medical field. The technical problems associated with this method are relatively easy to manage. Images acquired with the same technical settings (sensor-patient distance, table increment, slice thickness, pixel size, etc.) contain practically identical information, resulting in data sets with identical proportions. There is no need for an algorithm to correlate the data sets, and this should result in higher technical accuracy than in multimodal fusions. It is still necessary, however, to take into account differences in patient position. The stereotactic frames (Levin et al. 1988; Pelizzari et al. 1989) initially used for fusion of the data sets were replaced with noninvasive adhesive skin markers (Arun et al. 1987; Pelizzari et al. 1989; Berry et al. 2003) or data set correlation based on anatomical landmarks (Boesecke et al. 1990). The disadvantage of this noninvasive method is the poor reliability of adhesive skin markers and the considerable time needed when landmarks are used. The correlation of two CT data sets in one patient can be achieved relatively easily and reliably by means of "landmark correlation." Corresponding bony points are marked in both CT data sets, and then both images are superimposed by matching up the corresponding points (Fig. 22). This method is suitable for routine clinical use, as it enables the rapid fusion of pre- and postoperative CT image data sets from the same patient. In this way tumor volumes can be transferred and the results of reconstructions in the facial skeleton can be evaluated with millimeter accuracy.

Although the correlation of CT and MRI data sets based on anatomical landmarks is often a very difficult task for the therapist, the fusion of CT and MRI allows us to transfer soft tissue structures (e.g., tumors) that are clearly delineated by MRI to the CT scan, making it possible to combine soft tissue information and skeletal information in the same image.

When a noninvasive registration splint is used, the well-defined splint-based markers can be used for correlation. This requires the patient to wear the splint during the acquisition of both data sets (Fig. 23).

Splint-based registration is a repeatable process that allows us to transfer tumor boundaries from the MRI data set to the CT data set for pretherapeutic analysis and to compare pretherapeutic acquisitions with all further data sets that are acquired after chemotherapy, radiotherapy, or operative treatment (Fig. 24). The use of registration splints also makes it possible to fuse CT and MRI data sets since the markers can be identified in both modalities (Schramm et al. 2000c). This could also be achieved with invasive screw markers, but these devices could not be used due to the long treatment periods. Thus we may list the following advantages for clinical therapeutic settings:

- By transforming pretherapeutic data into posttherapeutic data sets, we can measure the efficacy of chemotherapy based on the quantitative determination and localization of the tumor mass.
- By transforming pretherapeutic data into posttherapeutic data sets, we can perform a navigation-guided resection that conforms to the original tumor boundaries.
- By transferring the preoperative tumor boundaries into the postoperative data set, we can conduct a precise follow-up evaluation for tumor recurrence and refine the planning of postoperative adjuvant radiotherapy.

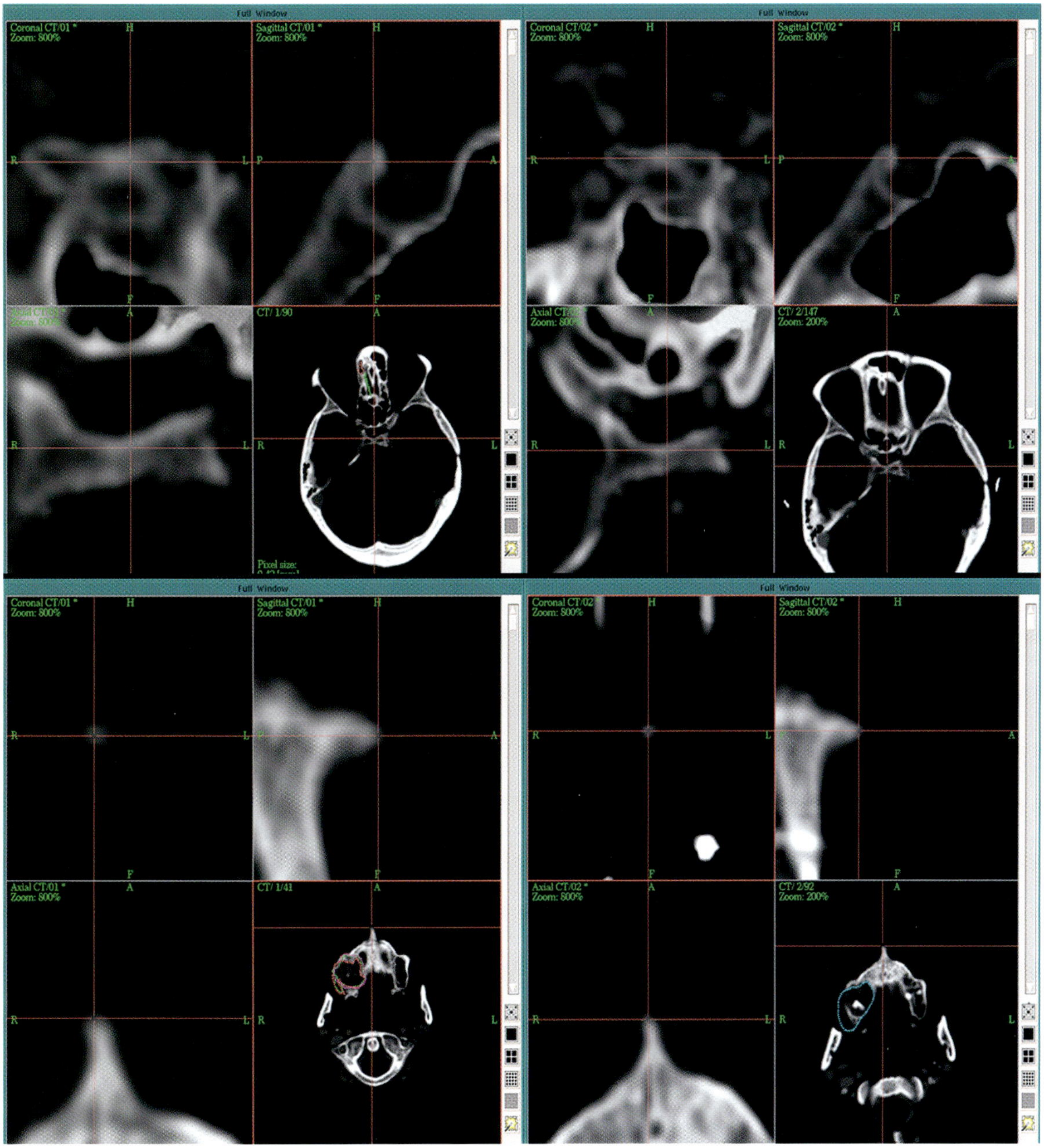

Fig. 22. Image fusion of two CT data sets based on the use of anatomical landmarks. The sella turcica (*above*) and the anterior nasal spine (*below*) are reproducible landmarks that are easy to locate and identify during the use of CT data sets. The data sets to be correlated (*CT 1* and *CT 2*) are displayed in the multiplanar mode (coronal, sagittal, and axial planes)

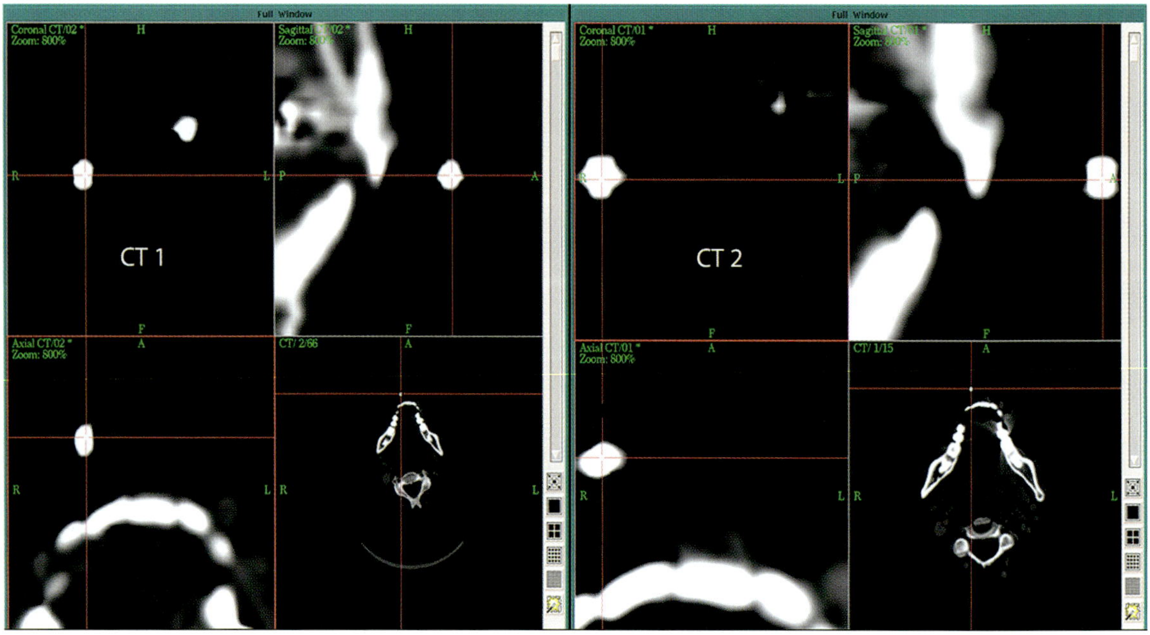

Fig. 23. Image fusion of two CT data sets based on the use of splint-based markers. The reproducible, well-defined markers on the arch splint allow for a rapid and precise fusion of the image data sets. The data sets to be correlated (*CT 1* and *CT 2*) are displayed in the multiplanar mode (coronal, sagittal, and axial planes)

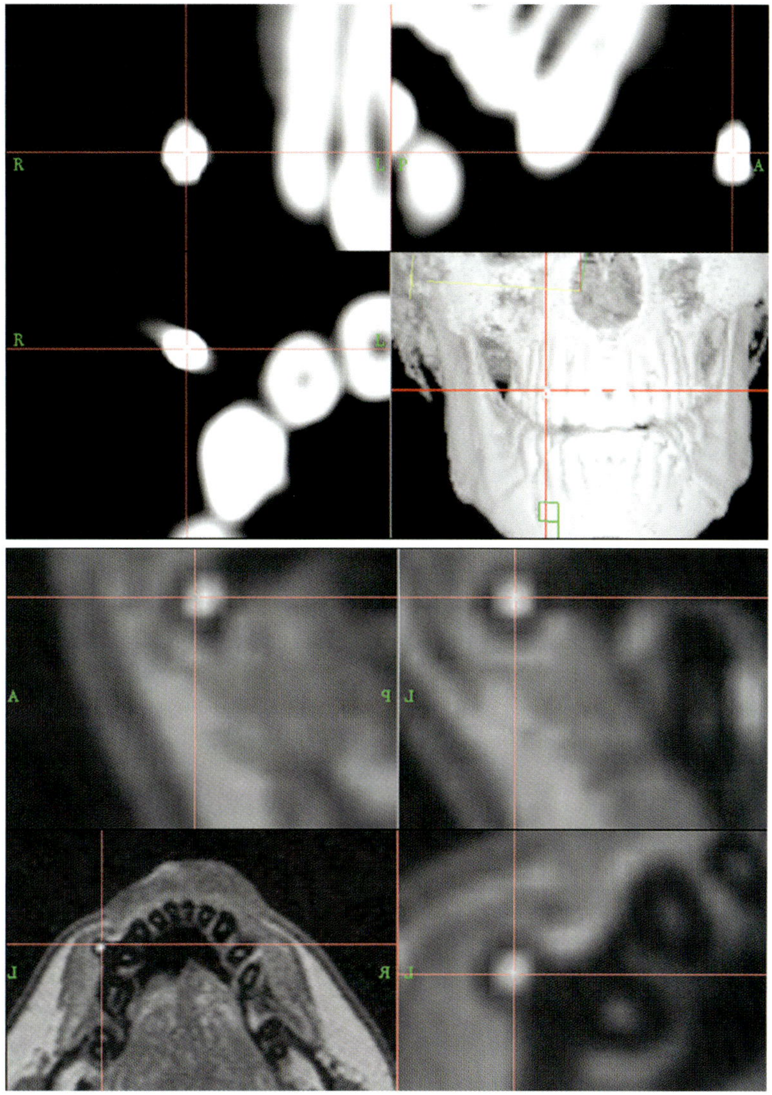

Fig. 24. Use of splint-based markers in the fusion of CT (*upper*) and MRI (*lower*) data sets. The reproducible, well-defined markers on the dental arch splint allow for the rapid and precise fusion of data sets, even those acquired with different imaging modalities. The data sets to be correlated (CT and MRI) are displayed in the multiplanar mode (coronal, sagittal, and axial planes)

Preoperative Preparations

Contents

Definition of the Reference Points 39
Intraoperative Setup 42
Registration 43

Definition of the Reference Points

After the patient has received the appropriate registration system, the acquisition of image data is carried out. When the examination is completed, the digital data from the CT or MR images is imported into the navigation system. Actual preoperative planning begins by defining the centers of the spherical markers in the CT or MRI data set (Fig. 25), as they will serve as reference points during the operation. Errors may result from faulty positioning of the registration splints by the therapist or patient. Vacuum-formed splints with an occlusal rest can reduce this source of error.

When the splint is fabricated, particular care should be taken that the markers are not imaged in the axial planes of artifact zones caused by dental filling materials or arch splints. Artifact problems may even render a marker useless for registration (Fig. 26).

Following a patient- and disease-specific analysis of the image data, the planning software is used to outline tumor boundaries, draw virtual lines and objects, define approach vectors, etc., depending on the nature of the planned procedure. A detailed description of the various forms of treatment is given under the headings for specific procedures.

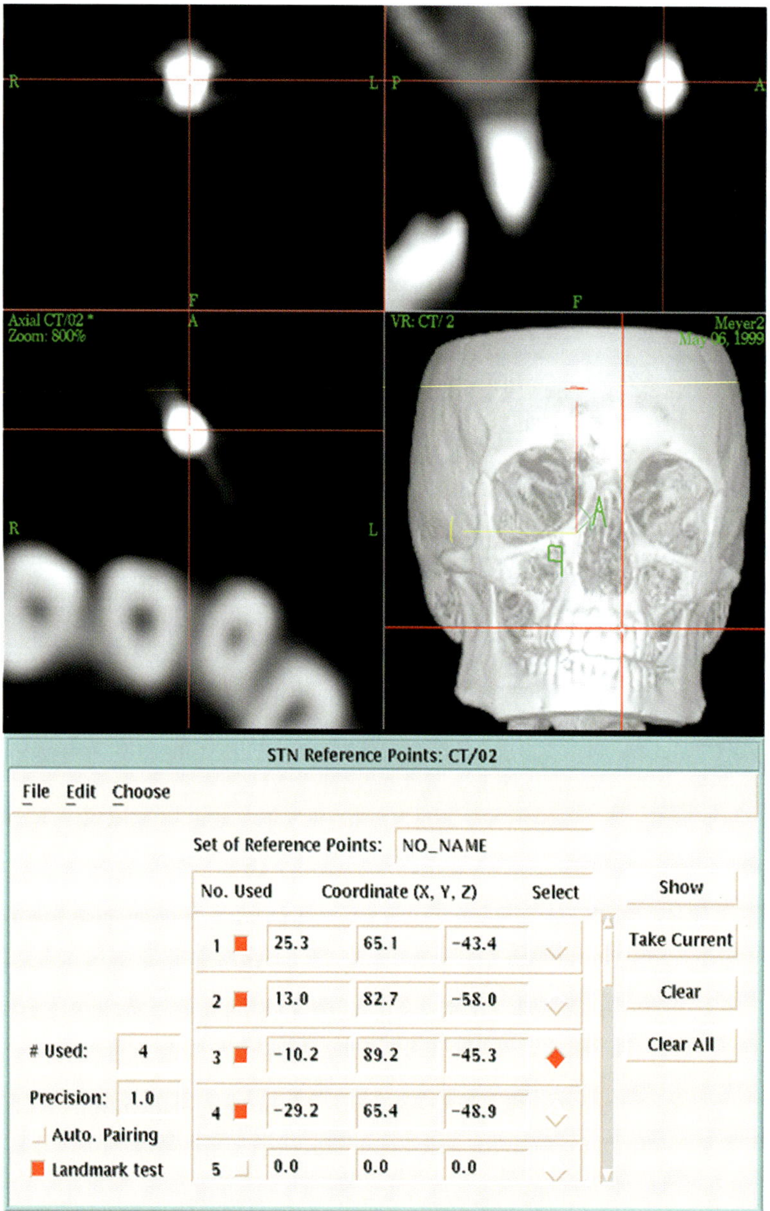

Fig. 25. Preoperative definition of the reference points. The centers of the reference markers in the dental arch splint are marked at high magnification (400–800%) in the multiplanar mode (coronal, sagittal, axial, and 3D)

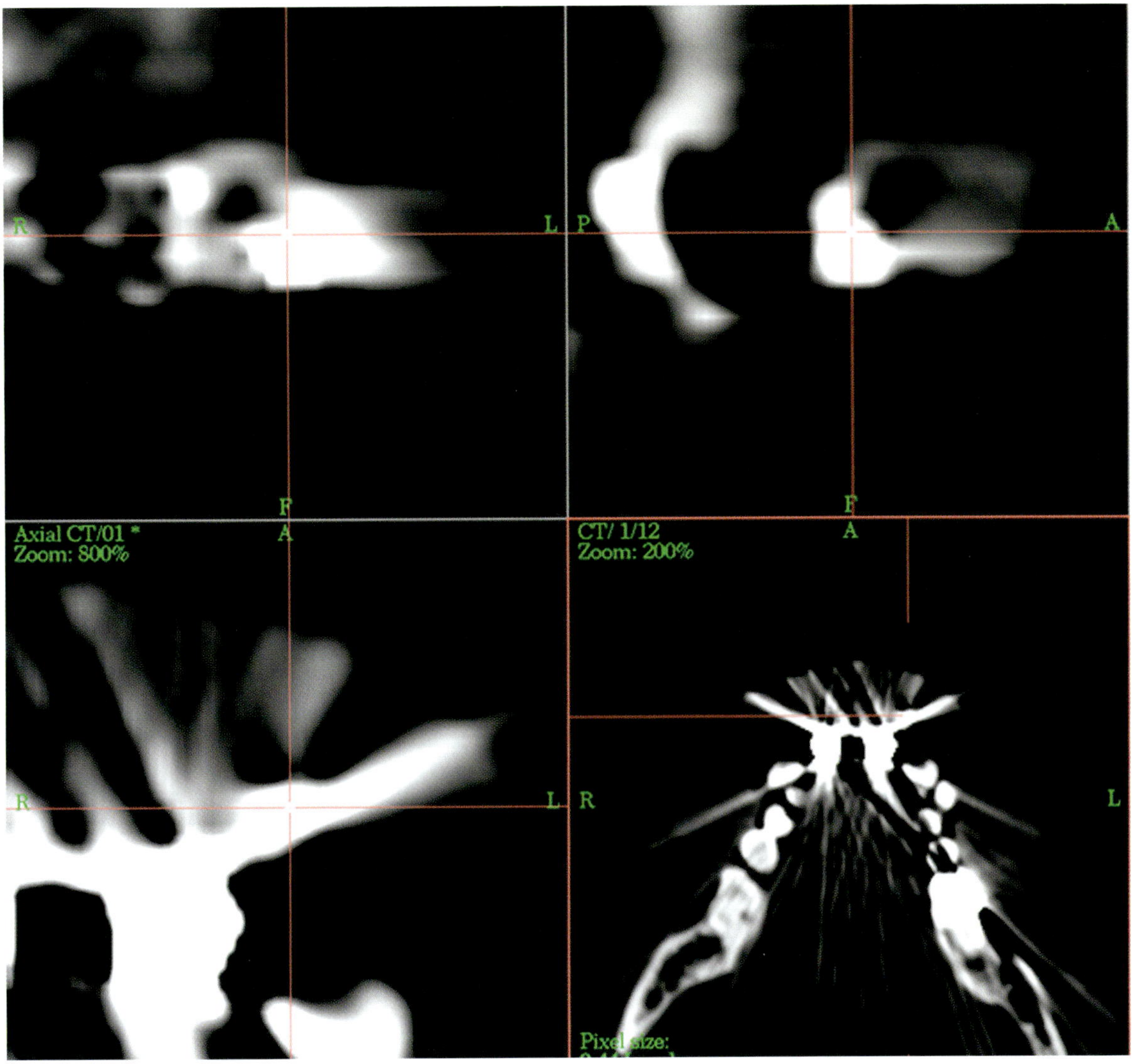

Fig. 26. Artifacts caused by dental fillings. The splint marker is located in a plane that is obscured by artifacts. As a result, the center of the marker cannot be accurately visualized, and that marker cannot be used for registration

Intraoperative Setup

After the navigation system has been set up in the operating room, the arm-mounted camera is positioned and any necessary instrument calibrations are performed. The DRF is attached to the Mayfield clamp or dental arch splint and is correctly aligned with respect to the camera (Fig. 27).

The infrared camera may be placed at the foot or head of the operating table as needed. Its placement should cause minimal interference with the surgeon, assistants, and instrumentation (Fig. 28).

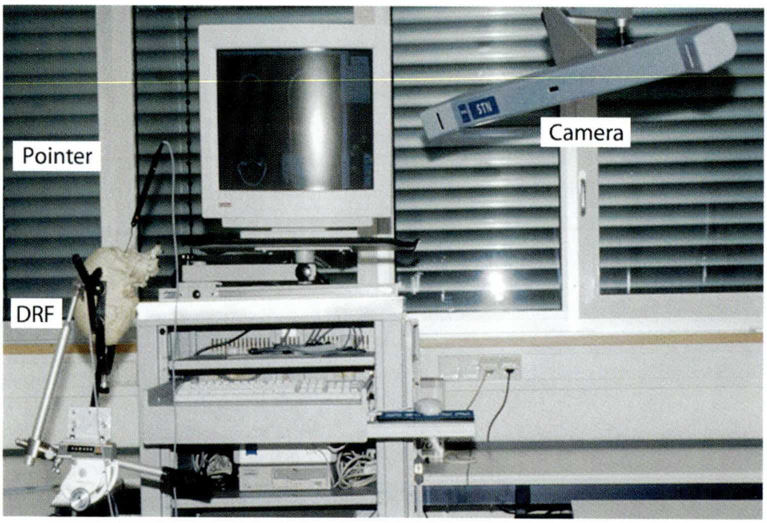

Fig. 27. Intraoperative setup of an active optical registration system. After the head is fixed in the Mayfield clamp, the registration system (*DRF*) and arm-mounted camera are correctly positioned. The pointer is prepared for registration

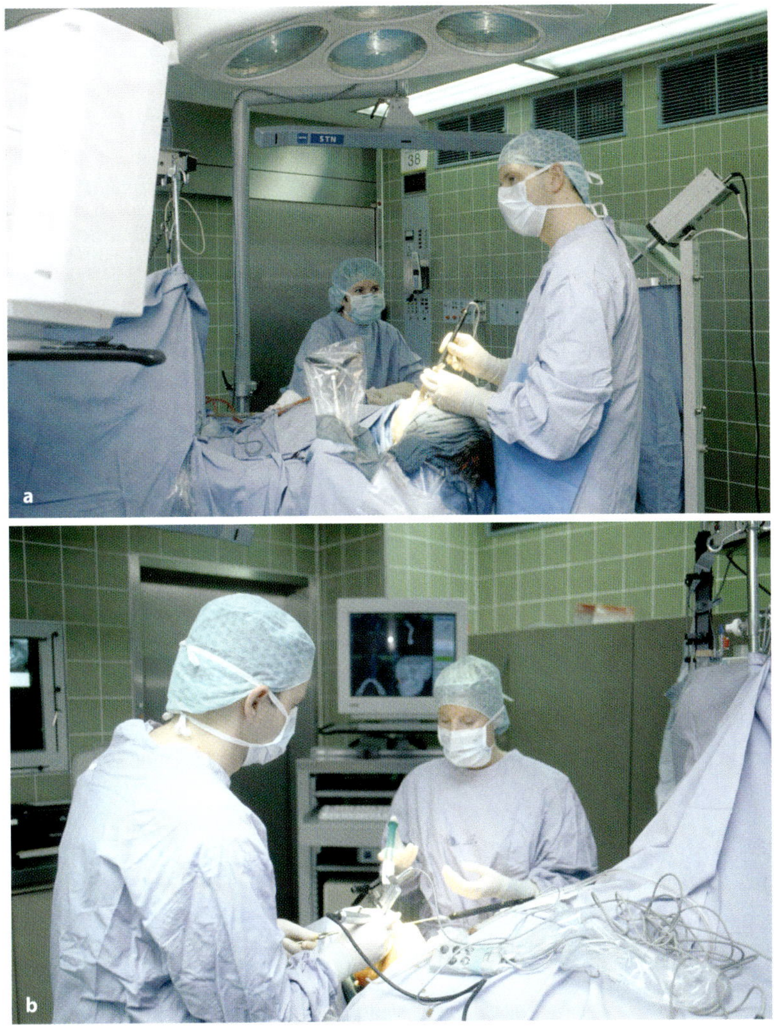

Fig. 28 a, b. Variations in the setup of the navigation system. The camera and monitor should be positioned to meet the requirements of the surgeon and of different treatment modalities

Registration

The first step in intraoperative navigation is registration. Generally a pointer is used to define the reference points, but in principle the tip of any trackable instrument can be used for reference point registration. The tip of the pointer is successively touched to the center of the hollow spheres on all the registration markers, and a correlation is established for each reference point (Figs. 29, 30). A minimum of three markers should be used for registration. Registration may be done before draping or under sterile conditions, and it can be repeated during the procedure as often as desired. The registration splint can be plasma-sterilized preoperatively or placed in disinfectant solution during the operation. It can be removed from the mouth after each registration. Preoperative registration before aseptic preparation of the operative field is preferred in neurosurgical operations owing to the separation of the registration field and operating field. Preoperative registration is unnecessary in procedures on the facial skeleton, and registration should be done under sterile conditions.

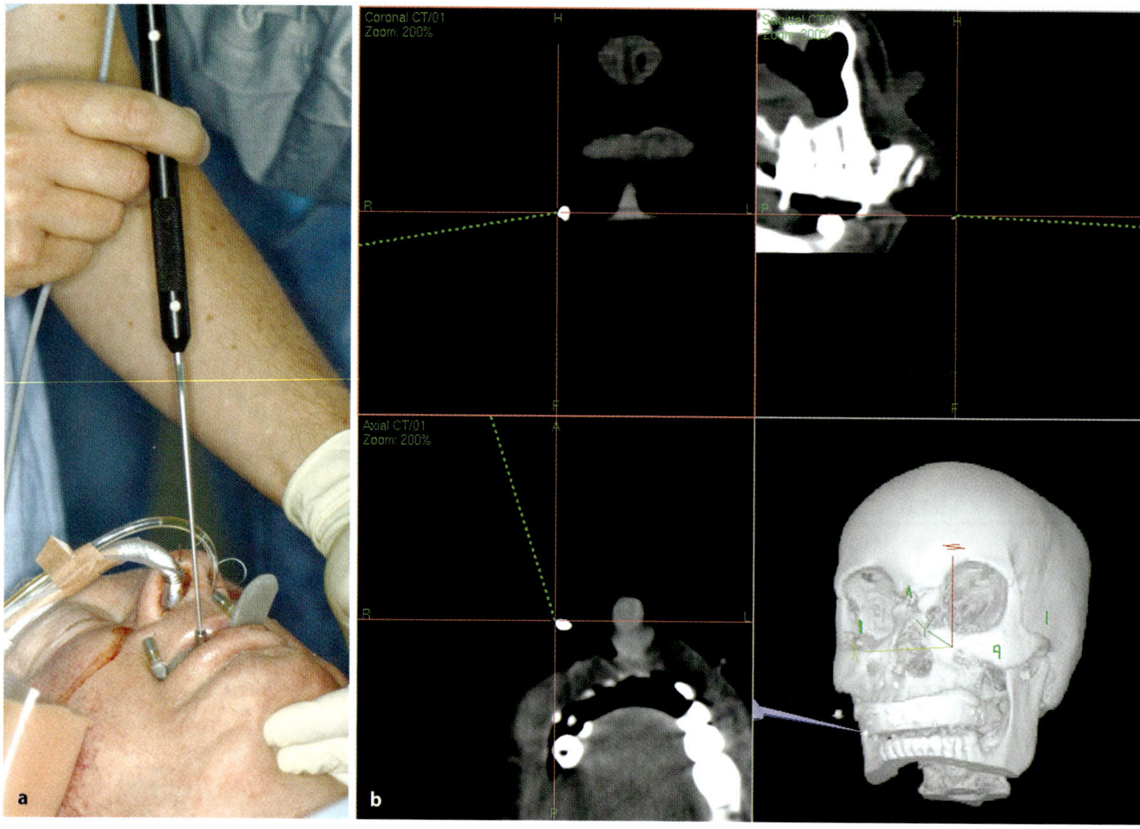

Fig. 29. Preoperative registration with a dental arch splint. The markers on the registration splint are individually touched with the pointer (a) and are checked for plausibility at the completion of registration (b). This process may precede the actual operation. The splint may be removed after successful registration

The coordinates of the reference points stored in the preoperative CT data set are compared with the coordinates of the reference markers registered during the operation and are checked for deviations. This deviation represents the internal reference point deviation (IRD) of the system. In our own laboratory studies, we found no correlation between the IRD and the intraoperative accuracy of registration, regardless of the registration method used. The result of the transformation is stated in millimeters as the internal deviation of the point coordinates of the markers in the CT or MRI data set and of the spatial coordinates of the reference markers on the patient. Values less than 1 mm indicate a successful registration, although they do not predict the attainable level of intraoperative accuracy because the IRD only reflects the agreement between the geometrical marker arrangement in the CT data set and the operative site. Nevertheless, the registration process should be repeated if the IRD is greater than 1 mm, as this most likely indicates faulty positioning of the registration system.

A clinical "landmark test" [placing the pointer tip on salient points of the facial skeleton: center of the glabella (Fig. 31), incisal point, lateral orbital rim, infra- and supraorbital foramina, external auditory canal] should be done to compare anatomical points on the patient with the virtual anatomy in the image data set. If this test is satisfactory, the registration process is complete.

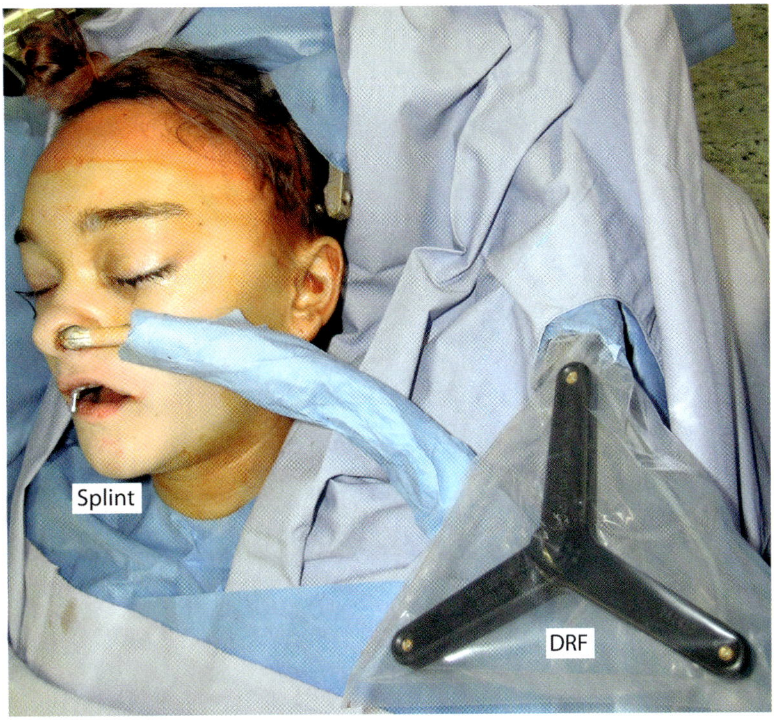

Fig. 30. Intraoperative registration with a dental arch splint. The markers on the splint can also be registered with the pointer under sterile conditions. The registration system can be plasma-sterilized or it can be covered with sterile film as shown

Intraoperative navigation can now be utilized during each phase of the operation. If the position of the DRF changes in relation to the operative field, however, a valid correlation can no longer be ensured. This problem may result from inadvertent slippage of the DRF in the holder or incidental movement of the patient's head in the Mayfield clamp (cranial osteotomy with a chisel, reduction maneuvers, etc.). Intraoperative reregistration should be performed in these cases. This process can be repeated as often as desired in cases where splint- and miniscrew-based registration is used. After successful clinical validation of the registration, the operation can be continued.

Besides the pure localization of structures with a pointer, the navigation system can be used to track endoscopes and any nonflexible operating instrument. Navigation-assisted microscopy is achieved by laser-based detection of the focal point, which can then be identified as a virtual image in the patient's image data set. The individual steps involved in navigation using a pointer, endoscope, and operating microscope are illustrated under the headings for specific surgical procedures.

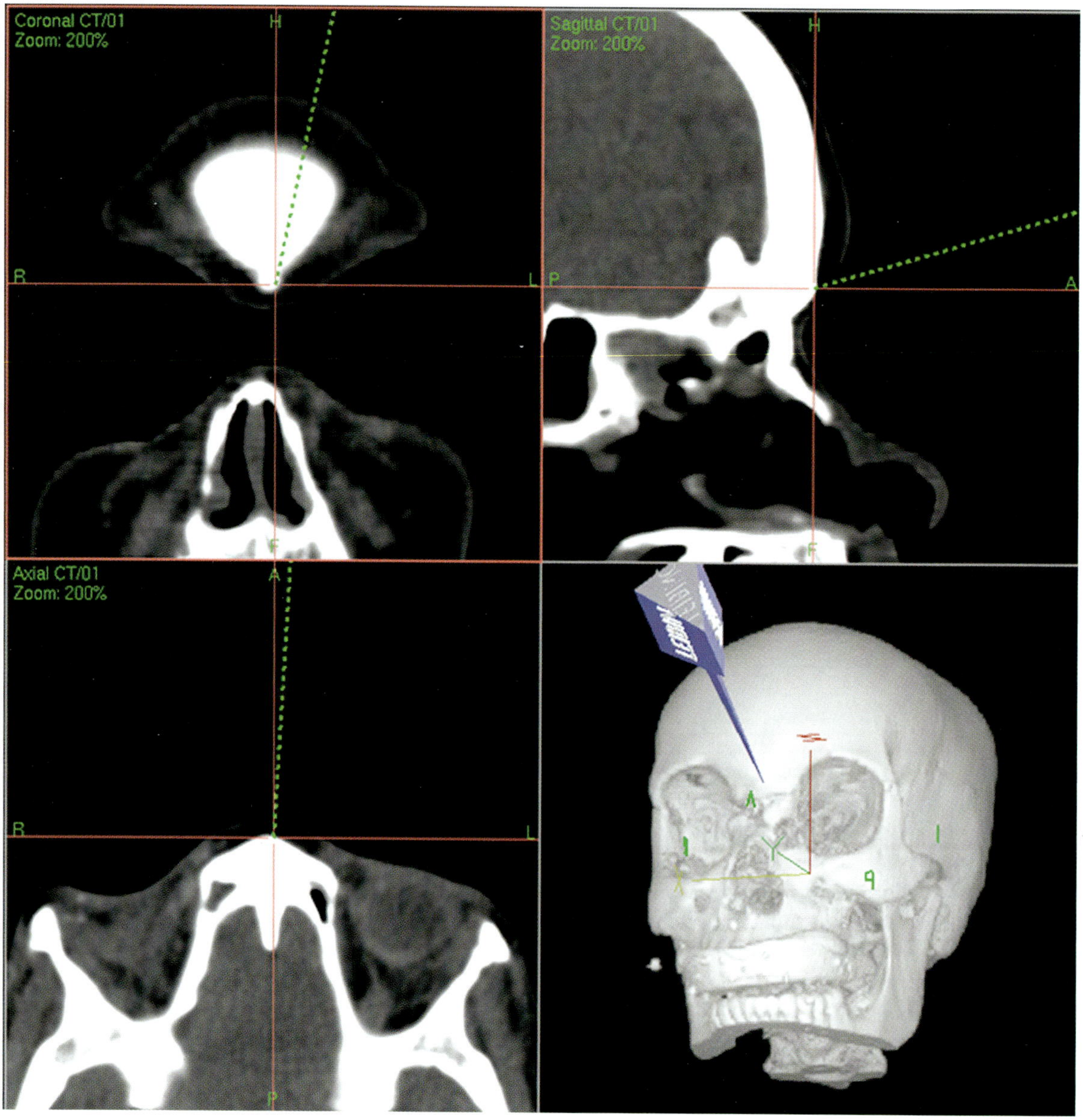

Fig. 31. Landmark test to validate the registration. An essential prelude to intraoperative navigation is validating the registration by touching reproducible landmarks (e.g., the center of the glabella) with the pointer. The position of the pointer tip in the CT data set is compared with the operative site

Intraoperative Accuracy

The accuracy (or inaccuracy) of intraoperative navigation depends critically on the following five factors:

1. Inaccuracy of the CT data set and its processing and visualization
2. Inaccuracy of the navigation system used
3. Inaccuracy of pointer localization
4. Inaccuracy in registering the patient's head with the registration system
5. Inaccuracy of the registration method used

The first four technical factors in this list can be kept below 0.2–0.3 mm with proper technique (Husstedt et al. 1999). The greatest variation in accuracy results from the type of registration method used. Because the intraoperative accuracy of navigation is the sum of all five factors, the accuracy of the registration system is considered to be the most important factor.

The mean positional accuracy of 2 mm recommended for surgical applications (Sandemann et al. 1994) can be reliably achieved through the use of bone-anchored screw markers (Hassfeld et al. 1997, 2000; Brinker et al. 1998). Their advantages are their reliability and reproducibly high accuracy. They are invasive, however, and this limits their usefulness in emergency and elective procedures (Hassfeld 2000). Nevertheless, for many years screw markers have been the only feasible method of intraoperative navigation in oromaxillofacial patients.

Because the maxillary splint is considered a bone-based method because of its attachment to the dental arch, it is the only noninvasive registration method that provides consistently high intraoperative accuracy (Schramm et al. 2001c; Eggers et al. 2005; Hoffmann et al. 2005b,c). In surgery of the facial skeleton and skull base region, a registration splint with four markers arranged in an optimum geometrical pattern is accurate to less than 1.5 mm, depending on the type of splint used (Naumann 2001; Nilius 2001; Fig. 32).

Splint-based registration is superior to invasive markers in the facial skeleton because the center of the reference points on the splint is closer to the center of the facial skeleton than when screw markers are used: The greater the distance of the operative field from the center of the reference markers, the poorer the accuracy of the registration (Fig. 33). For a distance of up to 10 cm between the reference center and marker point, the accuracy of invasive bone-screw registration and noninvasive splint-based registration is less than 2 mm. When this distance is increased, deviations of up to 8 mm occur when splints are used. This is directly attributable to the increasing distance of the markers from the operative field.

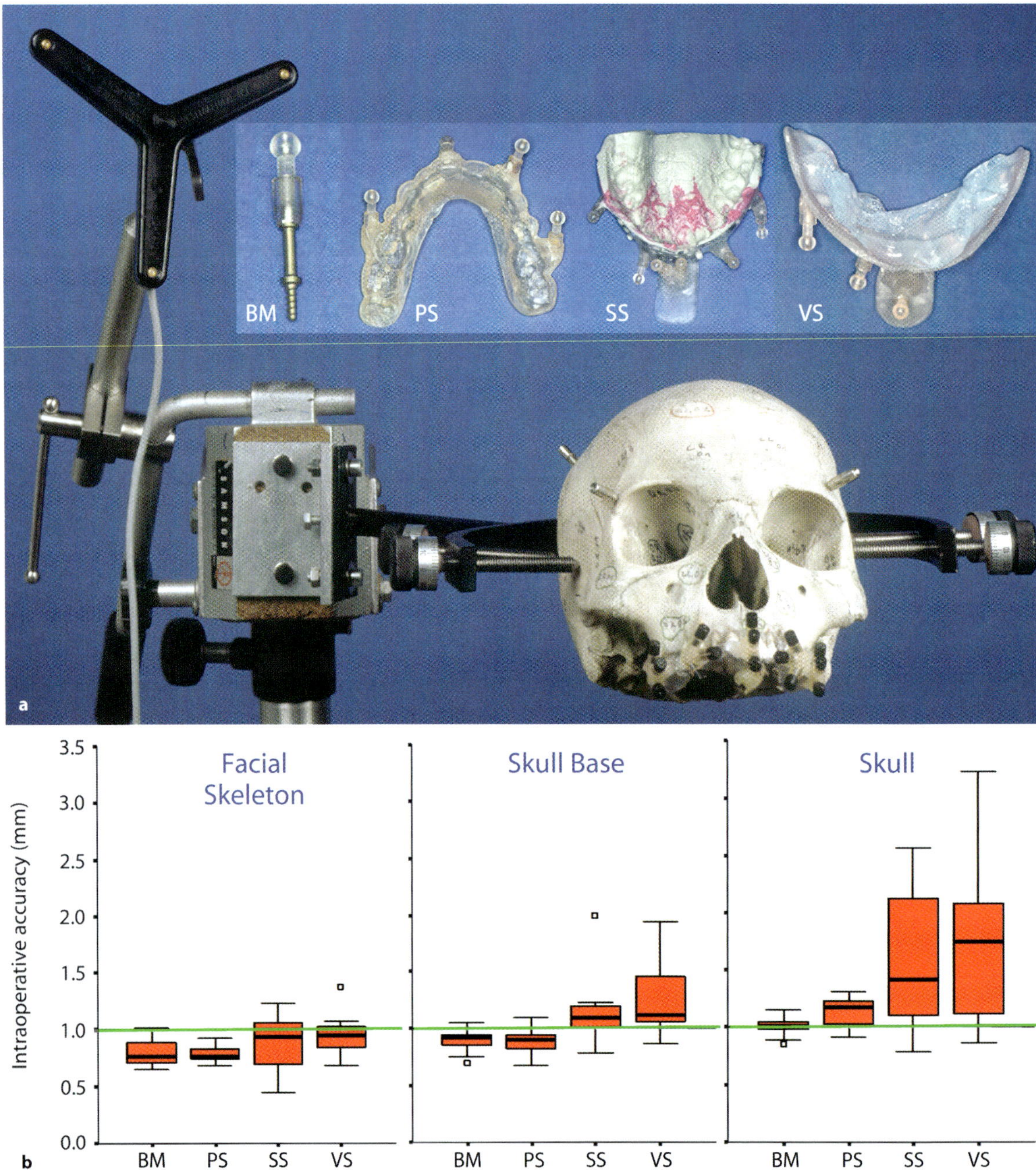

Fig. 32. Intraoperative accuracy of splint-based and screw-marker-based registration. The intraoperative accuracies of bone marker (*BM*), PMMA splint (*PS*), silicone splint (*SS*), and vestibular splint (*VS*) determined in laboratory tests can be directly compared based on their bony attachments (a). The vacuum-formed PMMA splints and screw markers provide a reproducible accuracy of 1 mm in all regions of the skull. The silicone impression splints show markedly higher values in the skull base and cranial vault (b)

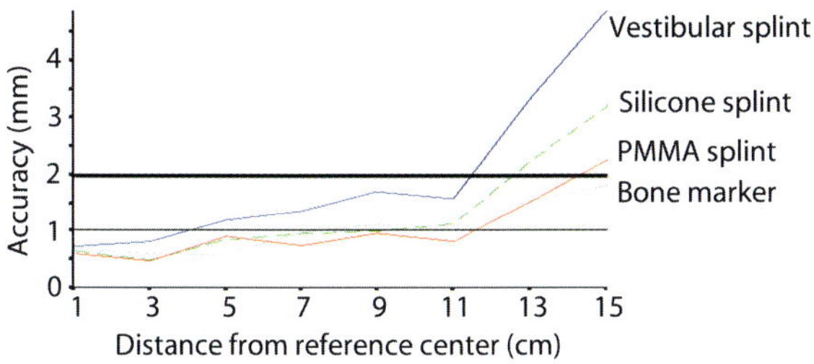

Fig. 33. Intraoperative accuracy as a function of distance from the reference center. The intraoperative accuracies of bone-screw markers (*bone marker*), vacuum-formed splints (*PMMA splint*), maxillary silicone impression splints (*silicone splint*), and vestibular silicone impression splints (*vestibular splint*) determined in laboratory tests are plotted as a function of distance from the reference center. When this distance is greater than 11 cm, the accuracy values of splint-based registration decline significantly. This is not the case with screw markers distributed symmetrically on the skull

Patient-friendly Navigation

Computer-based navigation in craniomaxillofacial surgery involves adjunctive measures designed to improve planning and spatial orientation. This means that patients are operated and treated according to the same principles as they would without the use of navigation. Application requires only thin-slice spiral CT scanning or DVT imaging prior to the operation: additional images are not required. Intraoperative registration does not cause additional risk or discomfort for the patient when a noninvasive method (splint) is used. Information on possible risks and precautionary measures and principles of informed consent are maintained in accordance with standard clinical practices. The application of computer-assisted surgery increases the safety and accuracy of the surgical procedure, and this should result in a better outcome for the patient.

Computer-assisted Therapy

Contents

Minimally Invasive Surgeries and Biopsies 53
Optic Nerve Decompression 66
Recommendations for the Treatment of Traumatic Optic Nerve Injury 67
Resections and Reconstructions 72
Lateral Skull Base and Temporo-mandibular Joint 73
Anterior Skull Base 86
Midface 86
Intraoperative Radiotherapy 104
Secondary Reconstructions after Tumor Resections 105
Traumatological Procedures 114
Primary Orbital and Midfacial Reconstructions . . 114
Secondary Orbital and Midfacial Reconstructions 126
Reconstruction with CAD-CAM Implants 135
Procedures for Midfacial Correction 142
Implant Insertions 154

Navigation-assisted procedures in craniomaxillofacial surgery can be grouped into the following categories:

- Minimally invasive procedures and biopsies
- Optic nerve decompression
- Resections and reconstructions
- Traumatological procedures
- Corrective osteotomies of the facial skeleton
- Implant insertions

Minimally Invasive Surgeries and Biopsies

Navigation-assisted biopsies were the first applications of computer-assisted surgery in the head and neck region (Watanabe et al. 1991). Since then, they have become widely practiced (Klimek et al. 1993a–c; Gunkel et al. 1997b; Siessegger et al. 2001; Postec et al. 2002; Kajiwara et al. 2003; Majdani et al. 2003; Casler et al. 2005) and are considered a domain of frameless stereotaxy (Grunert et al. 2002). It is particularly desirable to use a noninvasive registration method for these procedures. Splint-based registration satisfies this requirement and eliminates the need to use a head frame in endonasal endoscopic operations. The site of the intraoperative incisional biopsy (or biopsies) can be defined preoperatively and correlated with the postoperative histological diagnosis based on instantaneous views in the multiplanar display (Fig. 34).

Intraoperative navigation of the endoscopes is desirable in cases where significant anatomical changes are encountered and especially in posttraumatic paranasal sinus surgery. This enables the surgeon to correlate the visual impressions on the endoscope monitor with the position of the endoscope in the CT

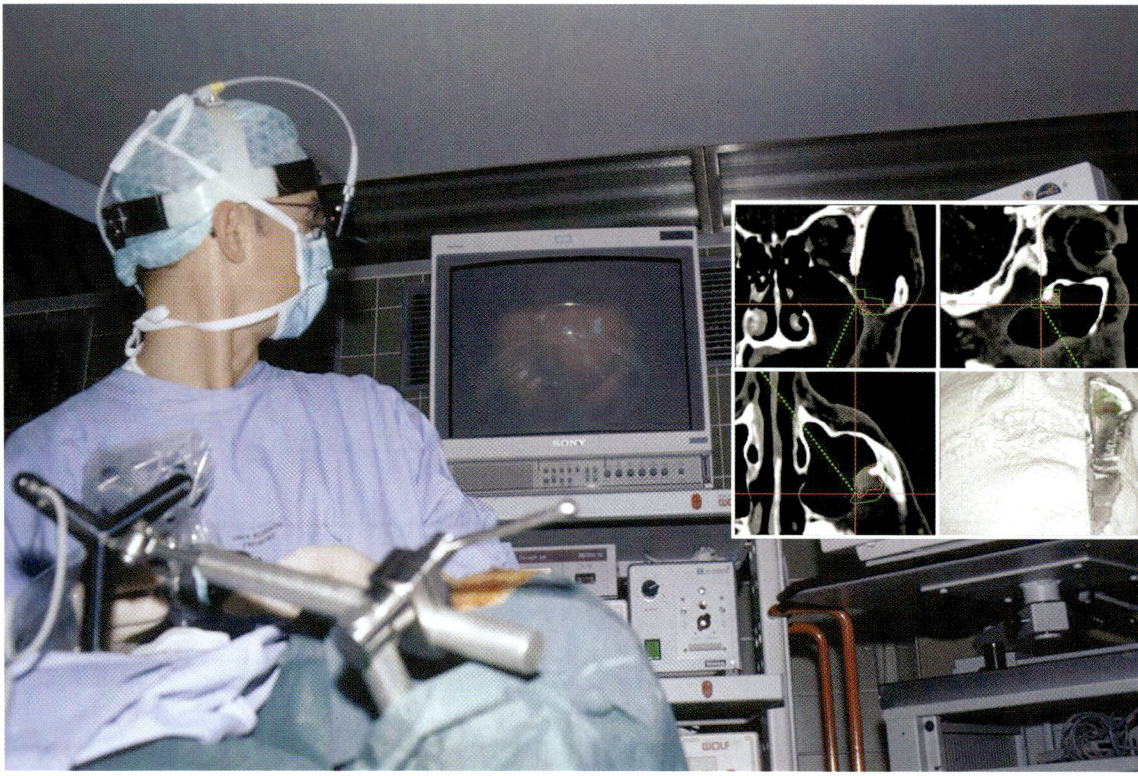

Fig. 34. Navigation-assisted endoscopic biopsy in the posterolateral portion of the left maxillary sinus (a). The area to be biopsied was marked preoperatively and can be identified intraoperatively in the multiplanar display of the CT data set (b, *red*)

data set and helps to eliminate the risk of injuring or displacing vital structures (Fig. 35).

In examinations to exclude a recurrent tumor and in oncological follow-ups, purely visual orientation at the operative site is unsatisfactory because of the surgically altered anatomy. The advantage of intraoperative navigation in these cases is that it provides a combination of pointer-based, endoscopically assisted microscopic treatment. When splint-based registration is used, a correlation can be established between the CT and MRI data sets, thus increasing the accuracy of the diagnostic studies (Fig. 36).

The correlated data sets can be used at any time for navigation-assisted surgery. Our illustrative case involves a mucocele of the right sphenoid sinus. Pituitary structures cannot be positively identified due to postirradiation changes (blue marking in Fig. 36), and a recurrence of the underlying disease cannot be excluded. In this case the noninvasive splint-based registration system makes it possible to perform a navigation-assisted operation without the need to acquire additional data sets. Intraoperative accuracy can be increased by combining the splint-based reference markers with extraoral orbital implants (Fig. 37), especially if the splint relies on soft tissue support.

During the operative procedure, the focal point of the operating microscope is tracked following successful registration. This facilitates the safe removal and biopsy of suspicious structures while avoiding injury to the pituitary gland. The route of approach and important vital structures can be outlined pre-

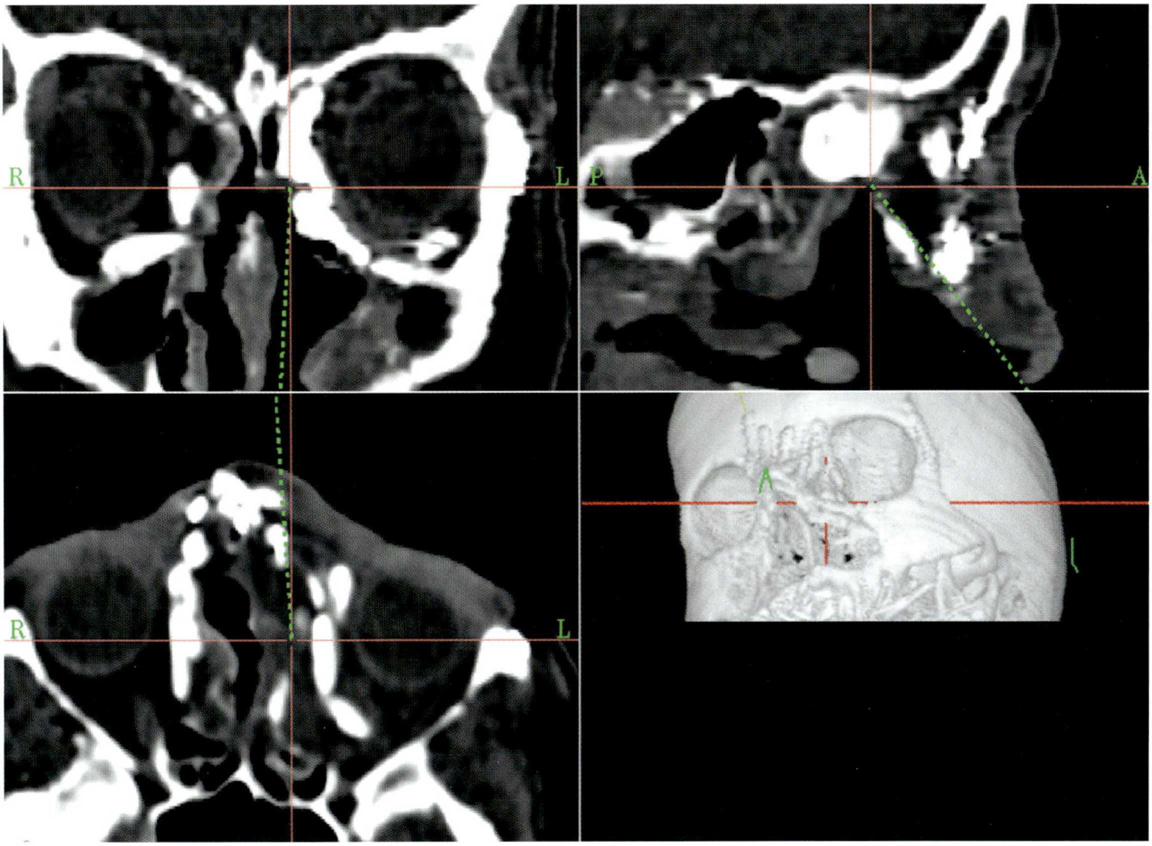

Fig. 35. Navigation-assisted endoscopic biopsy in the region of the left ethmoid cells in a patient with a methicillin-resistant *Staphylococcus aureus* (MRSA) infection following complex facial trauma

operatively and visualized during the operation (Figs. 38–40).

Another CT data set is acquired after the operation. When the registration splint is reused for this purpose, the splint-based markers can be used in correlating the pre- and postoperative data sets (Fig. 41).

The ability to accurately compare pre- and postoperative data sets permits a detailed evaluation of the operative result. The postoperative data set then establishes a baseline for further evaluations. Follow-up images taken at standard intervals should always be obtained with the registration splint in place to allow for accurate data set correlations and facilitate the early detection of changes (Fig. 42).

Navigation-assisted biopsies are appropriate in previously operated or previously treated areas and for multiple biopsies that require an objective means of correlating the biopsy specimens with their sites of origin. With splint-based registration, the same image data set can be used to perform any additional resections that may be needed.

The resection of neoplasms, especially benign tumors that would normally require an extensive exposure because of their relationship to vital structures, can often be done in a minimally invasive fashion by using navigation-assisted techniques. Navigation in these cases permits the tumor and adjacent structures to be identified, even if the tumor cannot be directly or indirectly visualized. Retromaxillary or

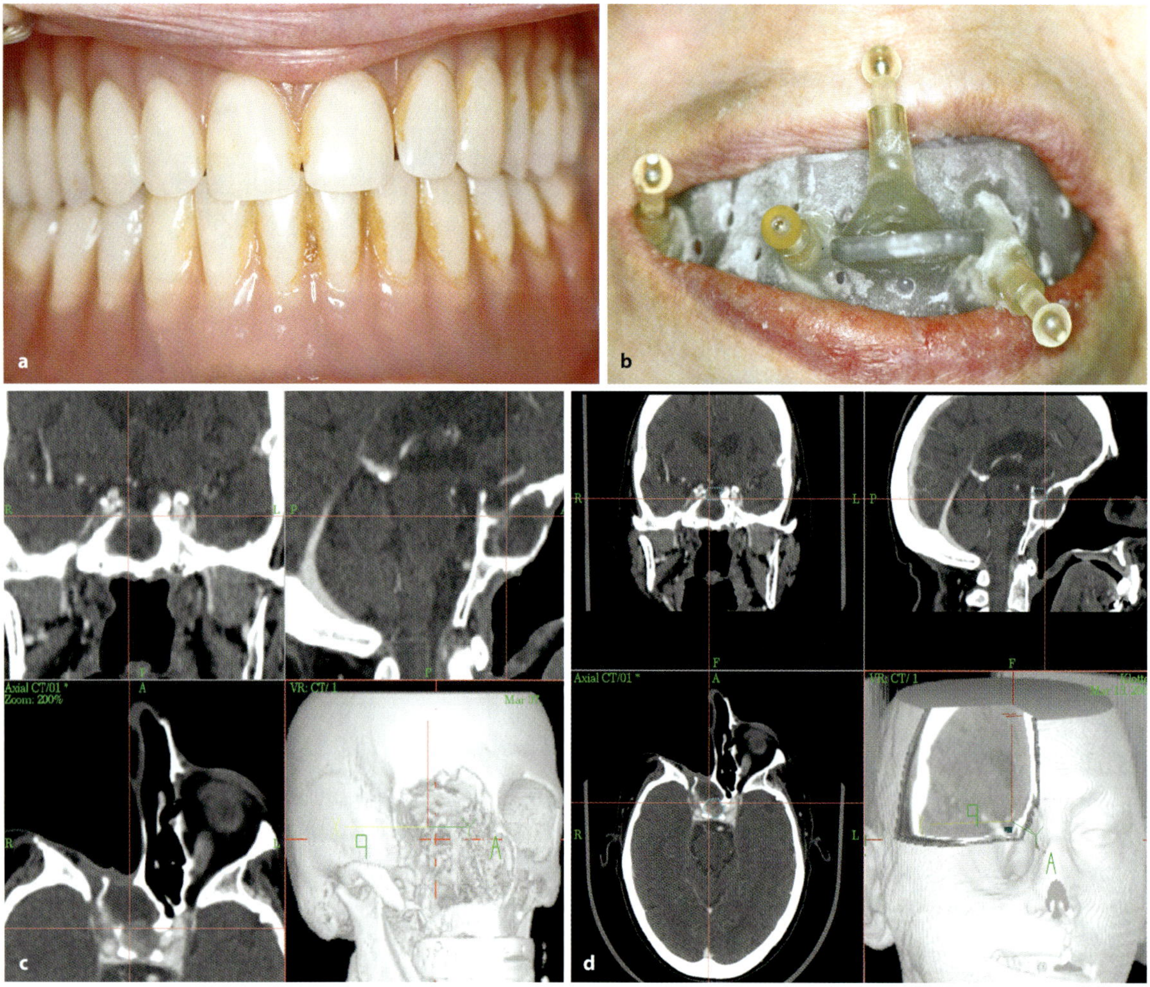

Fig. 36. Correlation of CT and MRI data sets for preoperative diagnosis. When splint-based registration is used (vestibular splint in a full denture wearer, **a, b**), a point-to-point correlation can be made between the CT (**c**) and MRI (**d**) data sets. This is a follow-up examination in a patient who underwent orbital exenteration and postoperative radiotherapy for squamous cell carcinoma of the right medial canthus

intraorbital osteomas are a particularly strong indication for the use of intraoperative navigation. For example, the retromaxillary space often must be approached by a preauricular or retromandibular route due to difficult visual conditions. By using infrared localization, however, the surgeon can reach the retromaxillary space through an intraoral route. This significantly reduces the morbidity of the procedure while increasing the safety and accuracy of the resection and preserving nearby structures (Figs. 43–45).

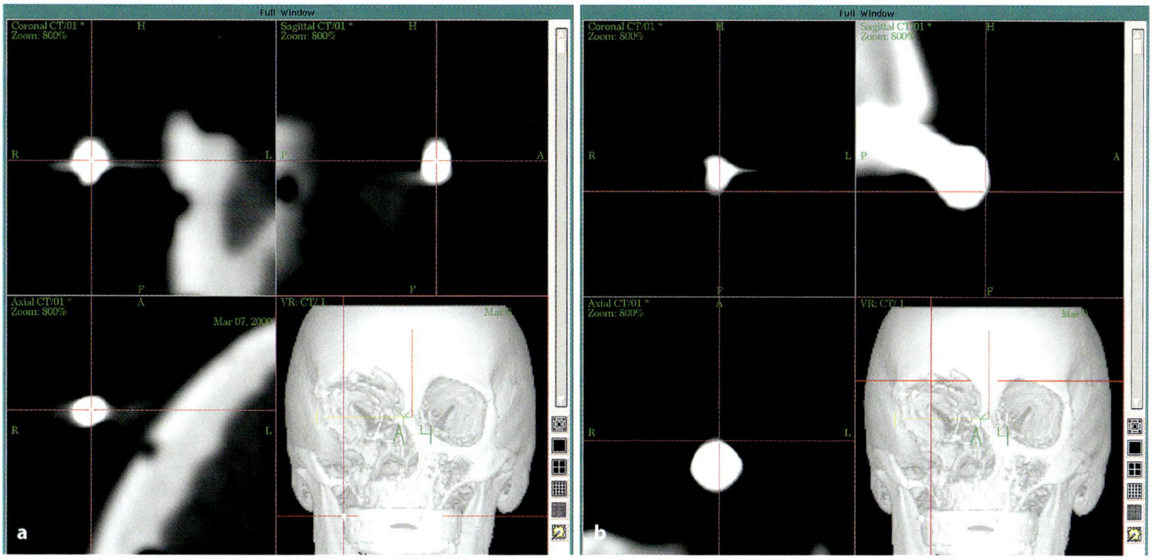

Fig. 37. Combination of splint registration markers and extraoral implants. The reference markers on the splint (a) can be combined with reference points on extraoral implants (orbital implant, b)

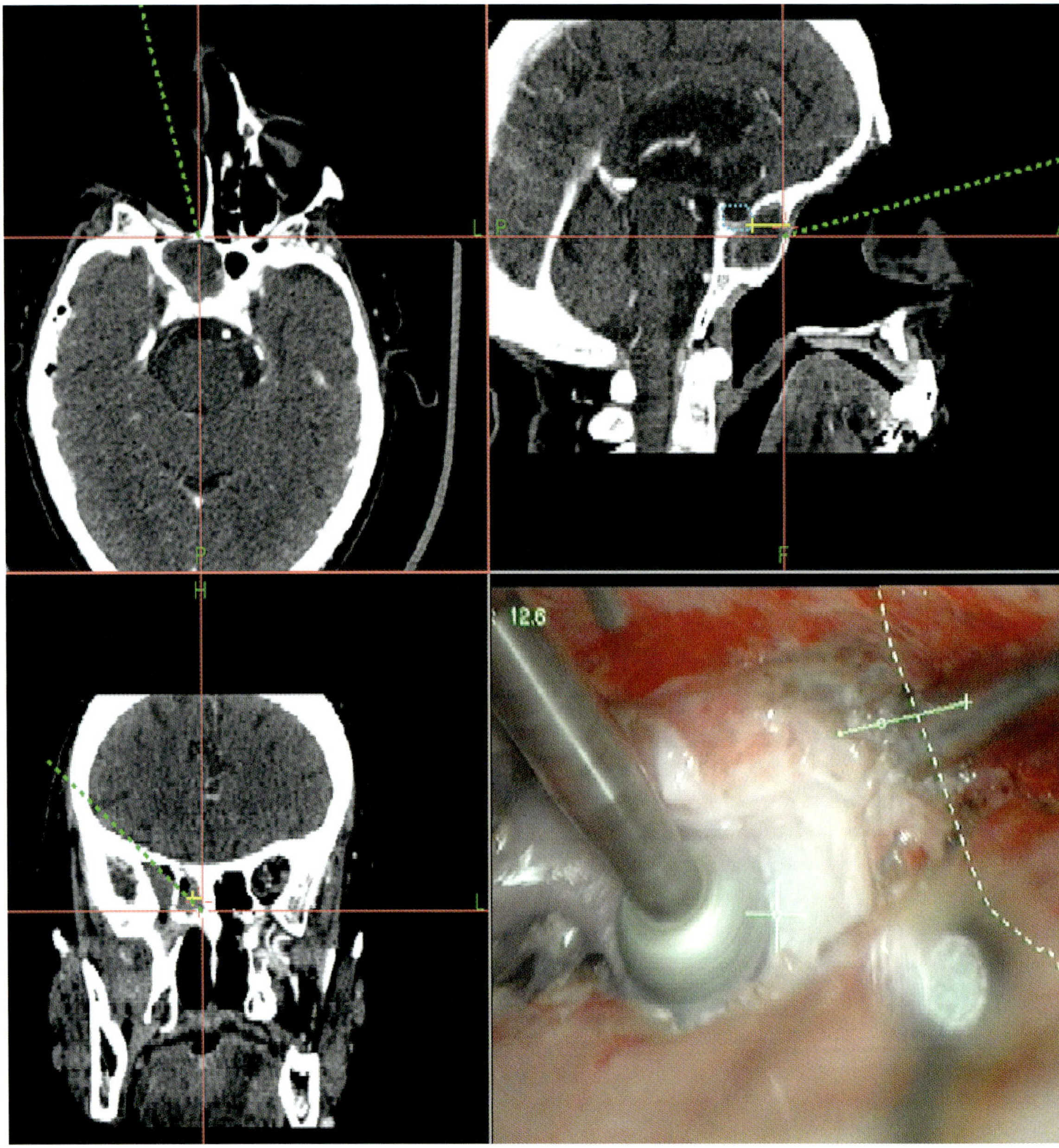

Fig. 38. Navigation-assisted technique for opening the anterior wall of the sphenoid sinus. As the anterior wall of the sphenoid sinus is opened (*lower right panel*), the position of the rotating instrument tip is shown in a multiplanar display (axial, sagittal, coronal) of the CT data set. The approach trajectory is marked in *yellow*, and the pituitary is outlined in *blue*. The *lower right panel* shows the field viewed through the operating microscope. The starting and end points of the instrument trajectory (*line in the upper right panel*) and the current tip position (*cross*) are superimposed as virtual structures

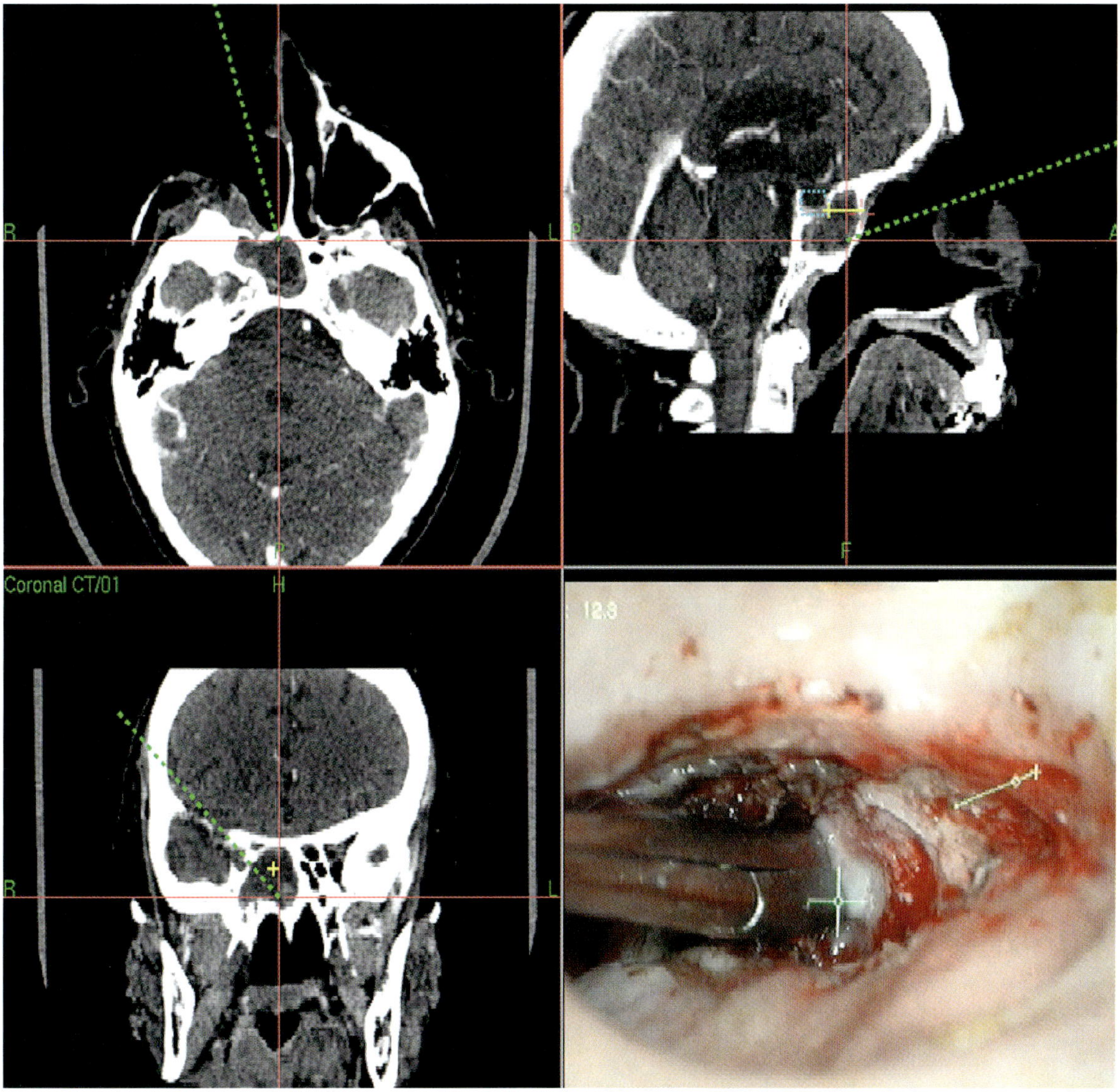

Fig. 39. Navigation-assisted forceps biopsy. The tip of the biopsy instrument is displayed in the multiplanar mode (axial, sagittal, coronal). The approach trajectory is marked in *yellow*, and the pituitary is outlined in *blue*. The *lower right panel* shows the view through the operating microscope. The focal point of the microscope is represented by superimposed *crosshairs*

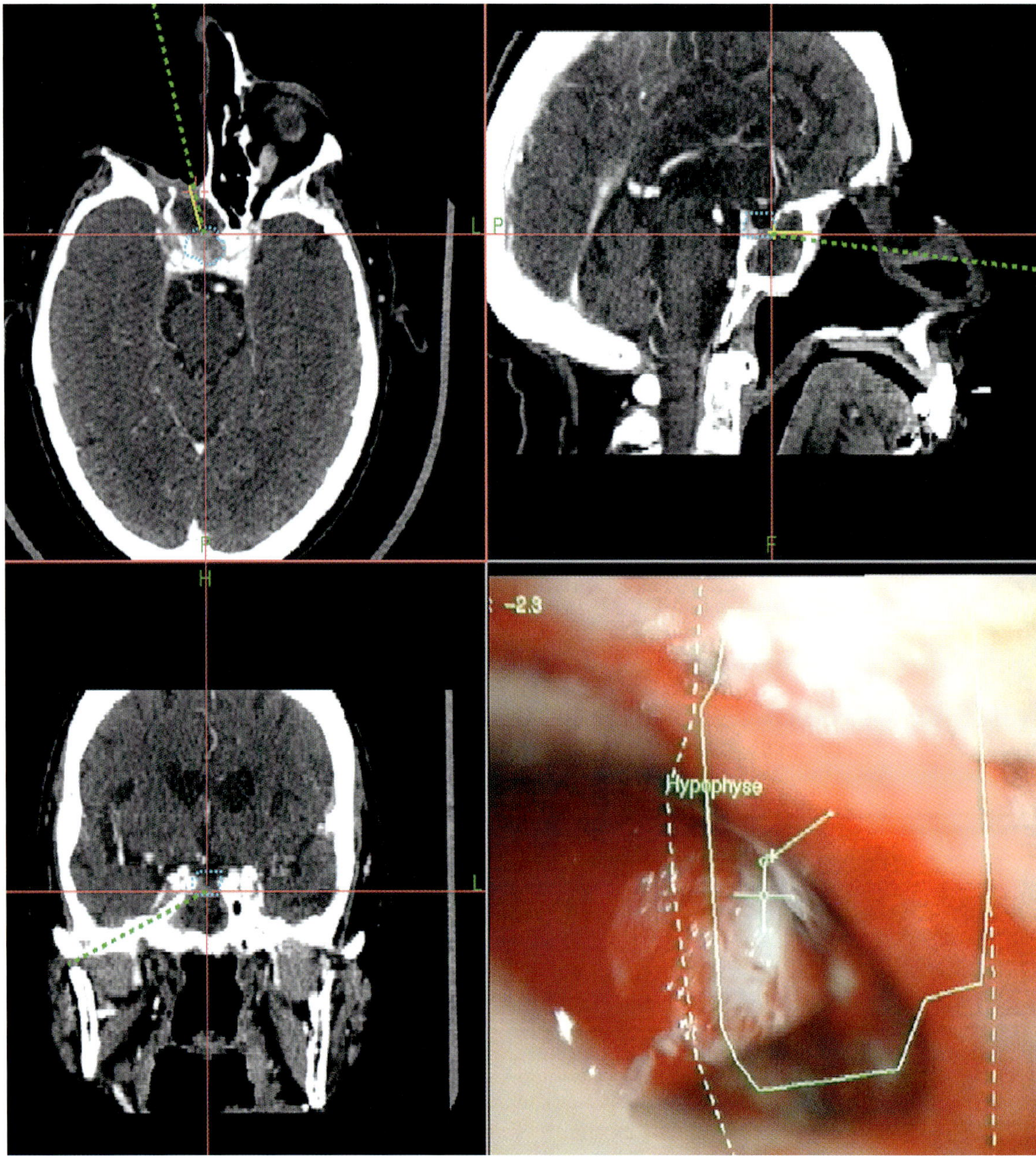

Fig. 40. Navigation-assisted exploration of the sphenoid sinus. The focal point of the operating microscope is displayed in the multiplanar mode (axial, sagittal, coronal). The approach trajectory is marked in *yellow*, and the pituitary gland is outlined in *blue*. The *lower right panel* shows the view through the operating microscope. The focal point of the microscope is represented by superimposed *crosshairs*. The starting and end points of the approach trajectory (*line next to the crosshairs*) and current position (*small cross on the line*) are superimposed as virtual structures. The *outline* marks the boundaries of the pituitary gland

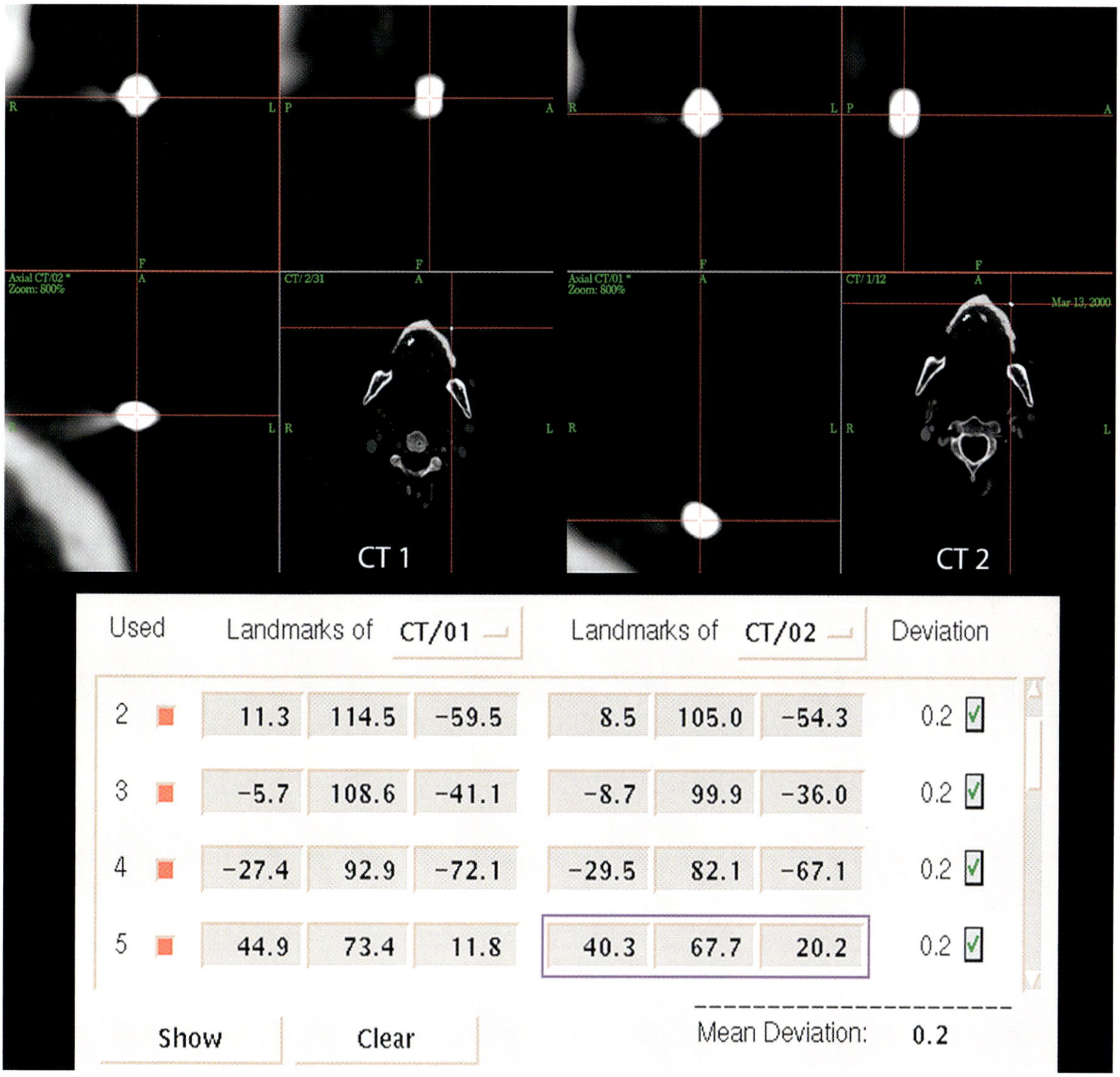

Fig. 41. Data set correlation using splint-based markers. The centers of the four splint-based markers are defined in the preoperative (*CT 1* in the *upper left panel*) and postoperative CT data set (*CT 2* n the *upper right panel*), whereupon the data sets are correlated based on the four corresponding points (*lower panel*). The deviation can be determined for each individual point, and the overall deviation can also be determined

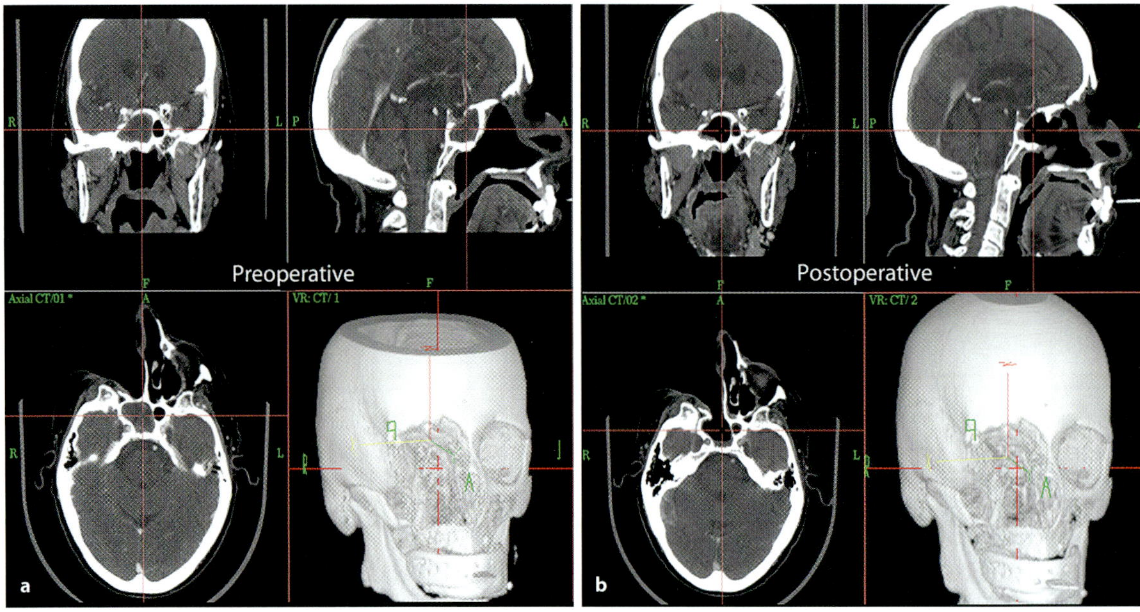

Fig. 42. Correlation of preoperative (**a**) and postoperative (**b**) CT data sets. Besides data set correlation using the splint-based markers (see 3D images), a point-by-point correlation of the data sets can also be performed. This provides a baseline for further examinations during oncological follow-up

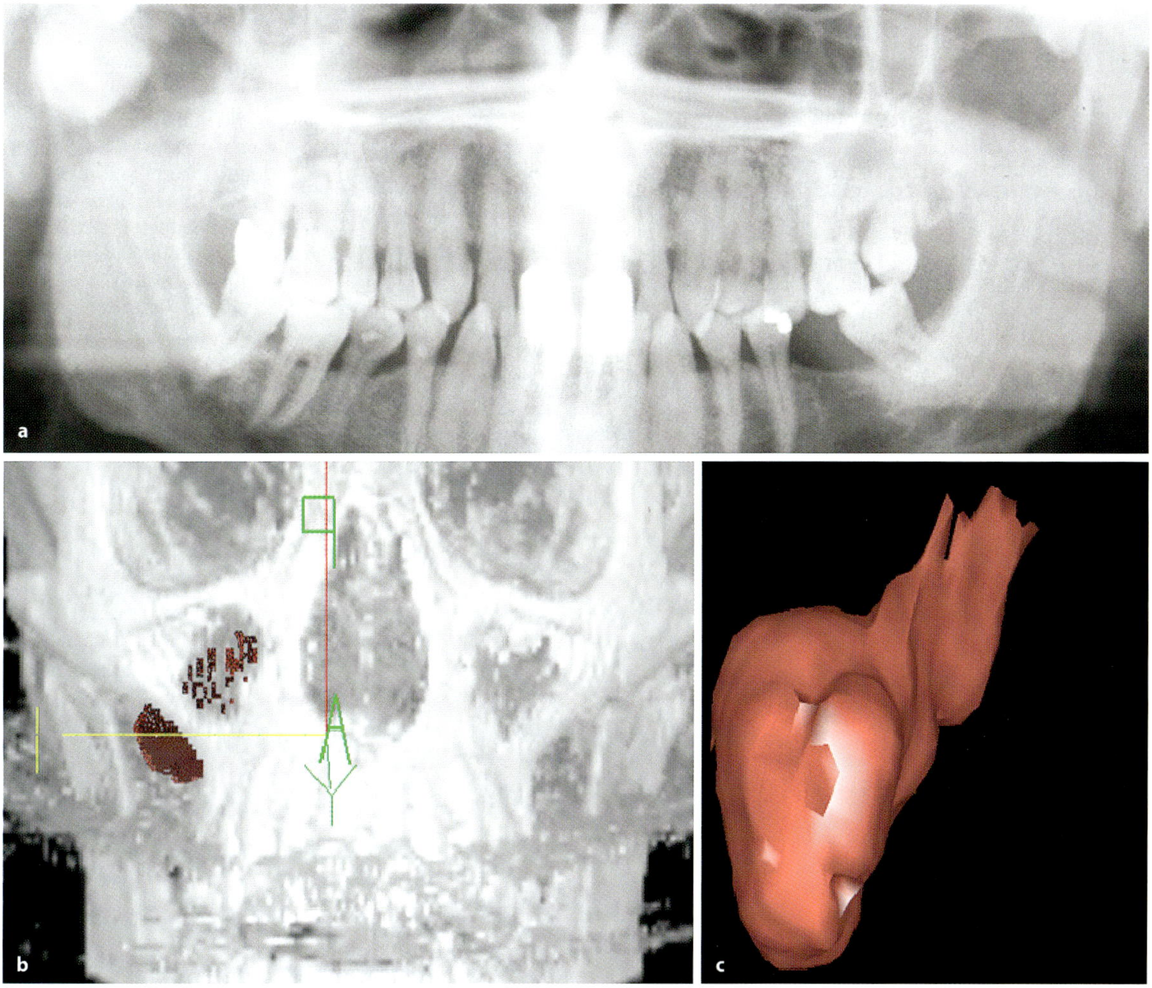

Fig. 43. Osteoma of the pterygoid process. The panoramic tomogram (a) shows an opacity at the level of the right temporomandibular joint, identified by CT as a bony expansion of the lateral plate of the pterygoid process of the sphenoid bone (b). The surface-rendered view after tumor marking (c) gives a 3D impression of the size and shape of the tumor

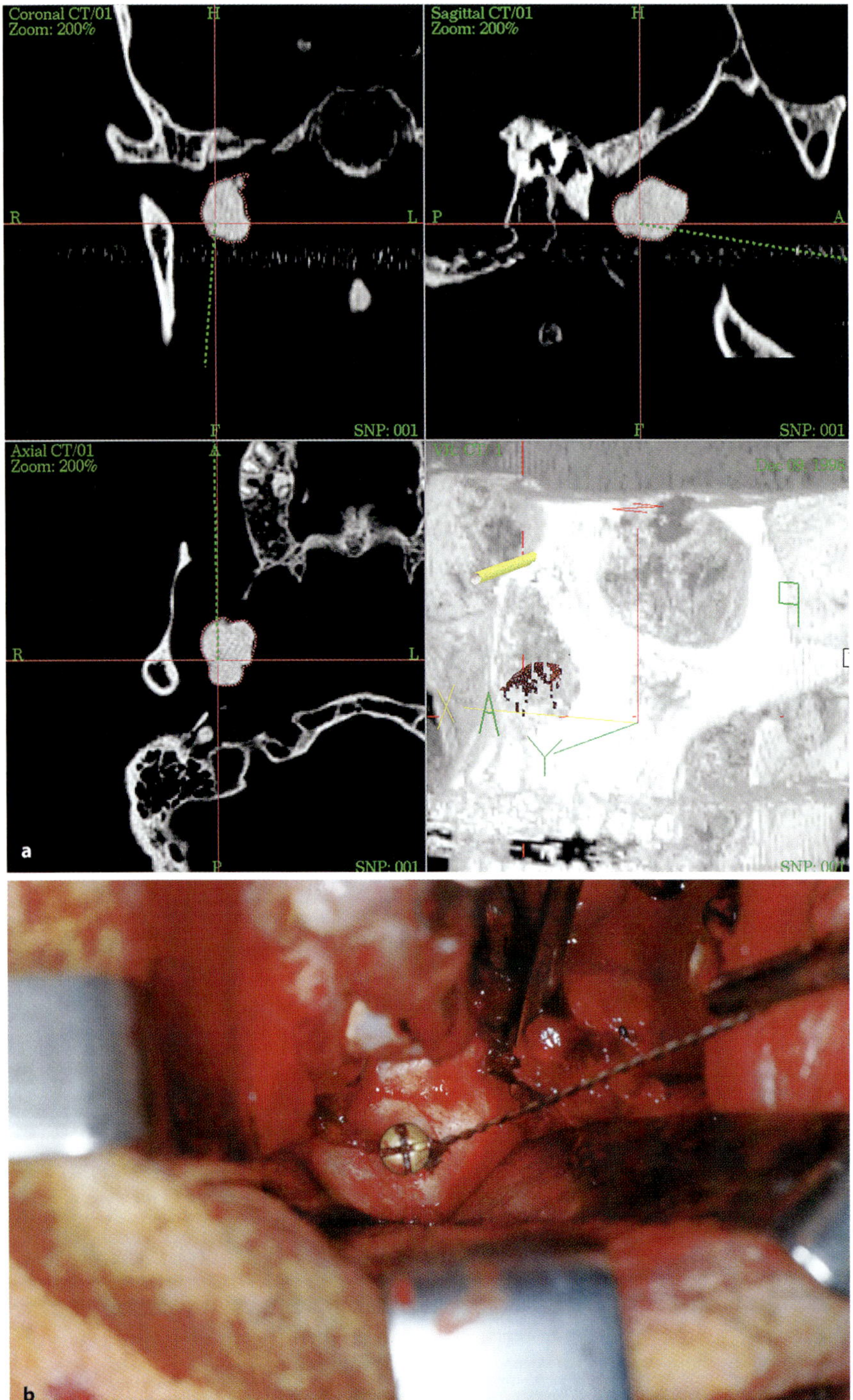

Fig. 44. Navigation-assisted resec-tion of an osteoma of the pterygoid process. a Navigation-assisted insertion of an internal fixation screw for attaching a retaining wire during the operation. c Navigation-assisted osteotomy of the unaffected part of the lateral plate. Clinical photographs show the tumor before (b) and after complete removal (d)

Fig. 44. (continued)

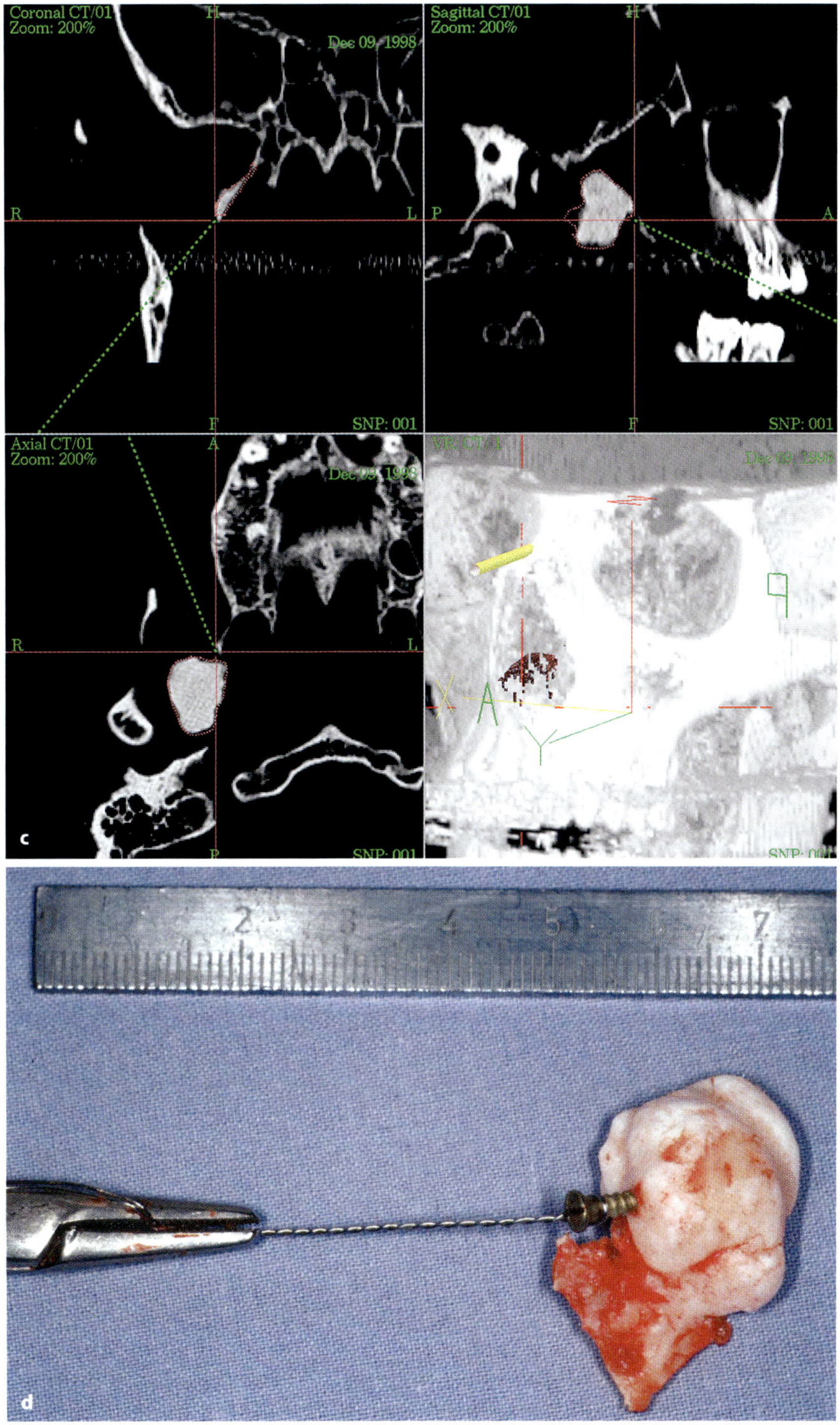

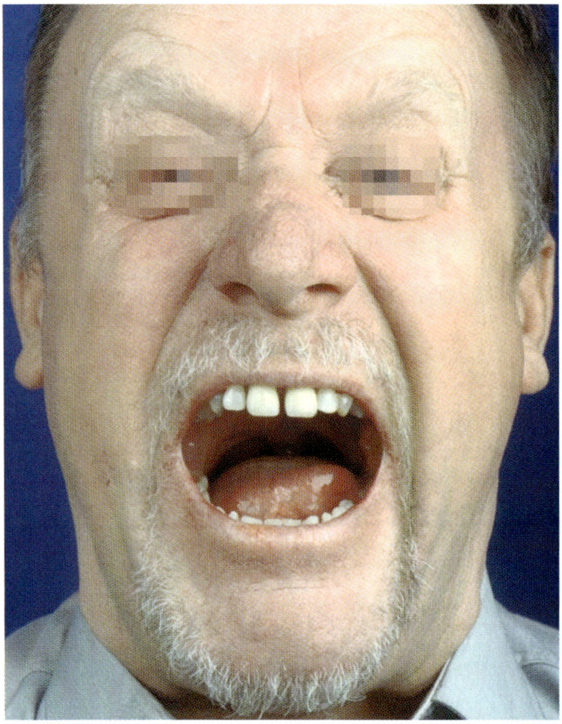

Fig. 45. Assessment of mouth opening after intraoral resection of an osteoma. Six weeks after the intraoral resection of an osteoma of the pterygoid process, the patient has regained a normal degree of mouth opening

Optic Nerve Decompression

The oromaxillofacial surgeon may come into contact with the prechiasmatic visual pathway during traumatological surgery, oncological surgery, and craniofacial reconstructions. A structured approach to recognizing and dealing with lesions of the visual pathway requires clearly delineated concepts and treatment strategies (Gellrich 1999). This includes a knowledge of the pathogenic mechanisms of possible visual pathway lesions as well as necessary primary imaging studies and further investigations. The treatment of lesions close to the optic nerve is a challenge for all disciplines that deal with head surgery, because an important goal in any intervention is to avoid damage to the visual system. The treatment of malignant tumors may be an exception to this rule, because adequate tumor clearance may require surgical interruption of the visual pathway. In traumatology and reconstructive plastic surgery, however, preservation of the visual pathway is an important priority, and visual loss would constitute a serious posttraumatic condition or complication (Lehnhardt 1973; Goldware et al. 1980; Raveh and Vuillemin 1988). In the past, the question of the predictability of a visual pathway lesion has not been adequately incorporated into primary diagnostic and therapeutic concepts, with the result that injuries of the visual pathway are generally considered a matter of fate. Often this is recognized at a later date when therapeutic options are no longer available. Beyond clinical tests of visual pathway integrity, which are often inconclusive, we have established flash visual evoked potentials (VEPs) and flash electroretinograms (ERGs) as reliable electrophysiological tests for confirming whether signal conduction through the visual pathway is intact, altered, or completely disrupted. These tests can be done during the primary workup and can also be used intraoperatively during a reconstructive procedure. Even the subjective and objective detection of unilateral blindness does not necessarily represent a definitive finding. Supported by multiplanar reconstructions of thin-slice CT scans, it is necessary to make an immediate (emergency) decision for or against the need to treat a visual tract lesion, particularly in terms of avoiding secondary damage to the visual pathway. The conservative treatment of choice for traumatic optic nerve damage is megadose methylprednisolone therapy (Urbason 30 mg/kg body weight i.v. and 5.4 mg/kg body weight per hour i.v. for another 48 hours). Surgical treatment consists of decompressing the orbital compartment in patients with a retrobulbar hematoma or exposing the intracanalicular segment of the optic nerve in cases with CT-confirmed trauma to the bony optic nerve canal or posterior orbit (Lehnhardt and Schultz-Coulon 1975). An analysis of our own cases and of the international literature shows that the time factor is greatly underestimated in the treatment of optic nerve trauma. Modern therapeutic concepts require a differentiated approach to the diagnosis and treatment of traumatic optic nerve injury, with the overriding goal of preserving visual function.

Traumatic damage to the intraorbital or intracanalicular segment of the optic nerve usually represents a multifactorial process consisting of:

- A bony lesion
- Ischemia due to microvascular spasms or vascular occlusion
- Reactive edema
- A hemorrhagic mass

Damage to the visual pathway may be caused by trauma lasting only a fraction of a second or may result from slowly progressive nerve compression initiated by a traumatic event. Frontonasoethmoid fractures are most commonly associated with damage to the afferent visual pathway (Ramsay 1979; Momose and Joseph 1991). In many cases it is not possible to clinically assess the severity of a presumed optic nerve injury during the acute posttraumatic period (Davidson 1938; Cook et al. 1951; Garston 1970; Stutzin et al. 1988).

An integral part of the primary clinical evaluation in head-injured patients is a preliminary assessment of the visual pathway with testing of pupillomotor function, vision, visual field integrity, and ocular motility. In cases where the clinical assessment of visual function is not possible or is equivocal (e.g., due to unconsciousness, morphine administration, or massive swelling), electrophysiological testing by flash VEP and ERG should be performed during the early posttraumatic period in order to make an objective assessment of visual pathway function. In cases where intraoperative tests are done immediately after the completion of an orbital reconstruction with autologous bone grafts or after optic nerve decompression, for example, the electrophysiological measurements are taken while the patient is under general anesthesia. In this case testing can be done with a mobile neurophysiological unit equipped with separate parallel leads for recording an ERG and VEP. The traces are immediately evaluated based on the amplitude and latency of the electrical signals. Since these amplitudes vary even within a normal population, more than a 50 % amplitude difference between the right and left sides is considered to indicate an abnormal result. The active electrode for recording the ERG consists of a fiber electrode placed in the lower conjunctival sac. It is important to obtain an ERG in patients with an absent or abnormal ipsilateral VEP to ensure that visual signals are not compromised by an opacity of the refractive media or at the retinal level. This arrangement can be used in examining both conscious and unconscious patients. The clinical and electrophysiological findings are supplemented by a spiral CT examination, which is performed immediately after the fabrication of a silicone impression splint for later registration. The definitive decision for or against treatment of the visual pathway is based on the clinical, electrophysiological, and CT findings.

Recommendations for the Treatment of Traumatic Optic Nerve Injury

1. The primary diagnostic workup of every midfacial and/or basal skull fracture should include an assessment of visual pathway function. If this cannot be accomplished by an ophthalmological examination, a flash VEP and ERG should be obtained for the detection or exclusion of posttraumatic damage to the visual pathway. This also applies to craniofacial procedures involving the orbits.
2. A normal light response is a reliable parameter for confirming an intact visual pathway in emergency settings. In most cases, however, a definitive assessment of visual pathway function cannot be made during the primary evaluation of head-injured patients (in 60 % of our cases), due for example to the suppression of pupillomotor response by morphine administration. Even anisocoria or maximum pupillary dilation does not necessarily indicate an afferent lesion in the affected eye, as the actual cause may be an efferent lesion (internal ophthalmoplegia), direct injury to the iris sphincter, or even brain edema or a midbrain lesion. Pupillomotor response was a reliable parameter for diagnosing an afferent lesion of the visual pathway in only 30 % of our patients.
3. In the case of a clinically established afferent lesion of the visual pathway with decreased or absent vision or in an unconscious patient with a questionable afferent injury, the flash VEP examination makes it possible to grade visual pathway

function as "normal VEP," "abnormal but reproducible VEP," or "nonreproducible VEP." In the absence of clear-cut neuro-ophthalmological findings, the flash VEP provides the basis for a working hypothesis that, when combined with clinical and radiological findings, can justify the decision to treat the patient for a visual pathway lesion. Especially in patients with abnormal but reproducible flash VEP tracings, immediate therapeutic intervention is recommended to prevent additional secondary damage to the optic nerve.

4. In all cases with a clinically detected afferent lesion of the visual pathway or an abnormal VEP, megadose methylprednisolone therapy is recommended for a 48-hour period, provided this therapy is not contraindicated by the general condition of the patient.
5. Decompression of the orbit is indicated as a primary emergency measure in patients with an afferent lesion of the affected visual pathway based on a retrobulbar hematoma and there is no evidence of a cerebrospinal fluid leak, no pulsatile exophthalmos (indicating a carotid-cavernous sinus fistula), and no contraindications relating to the overall pattern of injury.
6. Decompression of the optic nerve canal should be performed as soon as possible in a conscious patient who has been diagnosed with an afferent lesion causing progressive or complete visual loss and there is direct or indirect radiological evidence of trauma in the retrobulbar orbit or in the region bordering the optic canal. Although vision did not return after optic nerve decompression in our patients who also had a nonreproducible VEP, returning only in patients who had an abnormal but still reproducible VEP, it is nevertheless prudent to recommend operative intervention. This policy should be continued until such time as results in larger populations or animal studies have proven that optic nerve recovery definitely cannot occur in patients with a nonreproducible VEP.
7. Optic nerve decompression is recommended in unconscious patients if there is direct or indirect radiological evidence of trauma in the retrobulbar orbit or in the region bordering the optic canal and there is an afferent lesion of the visual pathway on the affected side. If the afferent lesion cannot be diagnosed clinically, the presence of an abnormal VEP (reproducible or nonreproducible) should warrant immediate surgical intervention.
8. Postoperative CT documentation should be obtained in all patients who have undergone optic nerve decompression in order to document the morphological result of the operation.

Examples are presented below to illustrate the technique of computer-assisted optic nerve decompression (Figs. 46–49). Relatively little time is needed to fabricate a silicone impression splint, making it possible to proceed with operative treatment within 1–2 hours after initial care (Schramm et al. 2000e). Despite the ability of navigated microscopy to provide a highly detailed intraoperative display, the navigation should be supplemented at intervals by pointer-based tracking in order to achieve maximum accuracy (Fig. 47). Postoperatively, the result of the operation can be evaluated by using the splint-based markers to correlate the pre- and postoperative data sets (Fig. 48). If a secondary reconstruction of the resected medial orbital wall is necessary to correct postoperative enophthalmos, it can also be carried out with computer guidance and evaluated postoperatively by transposing the original contours into the postresection data set (Fig. 49).

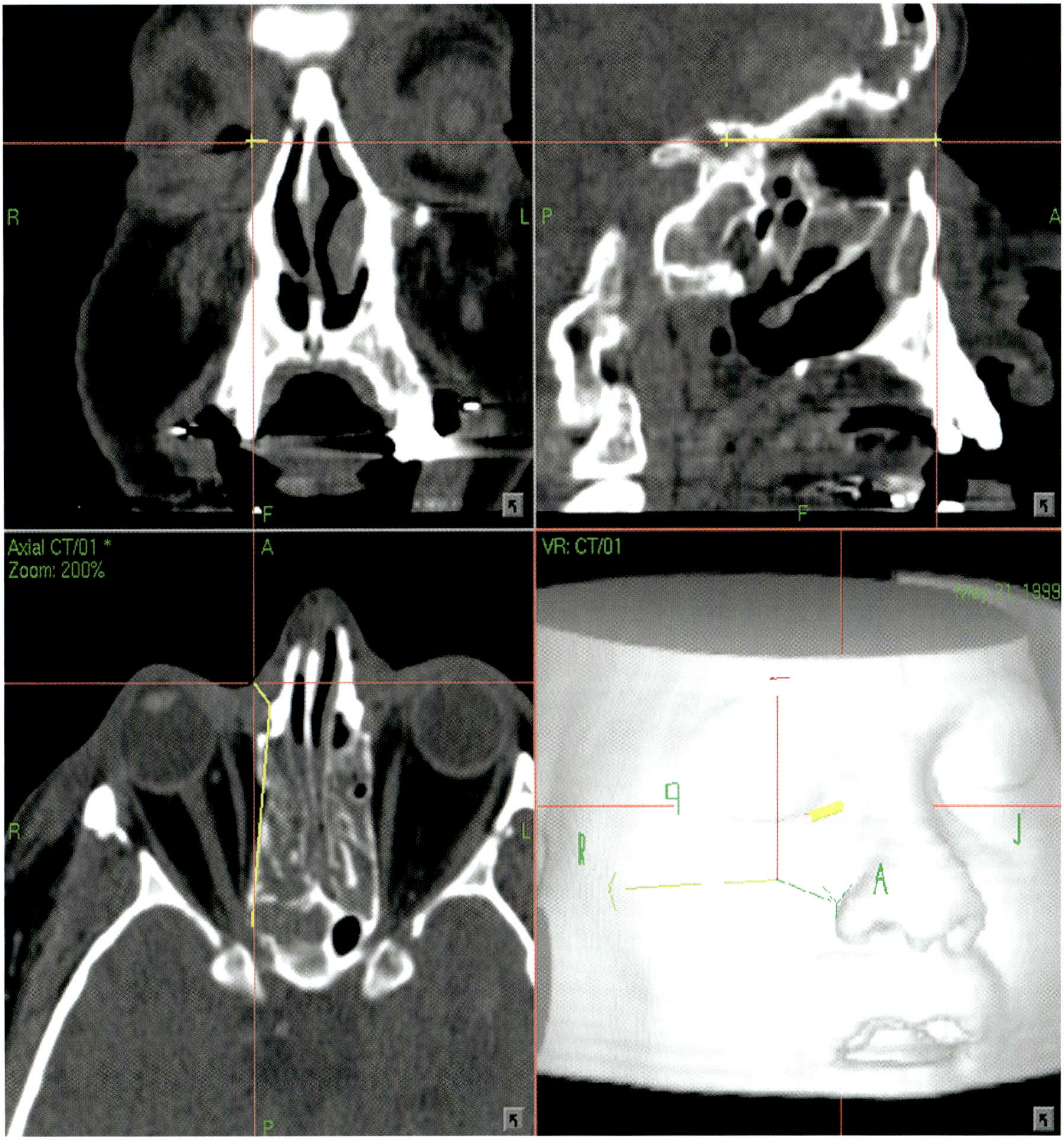

Fig. 46. Preoperative planning of optic nerve decompression. When using a prefabricated maxillary silicone impression splint (see 3D image), the surgeon can proceed at once with intraoperative navigation. The approach is determined in the multiplanar mode and marked with a *yellow line*. A transethmoidal approach was selected due to the traumatic etiology of the nerve compression

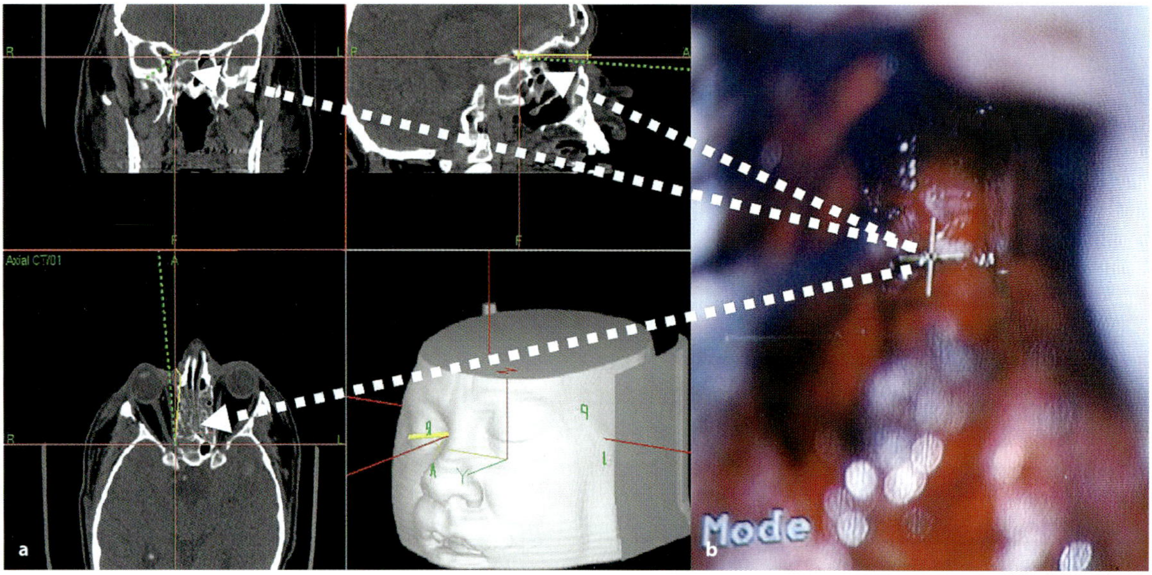

Fig. 47. Navigation-assisted microscopy for postoperative decompression of the right optic canal. The focal point of the operating microscope (*crosshairs in* b) is correlated intraoperatively with the preoperatively acquired CT data set using splint-based registration (a). The focal point is located at the center of the crosshairs in the sectional images

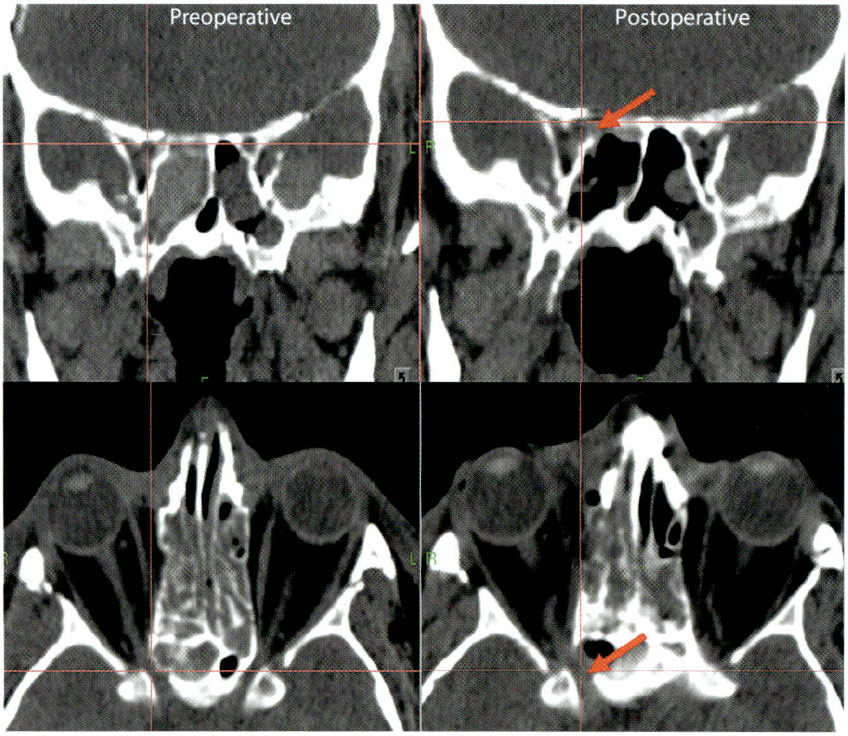

Fig. 48. Postoperative evaluation of optic nerve decompression. The splint-based reference markers are used in correlating the preoperative (*left*) and postoperative (*right*) CT data sets. The *arrows* indicate the resection sites for optic nerve decompression in the postoperative data set

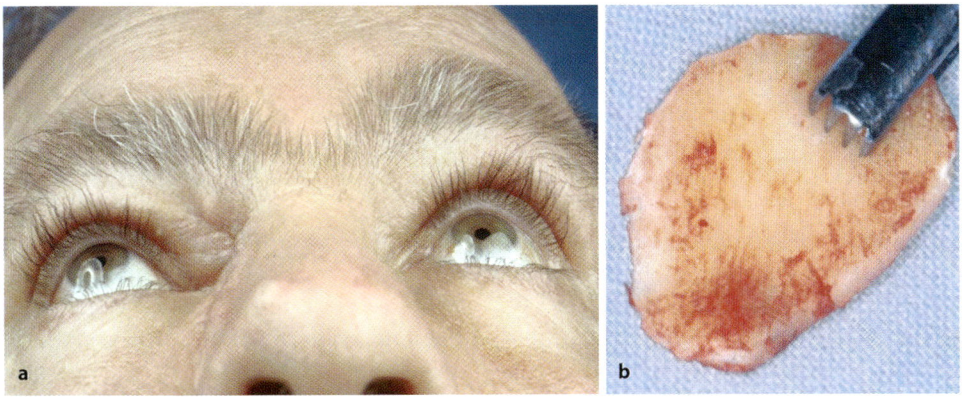

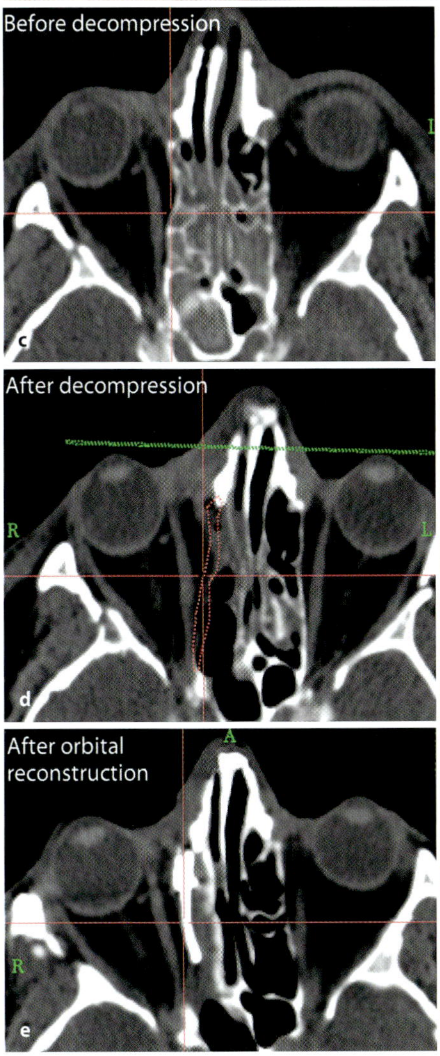

Fig. 49. Orbital reconstruction after optic nerve decompression. Enophthalmos of the right eye following resection of the medial orbital wall (**a, b**) was corrected by navigation-assisted orbital reconstruction with a calvarial graft. The original medial wall boundary was imported into the data set after optic nerve decompression in order to place the graft in the desired position during the reconstruction. CT scans before decompression (**c**), after decompression (**d**), and after orbital reconstruction (**e**). **f** Clinical appearance after reconstruction of the medial wall

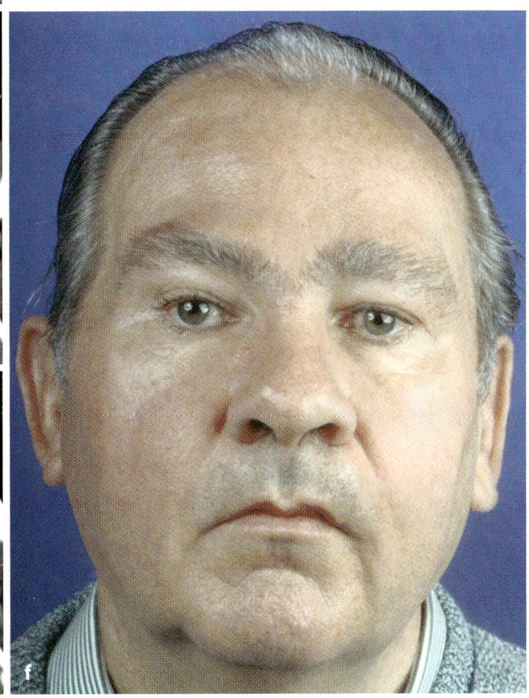

Resections and Reconstructions

Navigation-assisted tumor resections have already become almost routine procedures in clinical neurosurgery (Spetzger et al. 1996; Kajiwara et al. 2003; Raabe et al. 2003). In otorhinolaryngological surgery (Mann and Klimek 1998) and especially in oro-maxillofacial surgery, navigation systems have not been widely utilized in tumor resections and have mostly been limited to endonasal surgery (Truppe et al. 1996; Mann and Klimek 1998; Selesnick and Kacker 1999; Koele et al. 2002) and lesions in the skull base region (Carrau et al. 1996; Vaughan 1996; Hassfeld et al. 1998b; Caversaccio et al. 1999, 2002; Schramm et al. 1999c, 2000a; Hayashi et al. 2001; Heermann et al. 2001; Schmelzeisen et al. 2002a,b; Wang et al. 2002; Ecke et al. 2003). Preoperative planning usually consists of marking the tumor volumes and possibly the resection margins, outlining vital structures (e.g., vessels, nerves, meninges), and determining their intraoperative locations.

The treatment of malignant tumors near the skull base requires an accurate, 3D preoperative determination of the tumor extent, especially with regard to defining the resection margins while taking into account vital structures. But minimally invasive diagnosis in the form of incisional biopsies may also present a surgical challenge. The location, biological behavior, and extent of the tumor are crucial factors in selecting the surgical approach. As recently as the 1960s, tumors infiltrating the alar muscles, infratemporal fossa, and middle skull base were still considered inoperable due to the limited access, high blood loss, and unfavorable esthetic and functional outcomes.

As a result of interdisciplinary cooperation, particularly in operations on the skull base, operative techniques familiar in traumatology, craniofacial surgery, and orthognathic surgery have helped to improve surgical access to the skull base. While median and paramedian mandibular osteotomies in the setting of skull base surgery can give very good exposure of retromaxillary tumors and even the cranio-cervical junction in exceptional cases, lateral mandibular osteotomies have proven particularly useful for exposures of the middle cranial fossa. When median and paramedian osteotomies have been performed, it is essential to stabilize the bone segments in order to prevent the development of nonunion. Lateral osteotomies must respect the course of the inferior alveolar nerve. With vertical ramus osteotomies, the articular surfaces of the mandible must be replaced in an anatomically correct position in order to prevent postoperative functional abnormalities of the temporomandibular joint. In summary, we may emphasize the versatility of the temporary mandibular osteotomy as a safe, reliable method for gaining access to various regions of the skull base. When due attention is given to anatomical factors, mandibular osteotomies are associated with very little postoperative functional impairment.

A key problem, however, is the need to surgically encompass tumors with an adequate 3D safety margin, especially with tumors that have been downstaged by neoadjuvant chemotherapy or radiotherapy. This important goal requires accurate preoperative localization such as that provided by frameless stereotaxy. Computer-assisted surgery allows for preoperative planning and simulation, intraoperative localization and navigation, and postoperative follow-up. Through special adaptations of existing software, it is possible to correlate and transfer outlined tumor boundaries in various image data sets obtained from the same patient. This enables us to compare the volumes of tumor masses before and after chemotherapy and also transfer the original tumor boundaries into posttherapeutic data sets (Schramm et al. 2000c). These capabilities are useful not only for 3D preoperative planning and postoperative evaluations but also for the intraoperative infrared localization of virtually defined resection lines and proposed tumor clearance margins. Case examples will be presented to illustrate the advantages and possible indications of computer-assisted surgery in the treatment of lateral skull base tumors.

Lateral Skull Base and Temporomandibular Joint

A 45-year-old woman presented with lower facial deformity caused by fibrous dysplasia affecting the right lateral skull base and right mandibular condyle (Fig. 50).

Following the exclusion of an active process by scintigraphy, a navigation-assisted resection of the affected bony areas was carried out through a preauricular approach. The intraoperative instrument tracking allowed the safe and selective removal of the abnormal areas (Fig. 51).

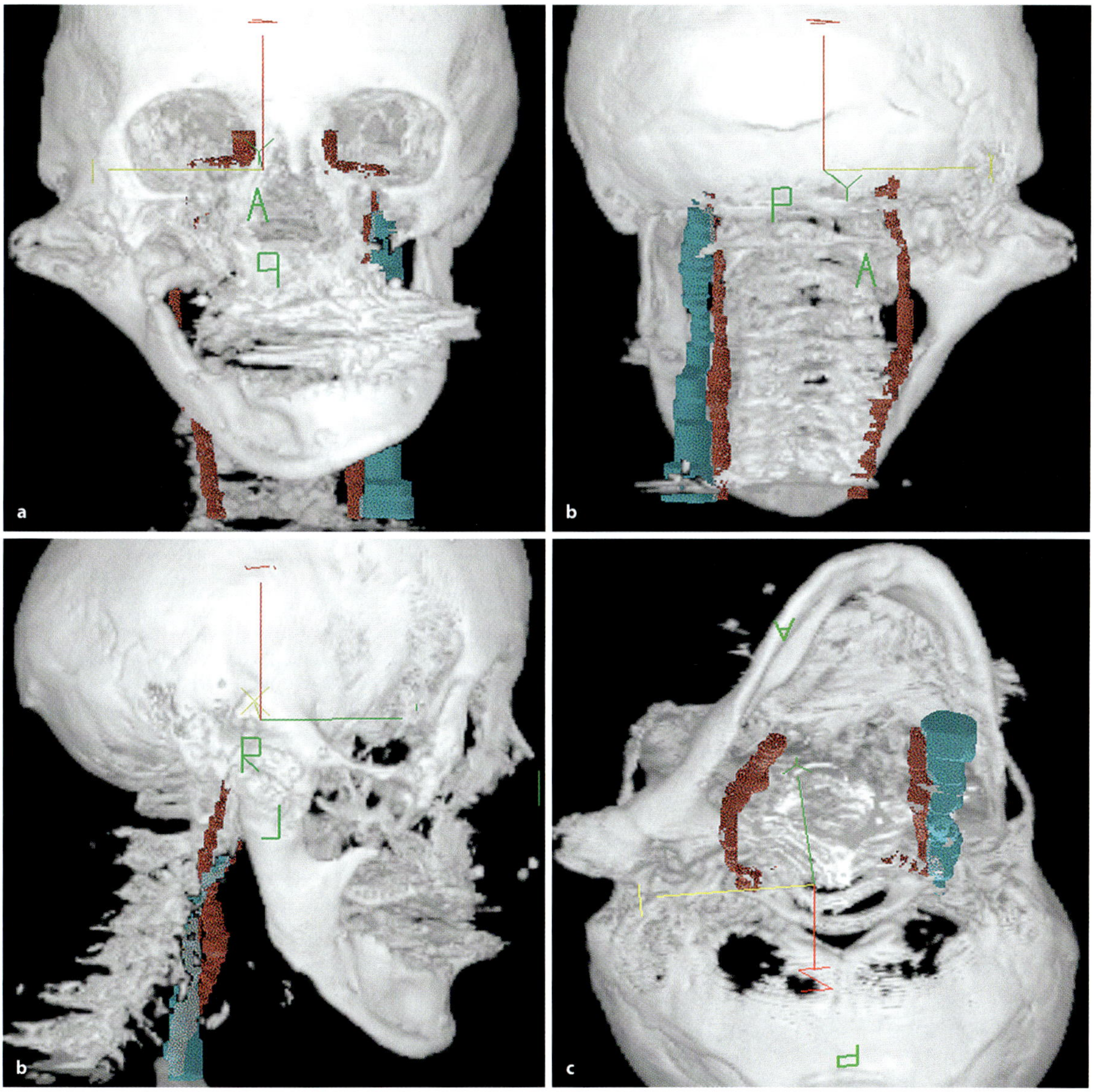

Fig. 50 a–d. Fibrous dysplasia of the lateral skull base. These images are 3D reconstructions of the preoperative CT data set. The two internal carotid arteries are shown in *red* and the left internal jugular vein in *blue*. The right internal jugular vein has already been obliterated. Note the proximity of the internal carotid artery to the mass

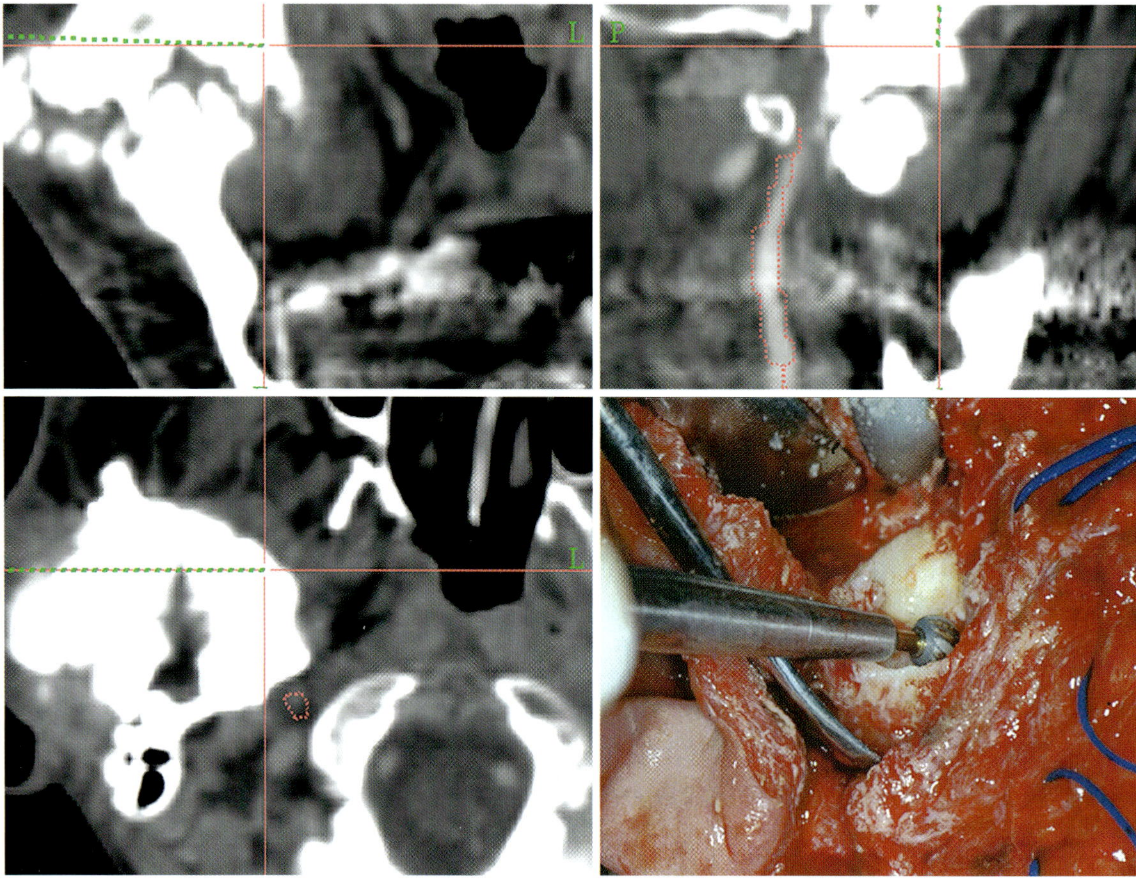

Fig. 51. Navigation-assisted removal of fibrous dysplasia of the lateral skull base. The tip of the rotating instrument (*bottom left*) is continuously displayed intraoperatively in real time in the multiplanar mode as the end-point of the *broken green line*. The internal carotid artery is marked preoperatively and superimposed on the image (*dotted red line*) to avoid inadvertent injury to that vessel during bone removal

Postoperative CT shows the extent of the resection after data set correlation using the navigation splint (Fig. 52). Because fibrous dysplasia is not a tumor mass, a complete or radical resection is not indicated because of the risk to vital structures. A contouring osteotomy is the treatment of choice (Fig. 53).

An example of bony ankylosis of the temporomandibular joint is presented in Fig 54. In this 34-year-old male a recidive occurred 10 years after joint resection and rib grafting. Because mouth opening was limited to 10 mm data set acquisition for navigation-assisted surgery was performed with an oral vestibular splint of a type that could be fabricated even in patients with a very limited degree of mouth opening (Fig. 55).

The operation consisted of a navigation-assisted osteotomy and contouring resection of the left temporomandibular joint. The proximity of the resection to the stylomastoid foramen made intraoperative imaging desirable (Fig. 56). The navigation splint was inserted for postoperative evaluation so that the data sets could be correlated with high precision (Figs. 57, 58).

An example of navigation-assisted resection of a meningioma is presented in Fig. 59. The result of the

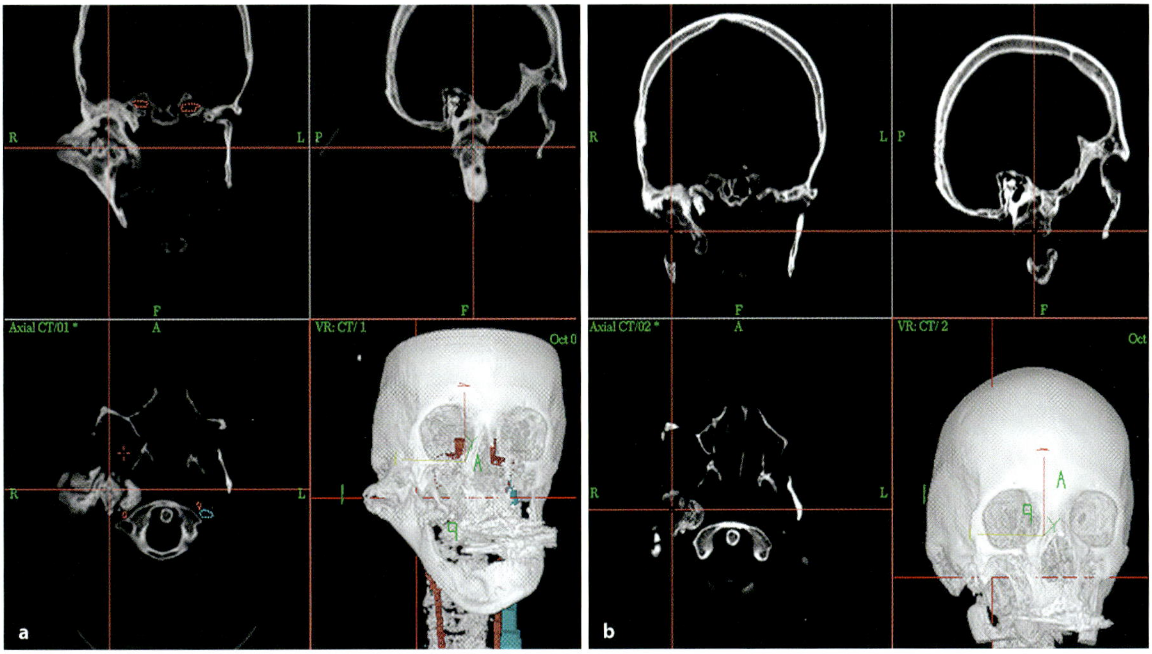

Fig. 52. Postoperative evaluation of a navigation-assisted contouring osteotomy of the lateral skull base (fibrous dysplasia). The preoperative (**a**) and postoperative CT data sets (**b**) are correlated with the aid of splint-based markers. The *red crosshairs* mark the corresponding points in both data sets in the multiplanar mode (coronal, sagittal, axial, 3D)

resection could also be validated with millimeter accuracy by correlating the pre- and postoperative image data sets based on the reference points of the removable maxillary splint (Fig. 60). Correlations of CT and MRI data sets with transfer of the preoperative tumor boundaries are essential for effective follow-up examinations, making it easier to distinguish between residual and recurrent tumor and surgery-induced scars.

A 66-year-old man underwent the navigation-assisted radical resection of an osteosarcoma of the lateral skull base. The preoperative acquisition of MRI and CT data sets with a navigation splint made it possible to correlate the data sets and also transfer and correlate the tumor boundaries (Fig. 61). Thus, the additional information contained in the MRI data set was imported into the CT data set used for intraoperative navigation to ensure that the soft tissue components of the tumor could also be identified. Tumor clearance can be significantly improved by the use of this technique.

Radical resection of the tumor along with large portions of the lateral skull base was facilitated by the intraoperative localization of tumor extensions. The primary reconstruction of the lateral skull base with a calvarial graft was matched to the initial situation with navigational assistance. By correlating the pre- and postoperative CT data sets with the navigation splint in place, the surgeon can transfer the tumor volume and confirm that an adequate resection has been accomplished (Fig. 62).

The transfer of the original tumor boundaries into the planning CT data set in preparation for postoperative radiotherapy increases the precision of radiotherapy planning (Fig. 63). In this way the radiotherapy field can be individually tailored to the postoperative anatomical relationships with regard to the original extent of the tumor. The traditional subjective comparison of images and operator drawings is replaced by an objective process. This eliminates the problem of making the dimensions of the radiotherapy field too large or too small.

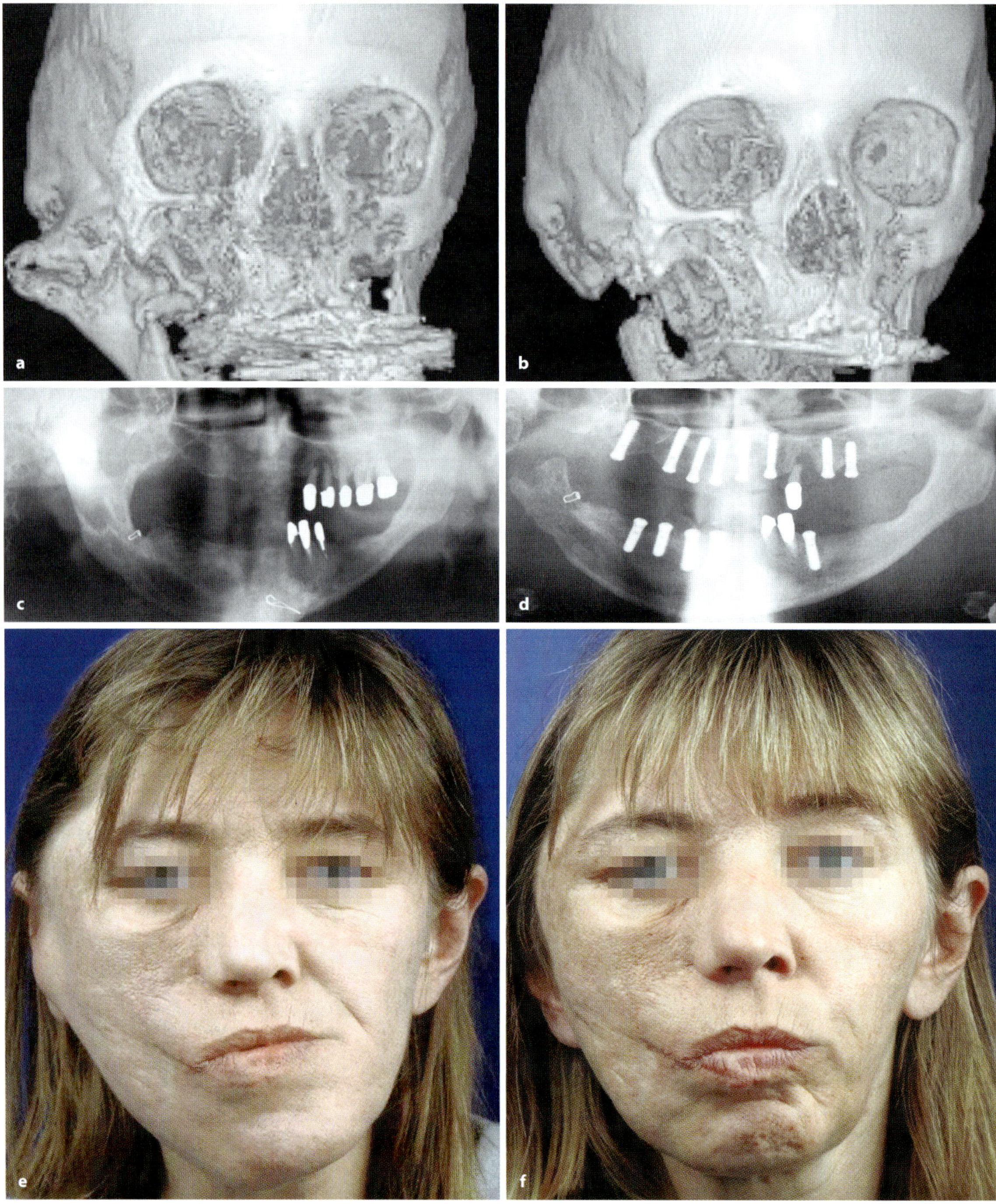

Fig. 53. Postoperative evaluation of a navigation-assisted contouring osteotomy of the lateral skull base (fibrous dysplasia). Preoperative (a) and postoperative (b) bony 3D reconstructions. Preoperative panoramic tomogram (PSCHA, c) and the tomogram following resection and reconstruction with a prosthetic implant (d). Clinical appearance before (e) and after (f) the end of treatment

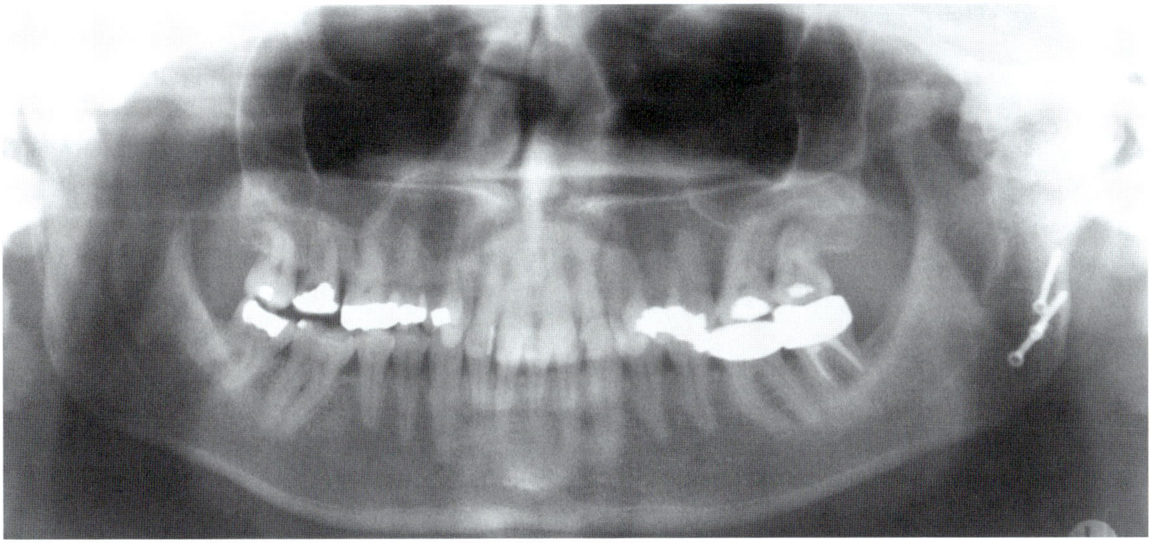

Fig. 54. Bony ankylosis of the temporomandibular joint (PSCHA). The patient presented with a recurrence of ankylosis 10 years after temporomandibular joint resection and primary reconstruction with a rib graft

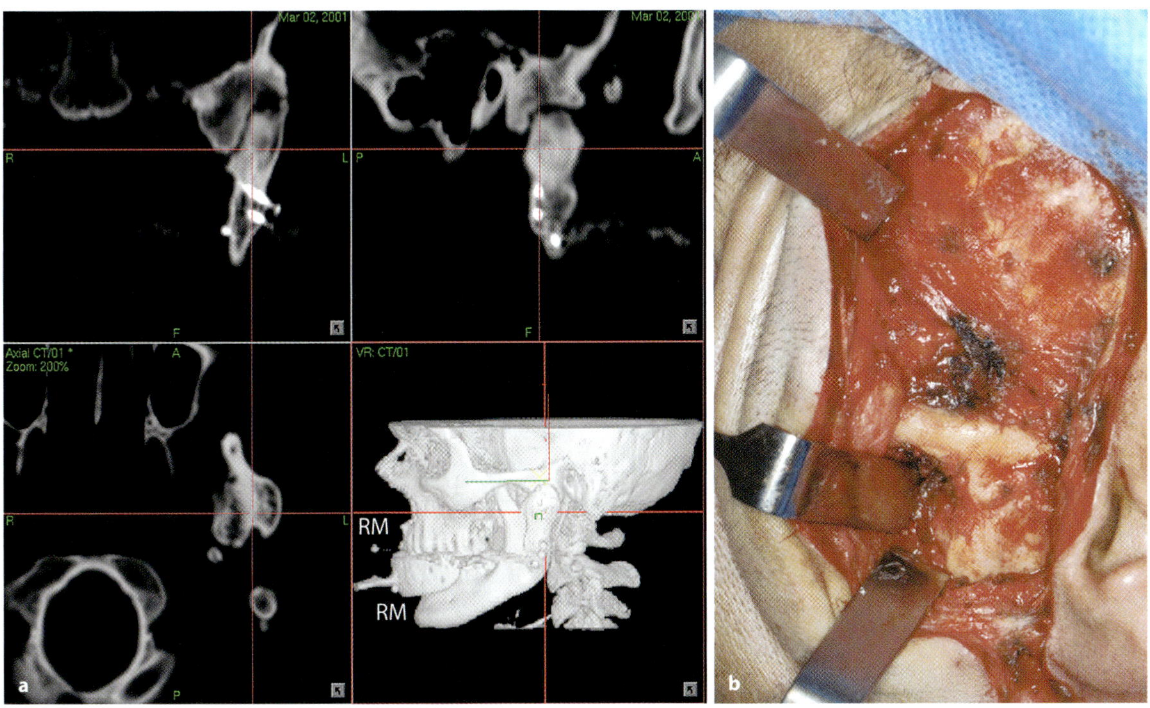

Fig. 55. Bony ankylosis of the temporomandibular joint (planning CT). The extent of the ankylotic transformation of the temporomandibular joint can be appreciated in the multiplanar display (a). The 3D reconstruction shows the navigation splint with the reference markers (*RM*). b Intraoperative view

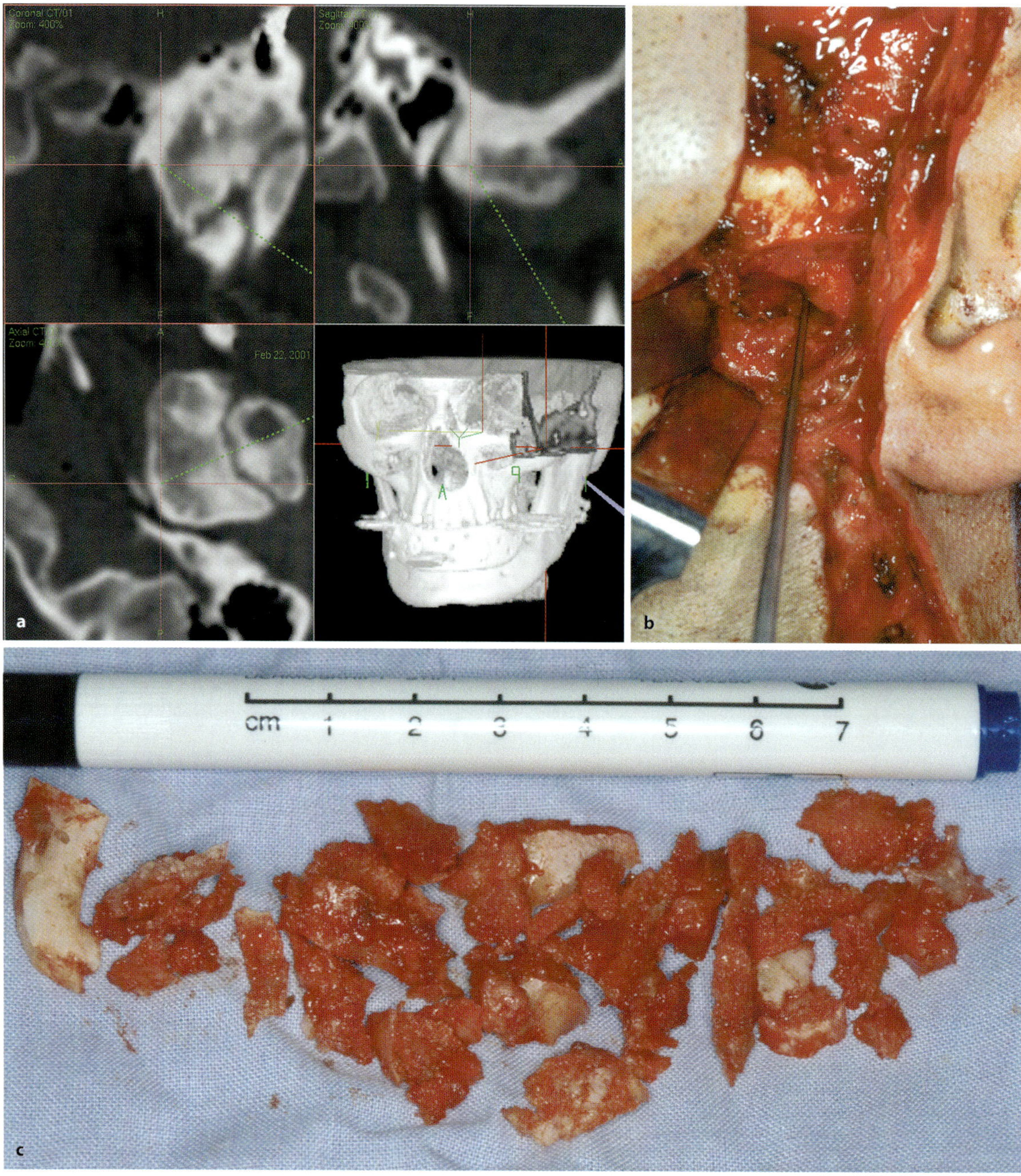

Fig. 56. Navigation-assisted resection of the temporomandibular joint. **a** Intraoperative image of the navigation-assisted osteotomy. **b** Navigation instrument being introduced through a preauricular approach. The multiplanar display (**a**) shows the proximity of the lesion to the site of emergence of the facial nerve. **c** Excision specimens

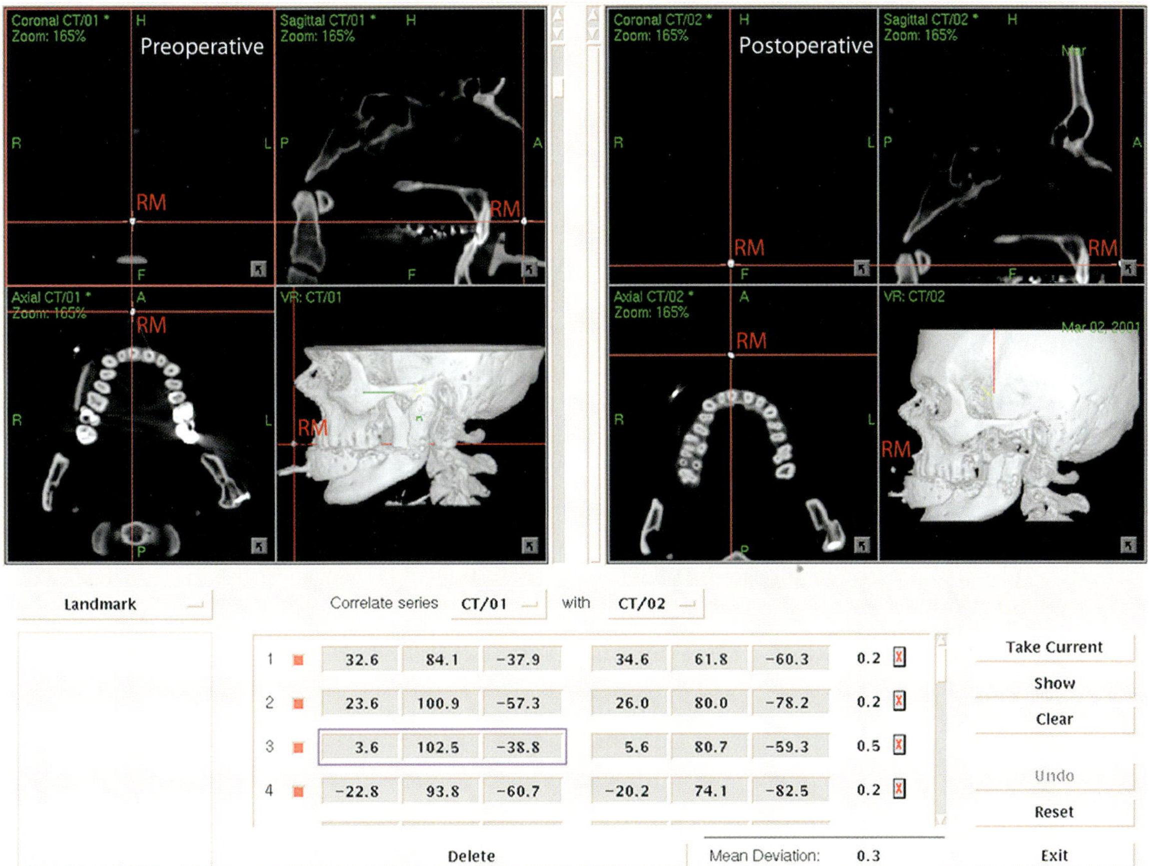

Fig. 57. Data set correlation with navigation splint markers. Correlation of the preoperative (*left*) and postoperative (*right*) CT data sets is done by correlating the four reference markers (*RM*) on the navigation splint. This can achieve a positional accuracy of better than 1 mm

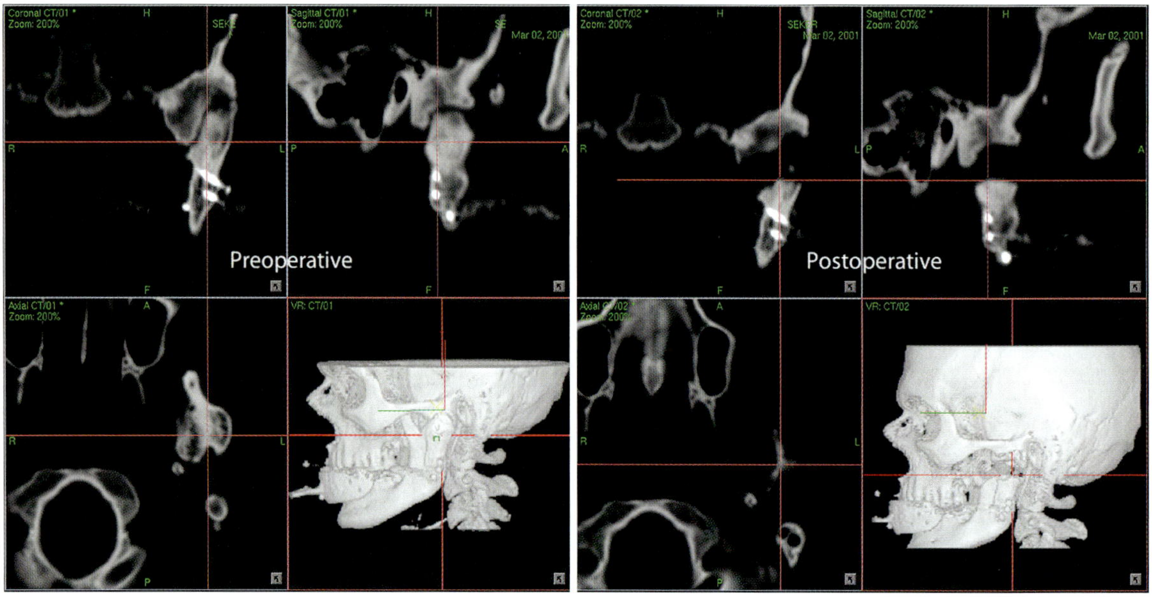

Fig. 58. Postoperative analysis after the resection of temporomandibular joint ankylosis. Correlation of the preoperative (*left*) and postoperative (*right*) CT data sets allows the postoperative result to be evaluated with millimeter precision

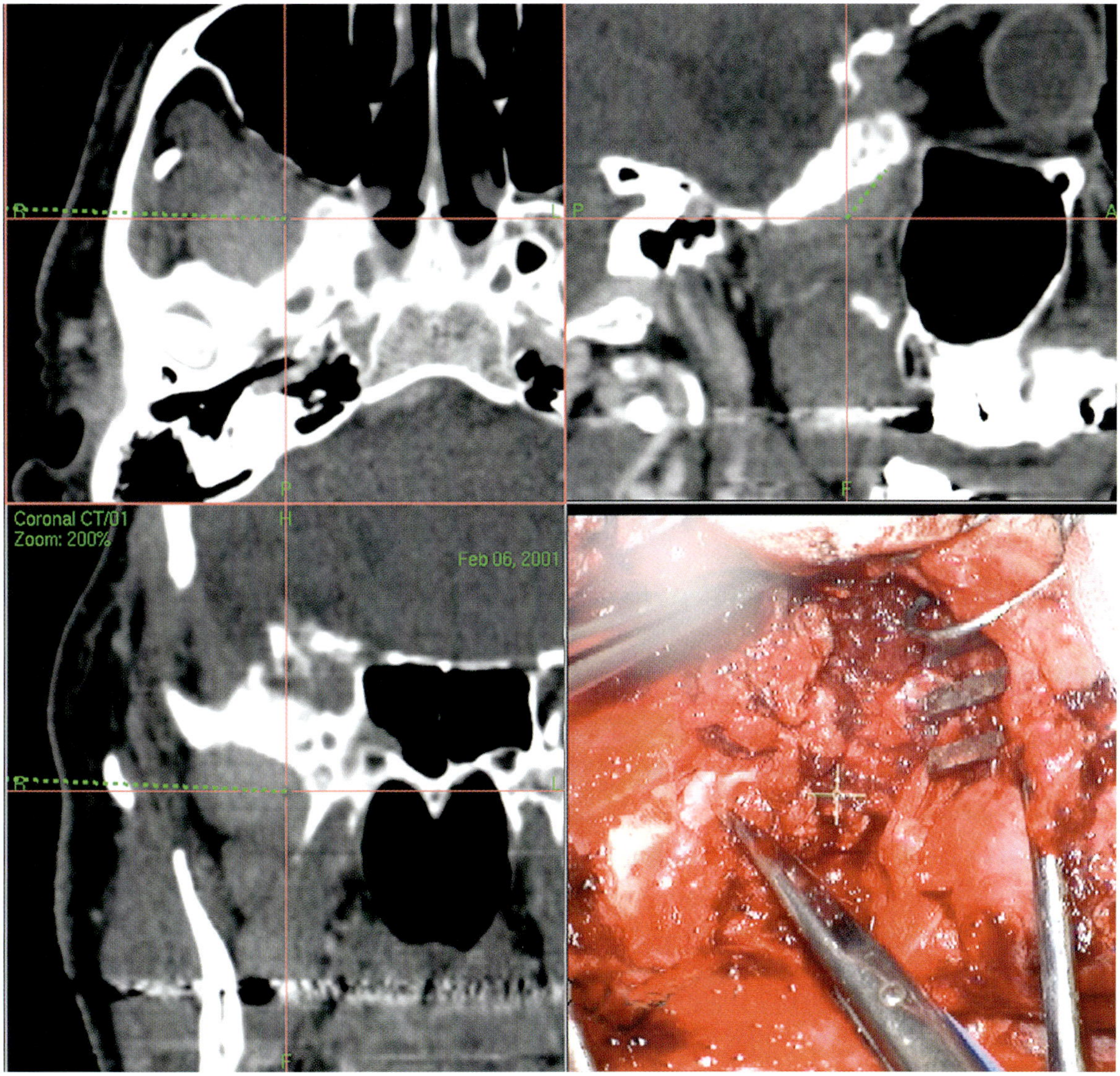

Fig. 59. Navigation-assisted resection of meningioma. The intraoperative view of the operative field in the multiplanar display of the CT data set enables the surgeon to achieve better tumor clearance by visualizing the tumor boundaries. *Lower right panel* shows the view through the operating microscope during the resection

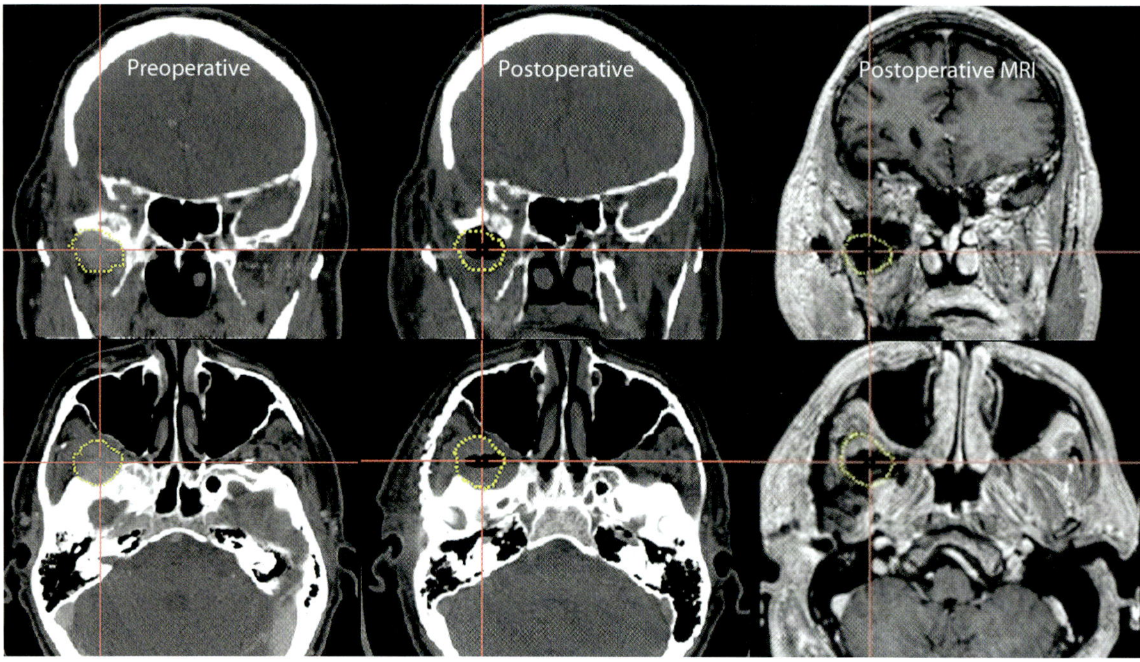

Fig. 60. Follow-up after meningioma resection. Correlation of the preoperative CT data set (*left*) with the postoperative CT (*middle*) and MRI (*right*) data sets makes it possible to transfer the preoperative tumor boundaries

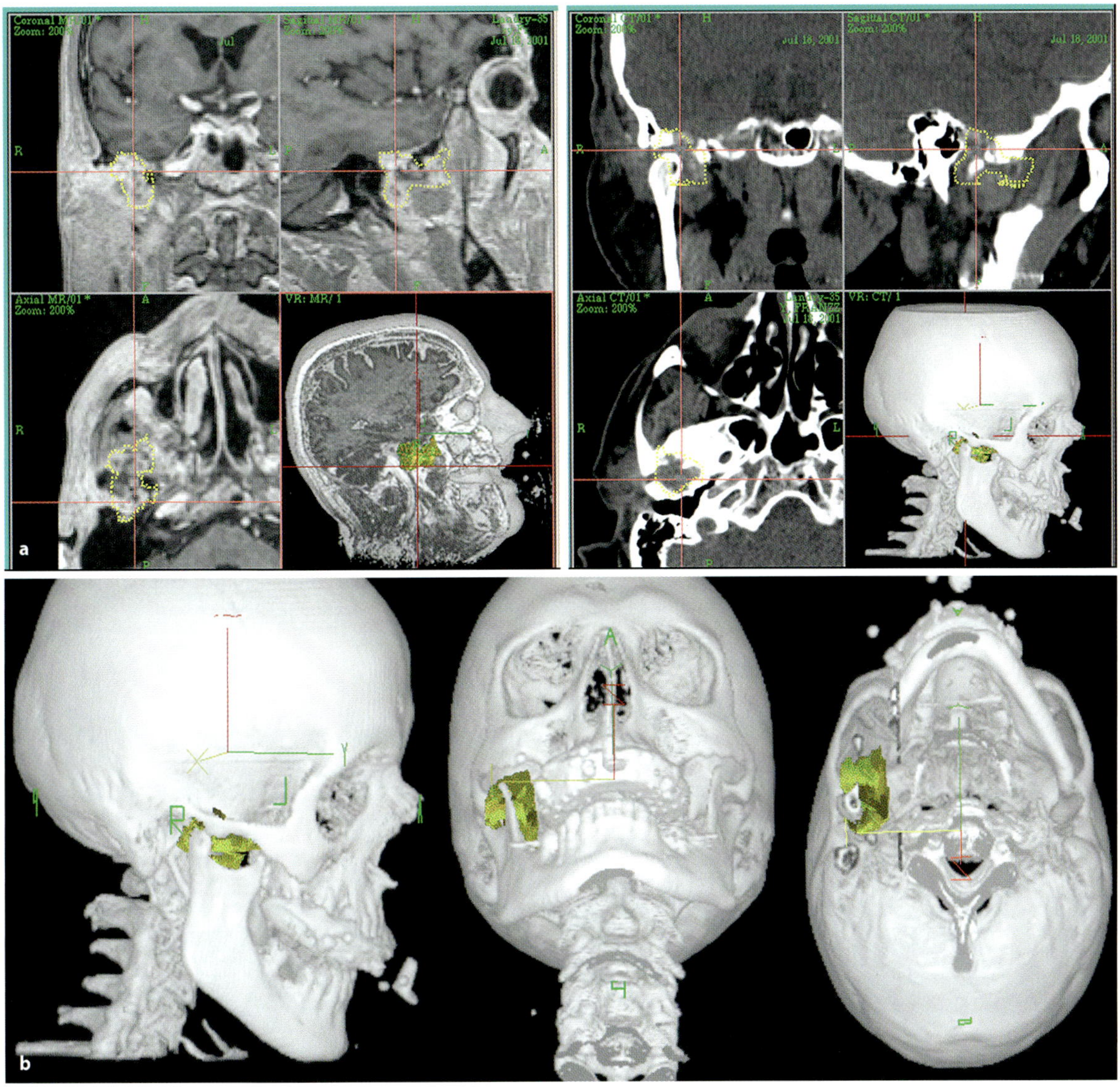

Fig. 61. Preoperative planning for the resection of an osteosarcoma of the lateral skull base. Correlating the preoperative MRI and CT data sets and transferring the tumor boundaries (a) makes it possible to combine the imaging information and improve tumor clearance using navigation-assisted technique. Superimposing the tumor volumes in the 3D reconstruction (b) makes it easier to select the route of approach and plan necessary osteotomies of the facial skeleton

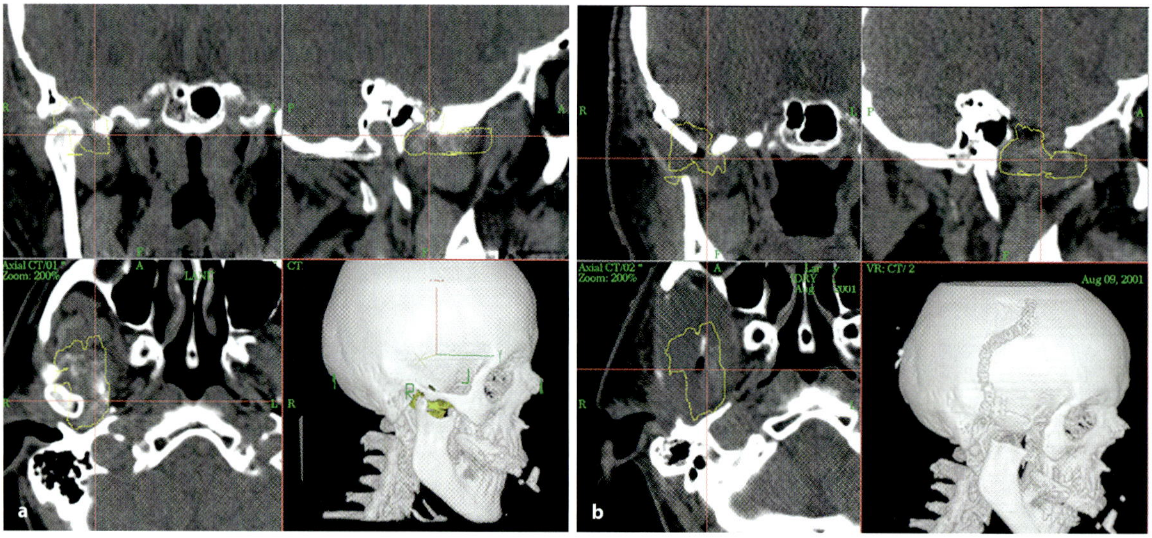

Fig. 62 a, b. Postoperative evaluation following the resection of a lateral skull base tumor. Correlation of the pre- and postoperative CT data sets makes it possible to transfer the tumor boundaries and evaluate the completeness of the navigation-assisted resection. The primary reconstruction with a calvarial graft is shown in the 3D image (**b**, *lower right*)

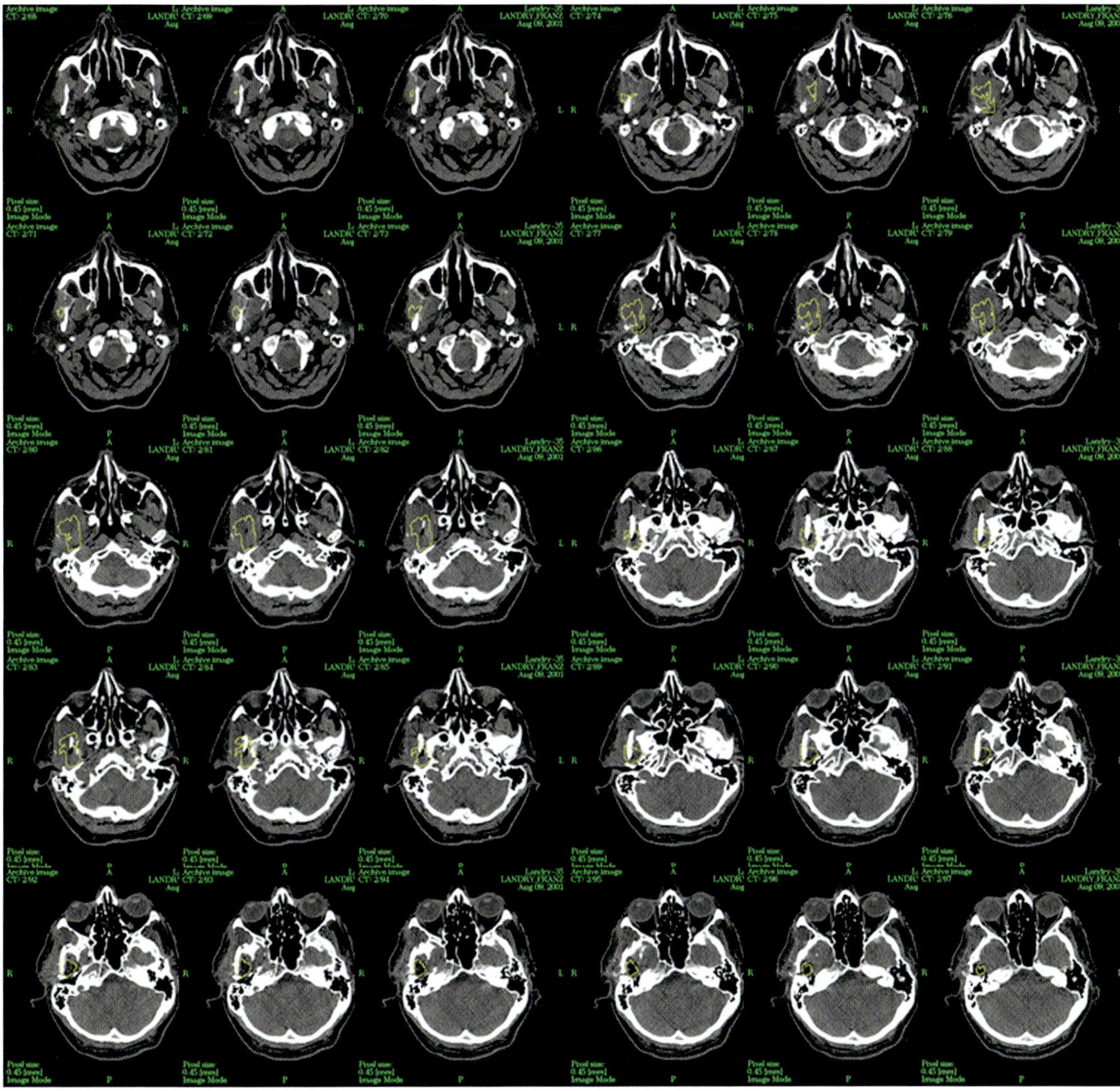

Fig. 63. Visualization of preoperative tumor volumes for the planning of postoperative radiotherapy. Correlation of the pre- and postoperative CT data sets makes it possible to visualize the original tumor boundaries to direct the planning of postoperative radiotherapy

Anterior Skull Base

Preoperative planning for tumors of the anterior skull base includes marking the tumor volumes based on the CT data set or transferring the margins from the MRI data set to the CT data set. Use of the registration splint permits the fusion of the CT and MRI data sets because the markers can be identified in both imaging modalities. In surgery done after preoperative chemotherapy, the pretherapeutic tumor boundaries can be transferred into the postchemotherapy data set (Fig. 64).

Through the transfer of pretherapeutic tumor volumes, a radical navigation-assisted resection can be carried out in accordance with the original tumor boundaries. Pointer-based navigation improves the adequacy of tumor clearance intraoperatively by demonstrating margins that are not clinically visible to the surgeon (Fig. 65).

Extensive resections in the naso-orbitoethmoid region are reconstructed with synthetic materials (titanium, polymers) or autologous bone grafts (calvarium, ilium, rib, etc.). A primary reconstruction is desired because of its functional advantages and quality-of-life benefits. Because intraoperative navigation makes available all information on the original facial skeletal contours before the tumor resection, the computer-assisted insertion and positioning of the synthetic materials or bone grafts can be more easily performed (Fig. 66).

Postoperative follow-ups can easily be correlated with the previous data sets by reusing the navigation splint. This allows the result of the operation to be validated in terms of radical tumor clearance and the quality of the reconstruction. At the same time, necessary postoperative radiotherapy can be individually planned and follow-ups can be maintained for several years, facilitating the early detection of recurrent disease (Figs. 67, 68).

Midface

Detailed, 3D planning of the resection and the functional-esthetic reconstruction is of critical importance in the treatment of midfacial tumors. Special attention is given to achieving an anatomical reconstruction of the orbital region and the rehabilitation of masticatory function (Fig. 69).

Primary reconstructions are generally preferred over secondary reconstructions because they tend to yield better functional and esthetic results. Primary reconstructions of the periorbital region involve the use of synthetic materials and autologous bone grafts as described above (Hammer et al. 1999). Comparing the reduction of tumor volume achieved after individual chemotherapy cycles provides a measure of tumor responsiveness to pharmacological therapy. If the tumor volume is found to increase during chemotherapy, the therapy should be discontinued at once and the patient referred for immediate surgical resection of the tumor (Figs. 70, 71).

Masticatory function after partial mandibular resections can be rehabilitated with an obturator prosthesis without the need for extensive bony reconstructions, which are rarely indicated given the low 5-year survival rates in these patients. The prosthesis can be attached to teeth or dental implants in the residual mandible. Dental implants anchored in the zygoma can provide stable abutments within the resected area. The titanium screw system developed by Branemark for anchoring bone-integrated screw implants in the zygoma (Zygomaticus fixture) allows for implant-based prosthetic reconstruction of the posterior maxilla without additional bone augmentation. Often no other treatment options are available, especially in patients with extensive tissue defects, and the solid bone of the zygoma provides the only foundation for stable implant attachment. In most cases these implants are inserted immediately after the tumor resection. If the position of the implant has already been planned and simulated preoperatively, both the resection and the implant insertion can be done under navigational guidance. In this way the placement of the implant can be planned in accordance with prosthetic requirements, and the planning can be accurately transferred to the patient at operation (Fig. 72).

The operative treatment of midfacial tumors consists of navigation-assisted radical surgical resection followed by a primary reconstruction of the periorbital region and prosthetic reconstruction using

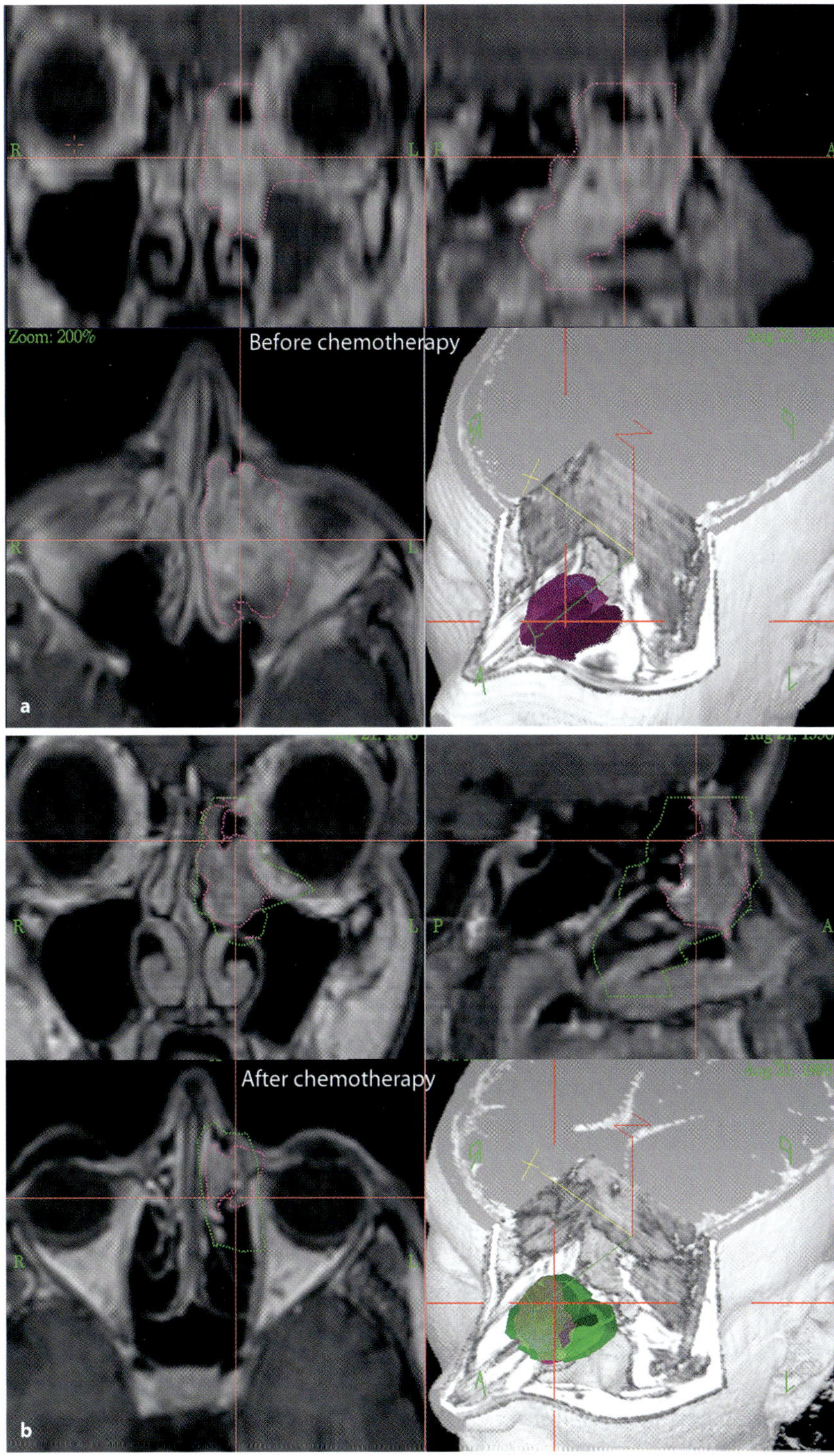

Fig. 64. Esthesioneuroblastoma of the anterior skull base before and after neoadjuvant chemotherapy. **a** MRI data set before neoadjuvant chemotherapy. **b** MRI data set after chemotherapy. The tumor boundaries are outlined in *purple*. By correlating the data sets with the markers on the navigation splint, the tumor boundaries can be transferred from the pretherapeutic MRI data set (*outlined in green* in **b**)

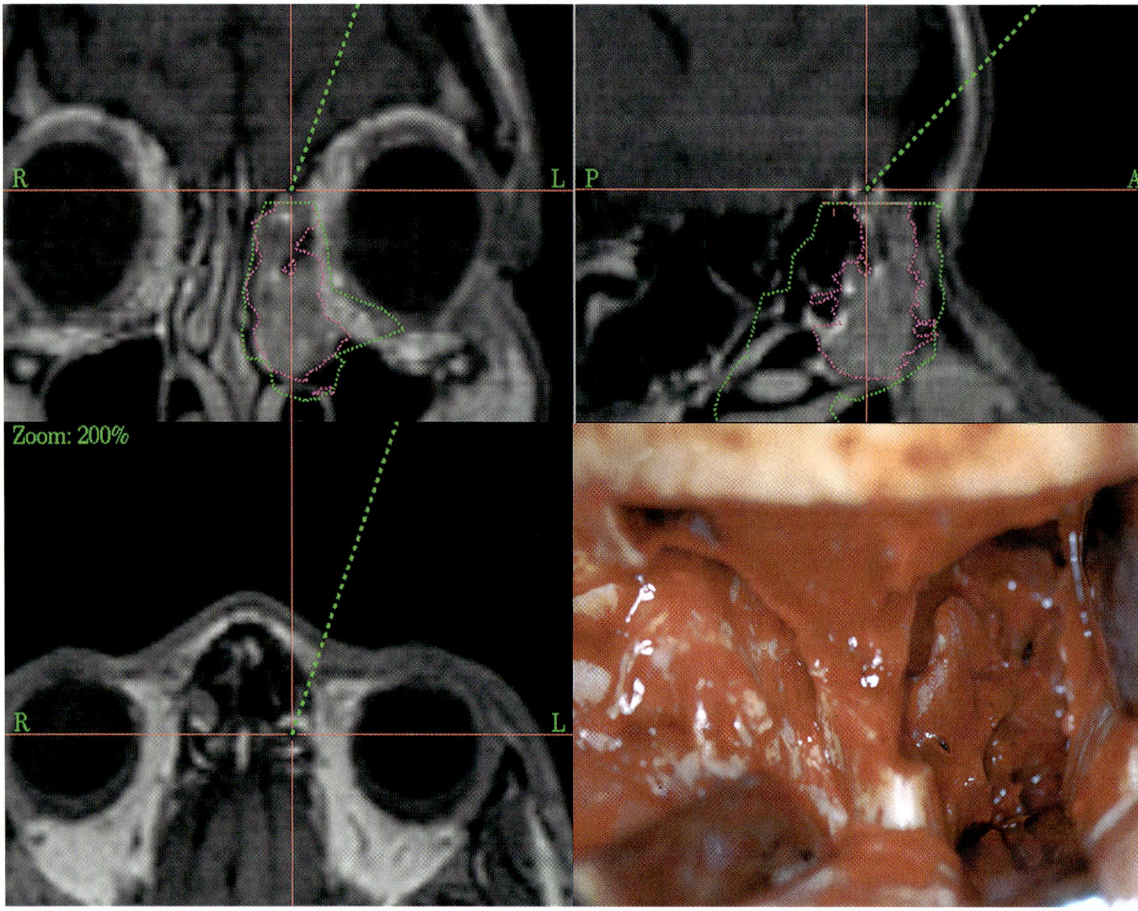

Fig. 65. Navigation-assisted radical resection of an anterior skull base tumor (esthesioneuroblastoma). The original tumor boundaries before chemotherapy (*outlined in green*) have been superimposed over the tumor boundaries after chemotherapy (*outlined in purple*) by correlating the pre- and post-therapeutic data sets. The images depict a moment during the pointer-based radical resection based on the virtual original tumor boundaries (*green*). These boundaries cannot be identified in the actual surgical field (*lower right panel*)

zygomatic implants (Gellrich et al. 2002c). Every phase of operative treatment is guided by intraoperative navigation. This increases radical tumor clearance while improving the quality and predictability of the reconstruction. Postoperative evaluation of the outcome by CT is an essential step in preventing postoperative complications and evaluating different operative methods. As in other settings, data set correlation is again of fundamental importance. It is easily accomplished by reusing the reference markers on the registration splint (Fig. 73).

Prosthetic rehabilitation of the maxilla can be performed after a period of 6–9 months. The use of zygomatic implants as abutments for the obturators improves the retention of the prosthesis, significantly improving the patient's quality of life (Fig. 74).

Navigation-assisted primary reconstructions have rarely been described in tumor resections (Schramm et al. 2000c). Accordingly, there have been no studies on the validation of orbital reconstructions in the setting of oncological resections. Positioning of the titanium mesh and bone grafts can be done accurately and reli-

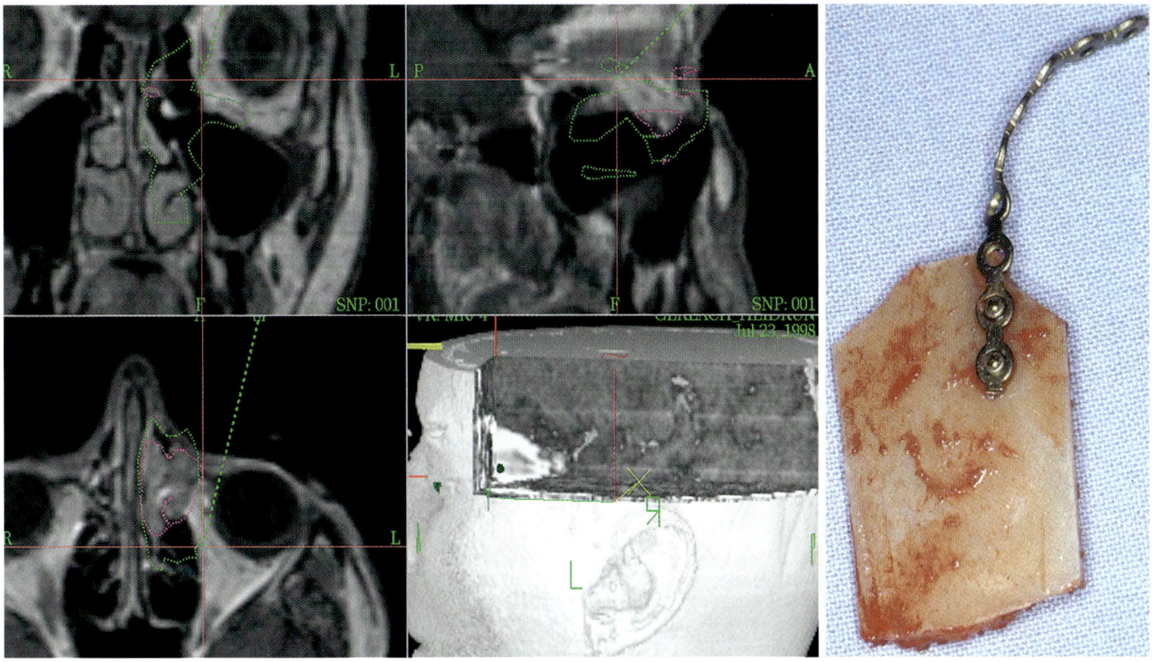

Fig. 66. Navigation-assisted primary reconstruction of the bony orbit following tumor resection. The images represent a pointer-based position check following the placement of a bone graft (*lower right panel*) for reconstructing the medial orbital wall. The reconstruction is guided by the original bony contours prior to resection of the anterior skull base esthesioneuroblastoma

ably by the use of splint-based registration (Schmelzeisen et al. 2000; Gellrich et al. 2002b). This is confirmed by the results of comparative volume measurements in our own patients. In validating our results, we observed a reduction in the postoperative orbital volume following the tumor resection and primary reconstruction, and this reduction can compensate for the soft tissue defect that is simultaneously created (Gellrich et al. 2002a–c). A navigation-assisted primary reconstruction was performed in ten patients with midfacial tumors. In all cases the titanium meshes and bone grafts used for orbital and midfacial reconstruction were positioned in accordance with the original bony contours prior to the tumor resection (Figs. 75–80).

Splint-based registration is a repeatable technique that allows the transfer of tumor boundaries from the MRI data set to the CT data set for pretherapeutic analysis and also from the pretherapeutic data set to all further acquisitions following chemotherapy, radiotherapy, or operative treatment. The use of registration splints also makes it possible to fuse CT and MRI data sets since the markers can be visualized in both modalities (Schramm et al. 2000c). This can also be achieved with invasive screw markers, but these devices cannot be used due to the long treatment periods.

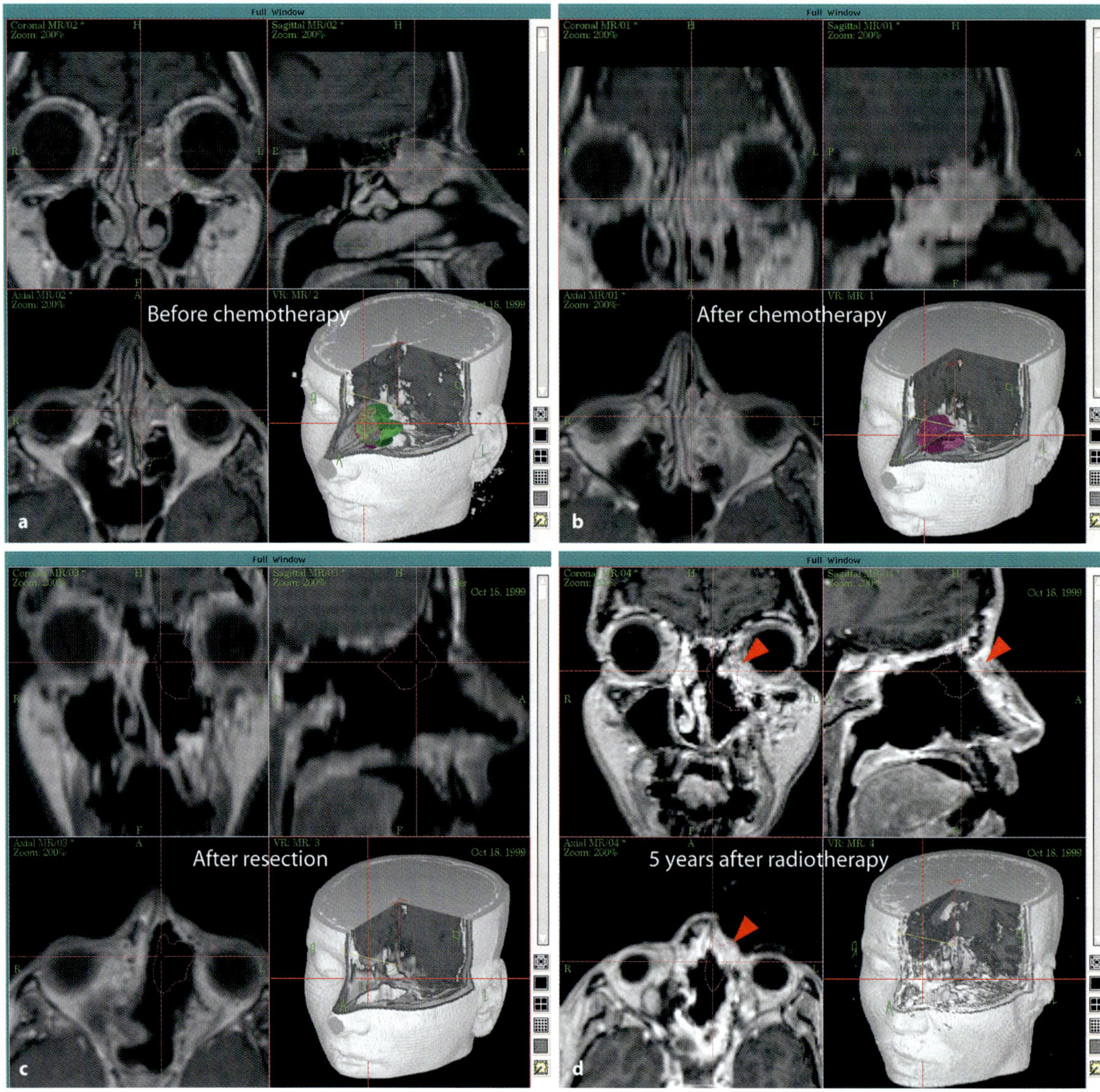

Fig. 67. Long-term follow-up after chemotherapy, tumor resection, and irradiation of an esthesioneuroblastoma of the anterior skull base. Follow-up examination for tumor recurrence 5 years after preoperative neoadjuvant chemotherapy, navigation-assisted radical tumor resection, and postoperative radiotherapy. **a** Before chemotherapy. **b** After chemotherapy. **c** After resection. **d** Five years after radiotherapy. The original tumor boundaries (*purple*) were transferred from the pre- to the posttherapeutic data set by correlation. The suspicious soft tissue structure in the former anteromedial portion of the tumor (*red arrows*) was identified by endonasal biopsy as reactive scar formation induced by the radiotherapy

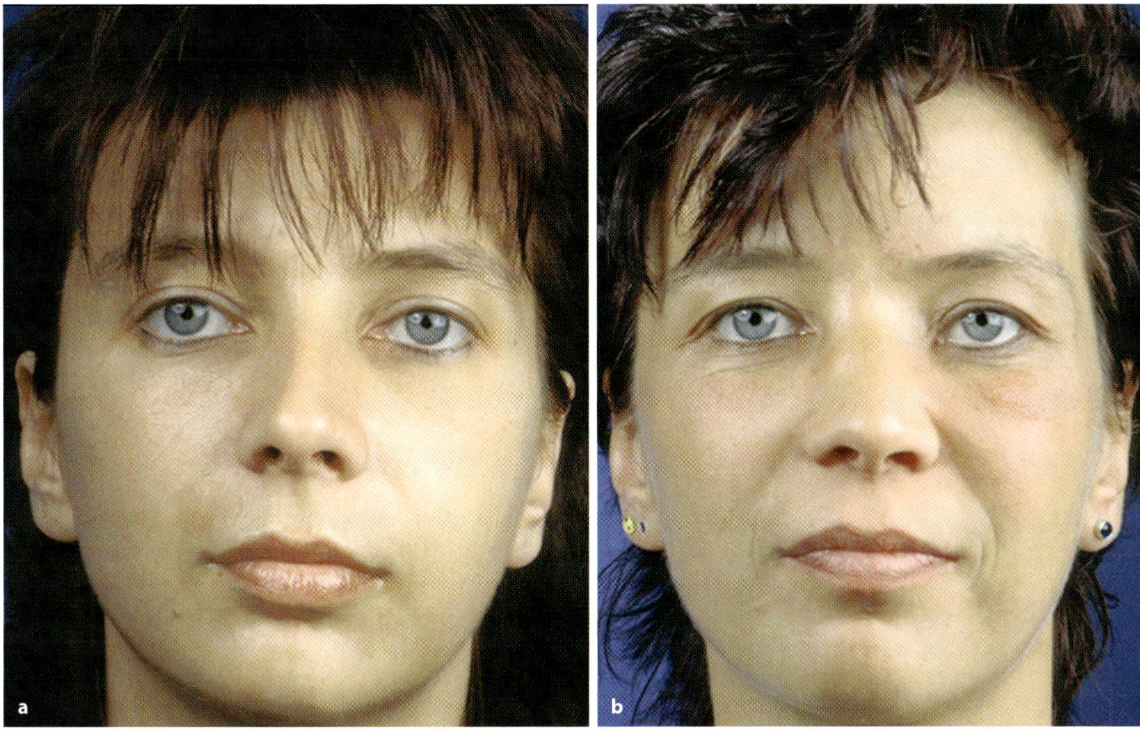

Fig. 68. Five-year comparison after chemotherapy, tumor resection, and irradiation of an esthesioneuroblastoma of the anterior skull base. a Before treatment. b Five years after treatment

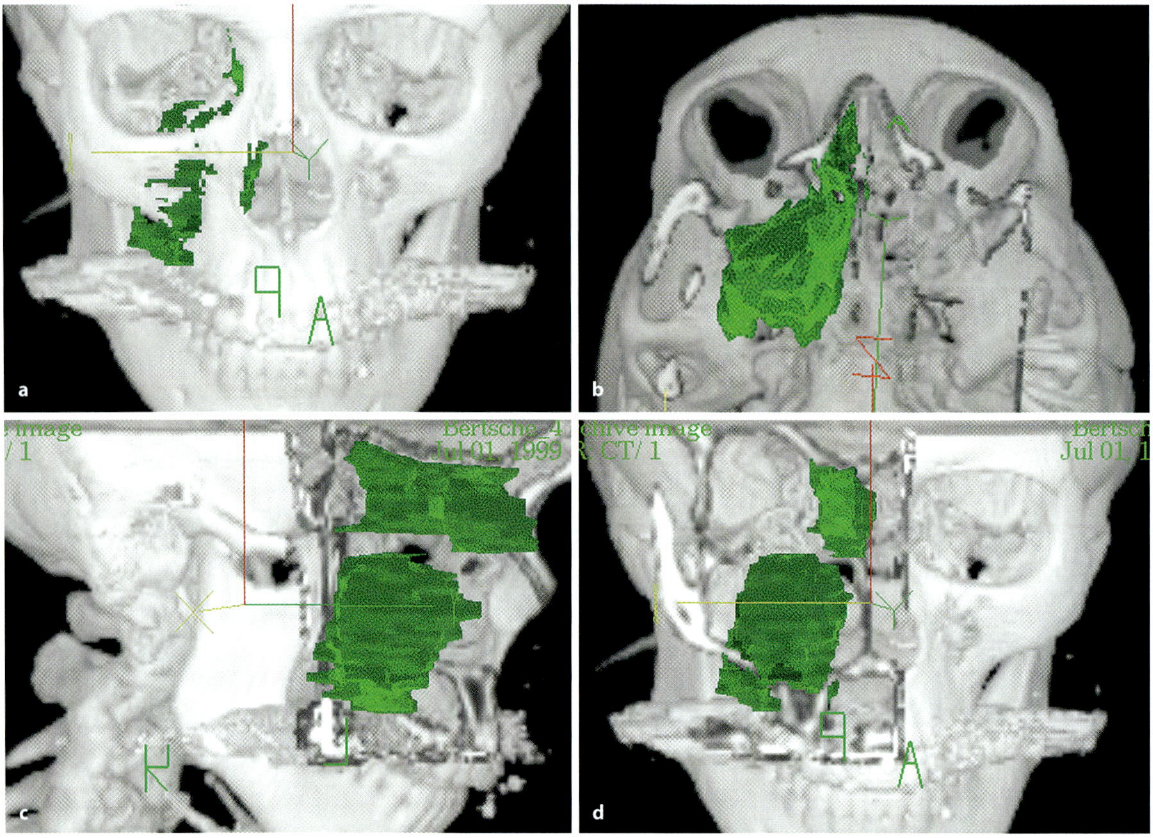

Fig. 69 a–e. Anaplastic carcinoma of the right maxillary sinus. Visualization of the tumor volume in a 3D reconstruction of the CT data set allows for detailed planning of the resection and reconstruction

Fig. 70. Follow-up of the chemotherapy response of an anaplastic carcinoma of the right maxillary sinus. **a** *Left* Initial situation (tumor volume 29.9 cm^3). *Right* After first cycle (tumor volume 17.8 cm^3). **b** *Left* After second cycle (tumor volume 10.2 cm^3). *Right* After third cycle (tumor volume 10.2 cm^3). **c** *Left* After fourth cycle (tumor volume 12.1 cm^3). *Right* Preoperative planning. Comparison of the tumor volumes before (*green*) and after preoperative neoadjuvant chemotherapy (*purple* after first cycle, *yellow* after second cycle, *blue* after third cycle, *red* after fourth cycle) indicates a reduction of tumor size after the first and second chemotherapy cycles, followed by enlargement of the tumor during the third and fourth cycles. This finding warrants the discontinuation of neoadjuvant therapy and should prompt immediate surgical treatment. Planning of the radical resection is aided by transferring the original tumor boundaries (*green line* in **c** *right*)

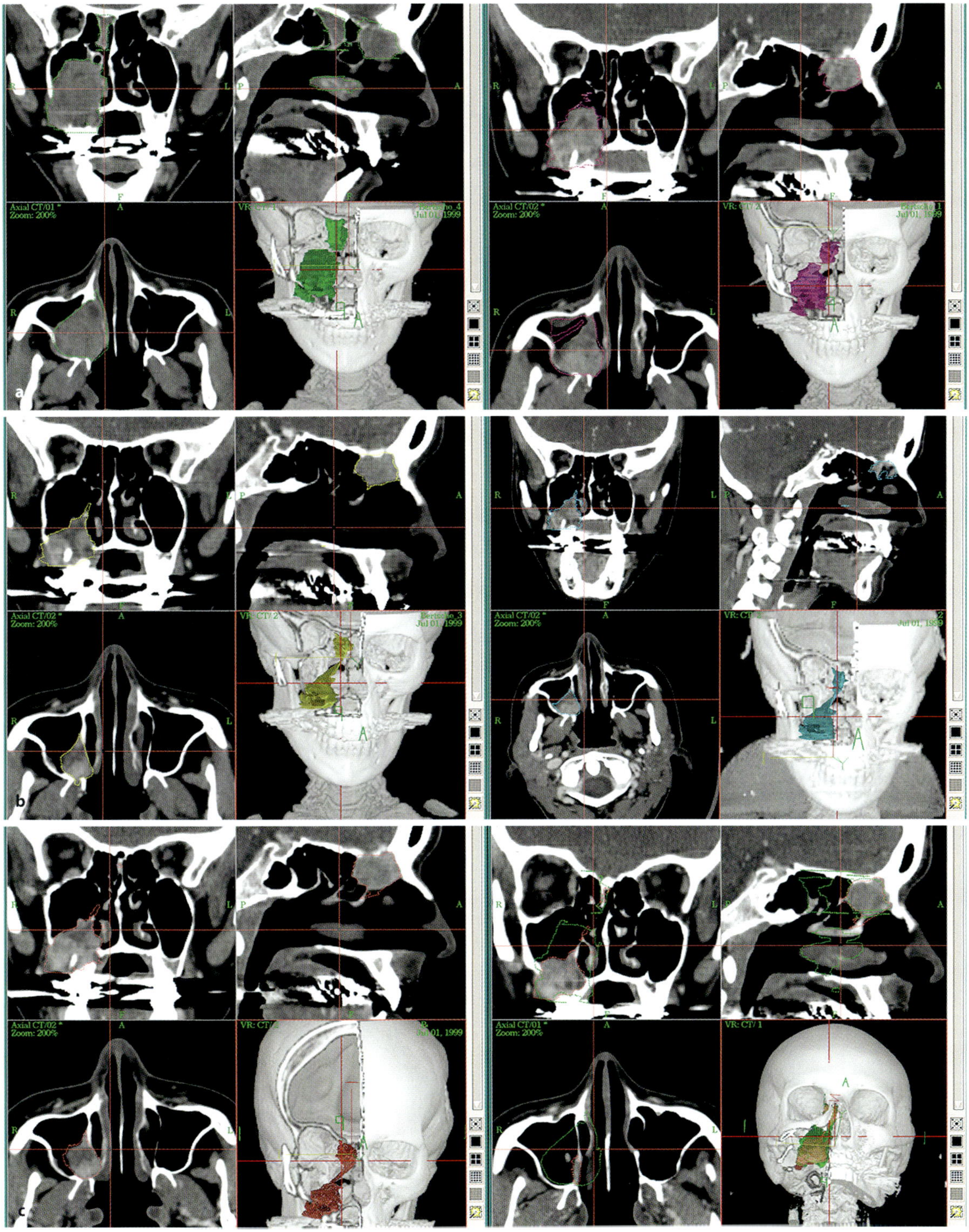
Axial CT/01 *
Zoom: 200%
VR: CT/1
Jul 01, 1999
a
Axial CT/02 *
Zoom: 200%
VR: CT/2
Jul 01, 1999
b
Axial CT/02 *
Zoom: 200%
c
Axial CT/01 *
Zoom: 200%
VR: CT/1

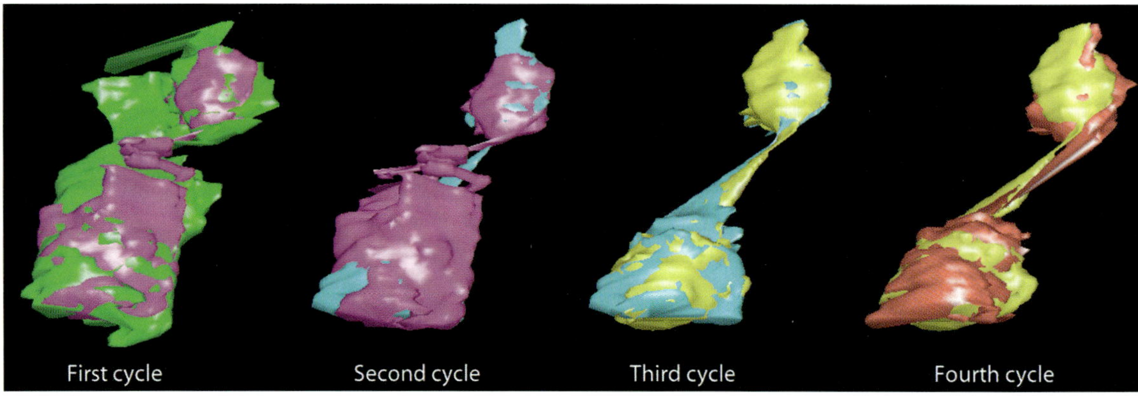

Fig. 71. Follow-up of tumor volumes during chemotherapy for anaplastic carcinoma of the right maxillary sinus. Comparison of the tumor volumes before (*green*) and after preoperative neoadjuvant chemotherapy (*purple* after first cycle, **a**; *blue* after second cycle, **b**; *yellow* after third cycle, **c**; *red* after fourth cycle, **d**) indicates a decrease in tumor size after the first and second chemotherapy cycles to 74% and 43% of the initial value (29.9 cm^3). Tumor size did not change during the third cycle but increased after the fourth cycle to 51% of the initial value

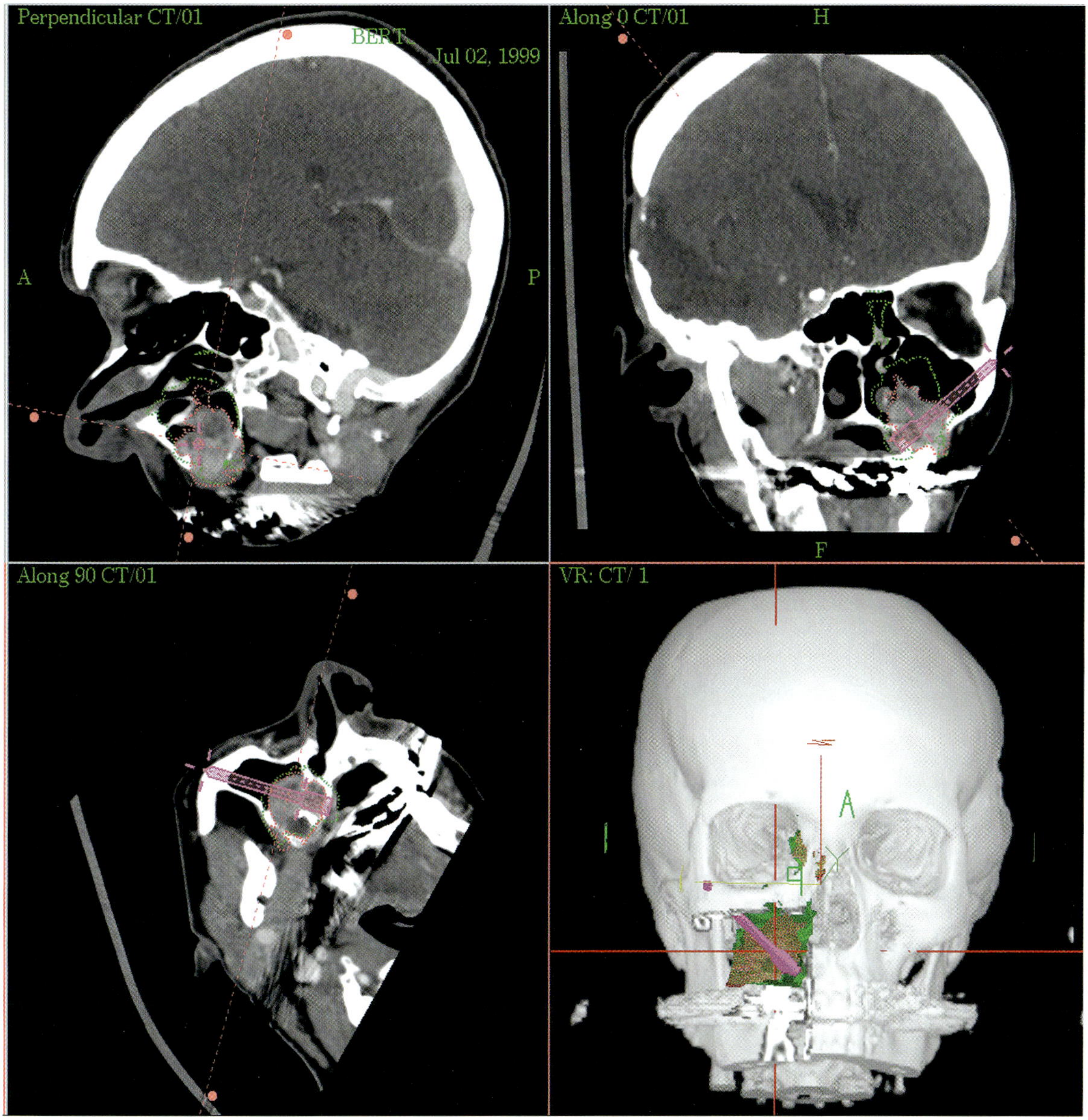

Fig. 72. Planning and simulation of a radical resection and the insertion of a zygomatic implant. The radical surgical resection is planned by transferring the original tumor boundaries (*green line*) into the CT data set after the completion of chemotherapy. With a partial resection of the maxilla, the surgeon can simulate the insertion of a zygomatic implant for a delayed primary prosthetic reconstruction

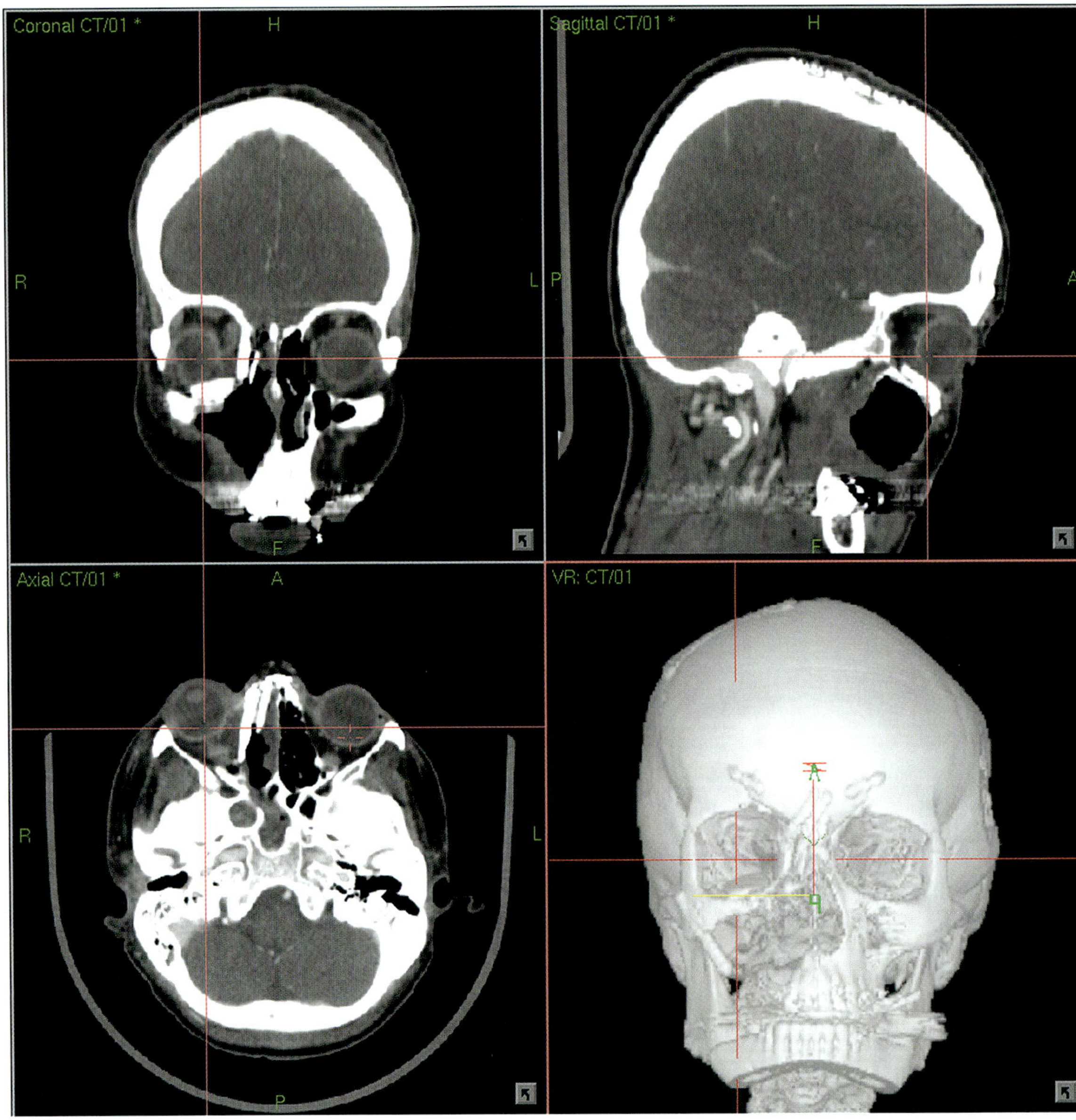

Fig. 73. Postoperative evaluation of a partial resection of the midface and orbit followed by primary reconstruction. The images show a primary reconstruction of the bony orbit. The zygomatic implant provides an abutment for an obturator prosthesis

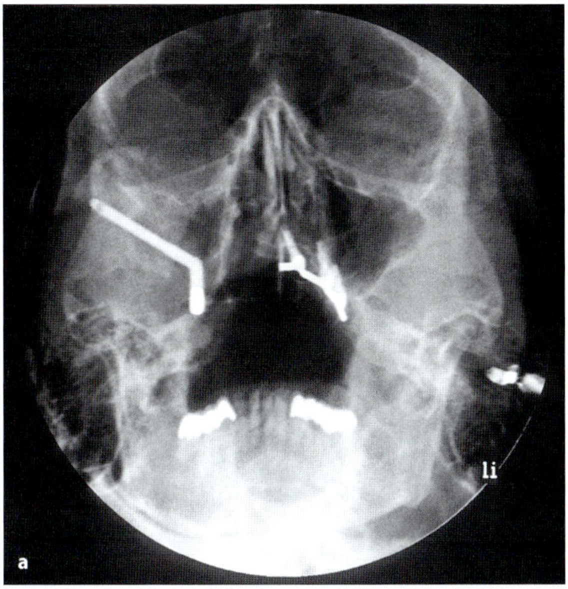

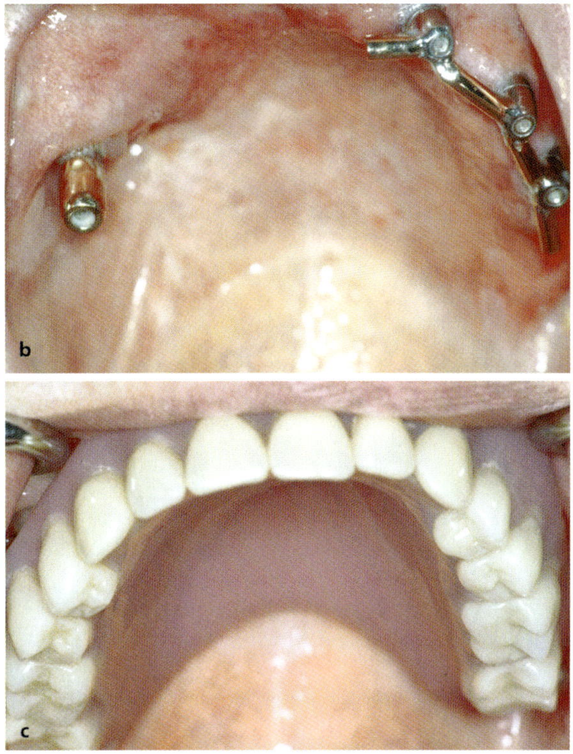

Fig. 74. Zygomatic implant and three dental implants for treatment with an obturator prosthesis. The radiograph (a) is a paranasal sinus projection taken after the insertion of an obturator prosthesis following a partial resection of the mandible for a malignant tumor. b Abutments. c Inserted prosthesis

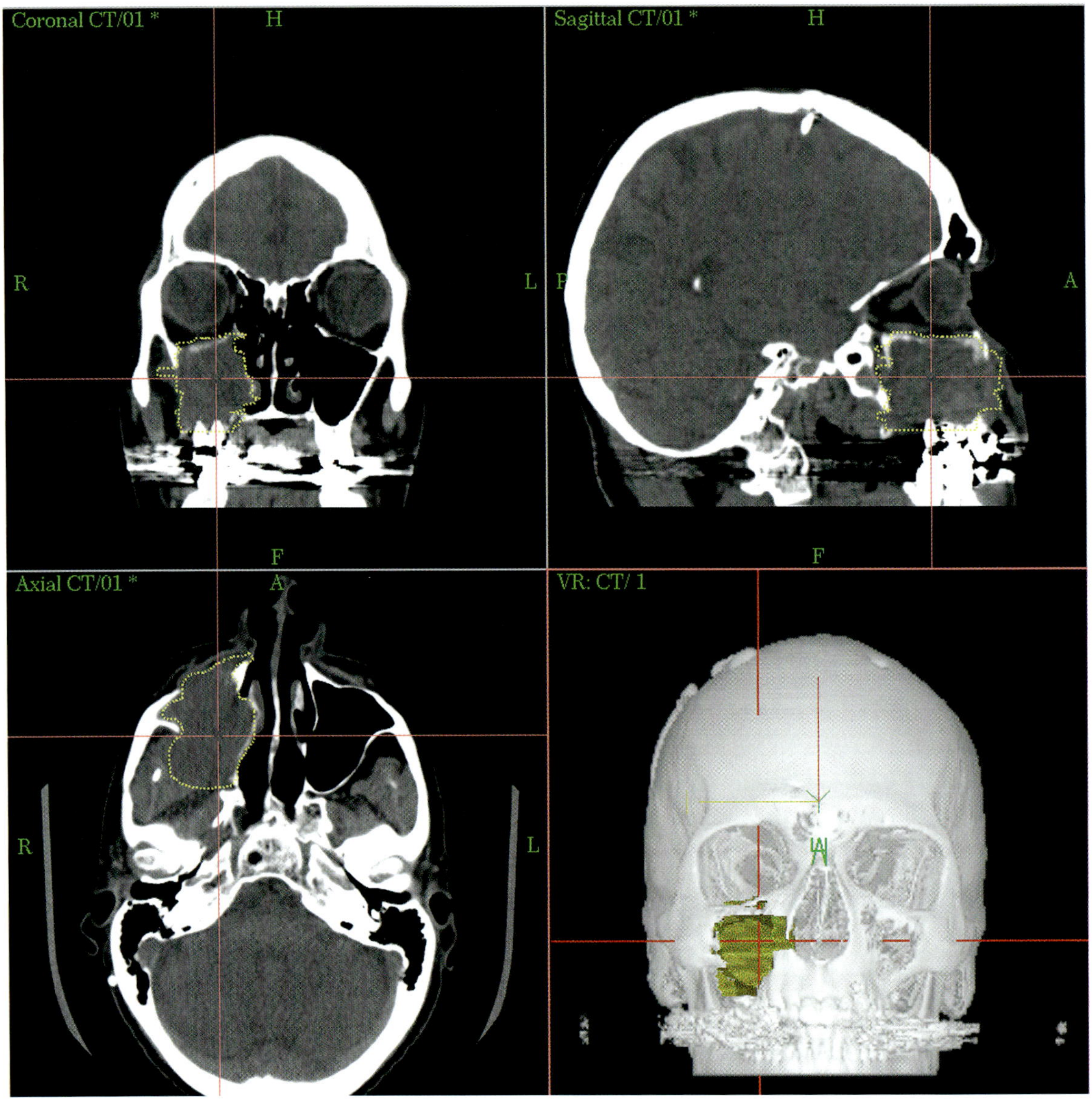

Fig. 75. Squamous cell carcinoma of the right maxillary sinus. The multiplanar mode demonstrates the extent of the tumor, whose boundaries have been outlined (*yellow*)

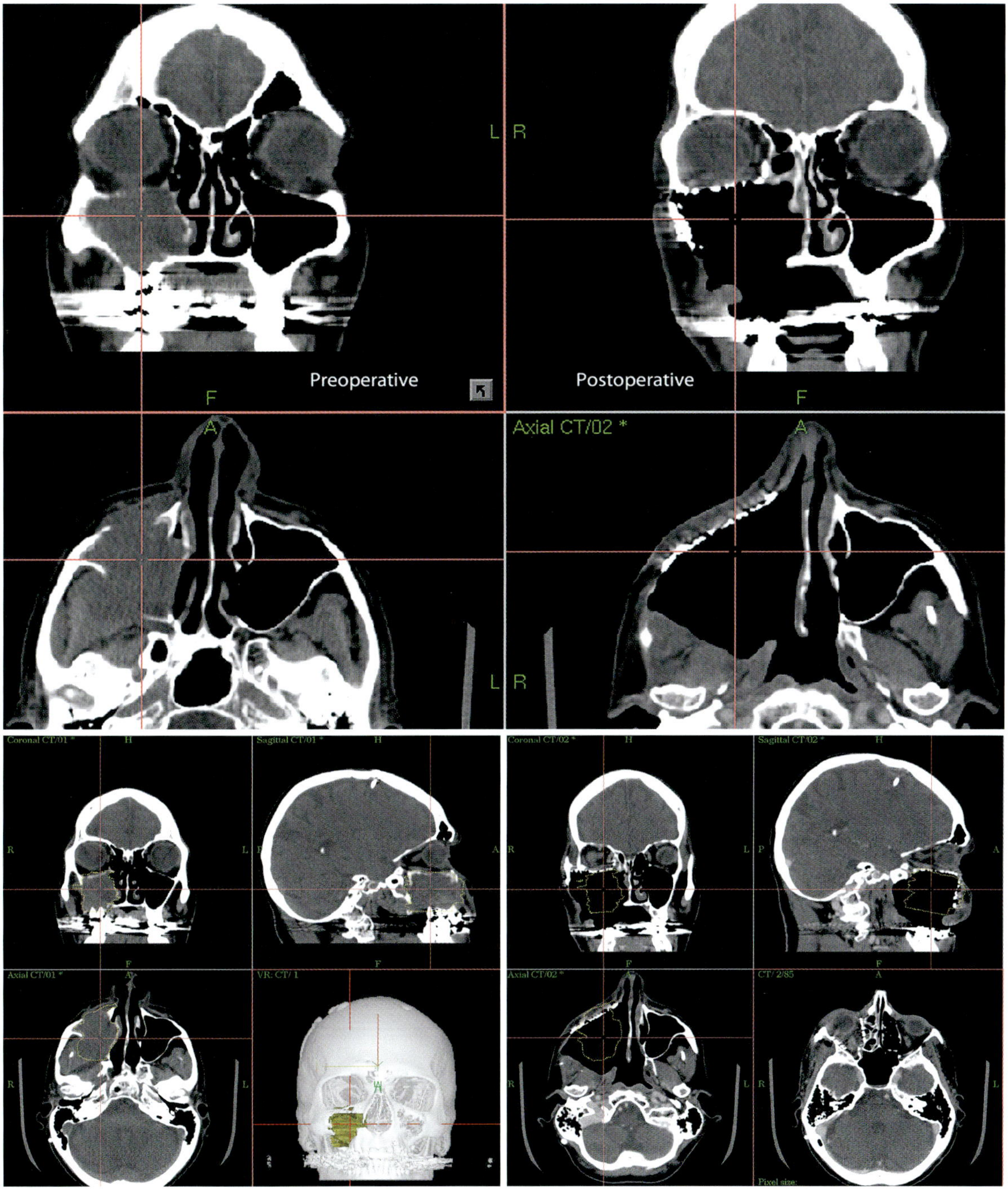

Fig. 76. Postoperative evaluation of a partial midfacial resection. The images represent the correlation of preoperative (*left*) and postoperative (*right*) CT data sets after the resection of a right maxillary sinus carcinoma followed by a navigation-assisted primary reconstruction of the midface and orbit with titanium mesh (*top*). After correlation of the image data sets, the tumor boundaries are transferred from the preoperative data set to the postoperative data set to better evaluate the adequacy of the resection (*yellow line at bottom*)

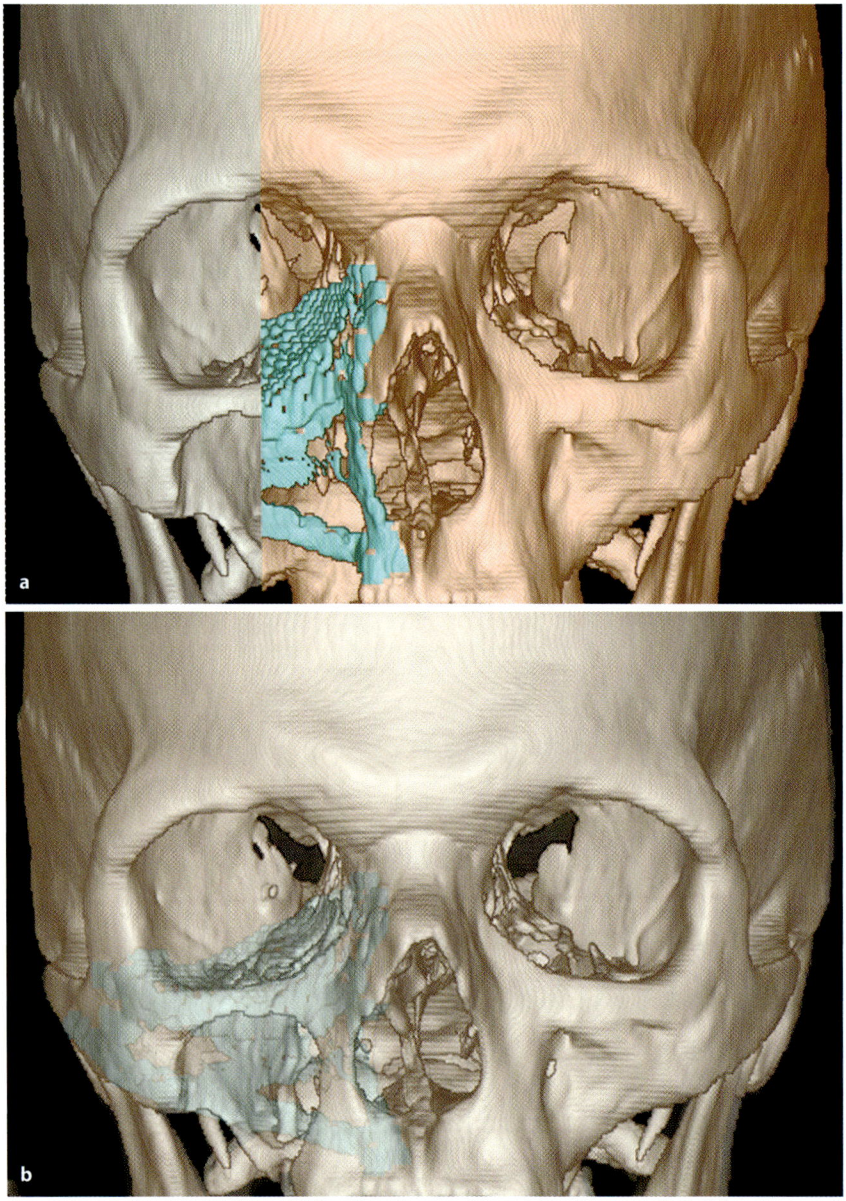

Fig. 77. Image fusion for the postoperative evaluation of a partial midfacial resection. The 3D images represent a 50% fusion (a) and a complete fusion of pre- and postoperative CT data sets after the resection of a right maxillary sinus carcinoma (b). The resection was followed by a navigation-assisted primary reconstruction of the midface and orbit with titanium mesh

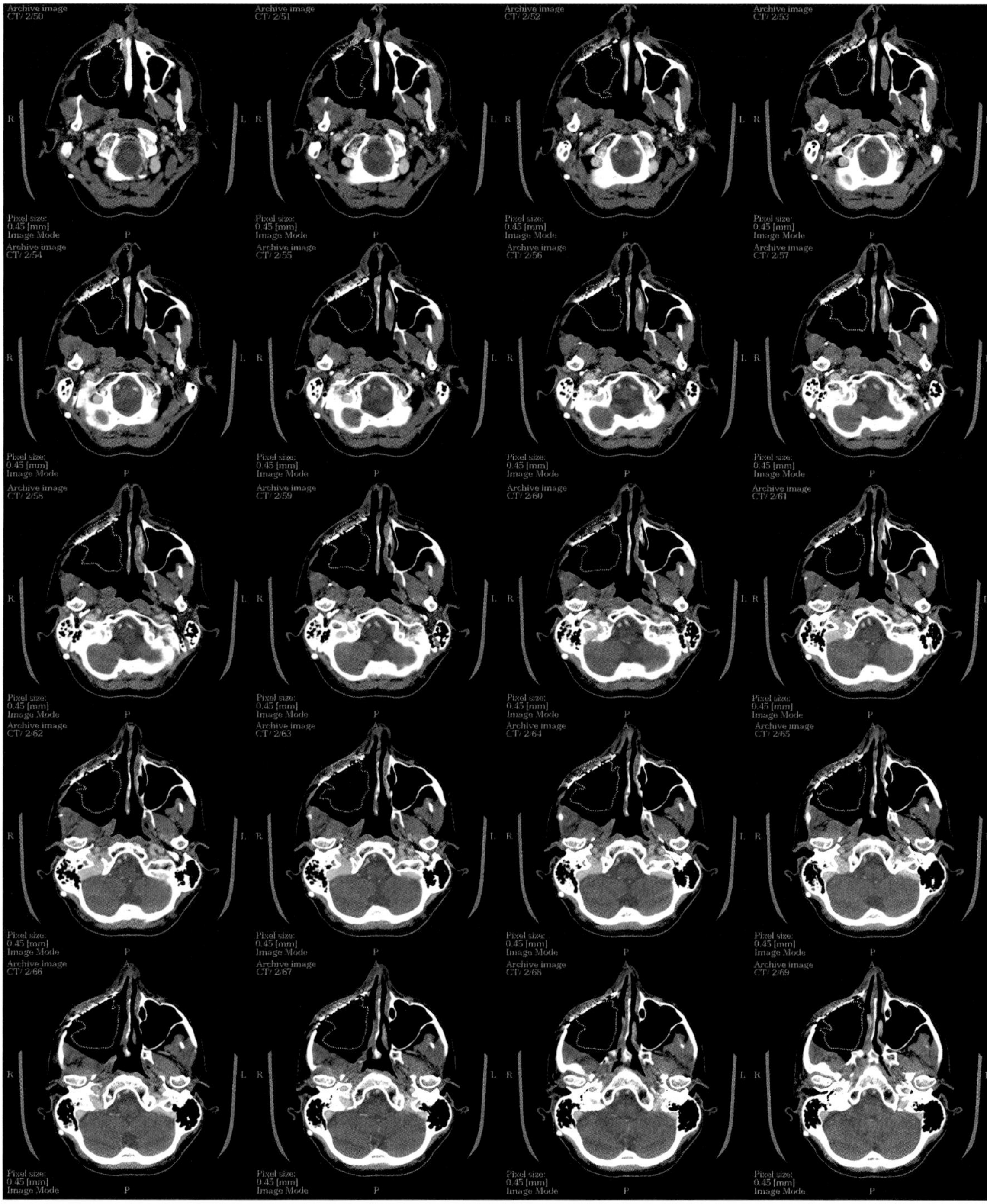

Fig. 78. Postoperative evaluation of the resection and radiotherapy planning. Transferring the tumor boundaries from the preoperative to the postoperative CT data set (*yellow line*) is useful in evaluating the adequacy of the resection and planning the postoperative radiotherapy field

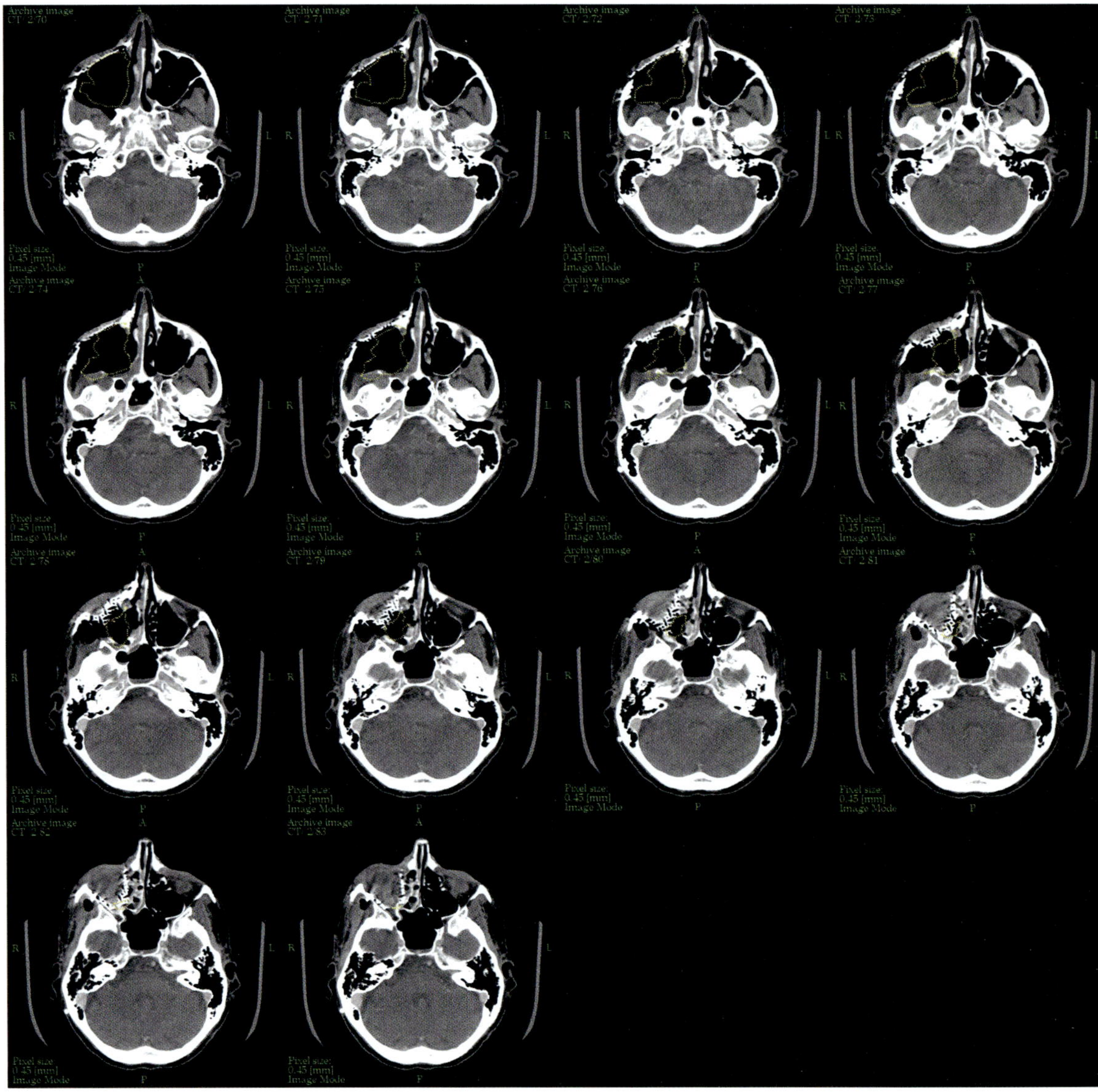

Fig. 78. (continued)

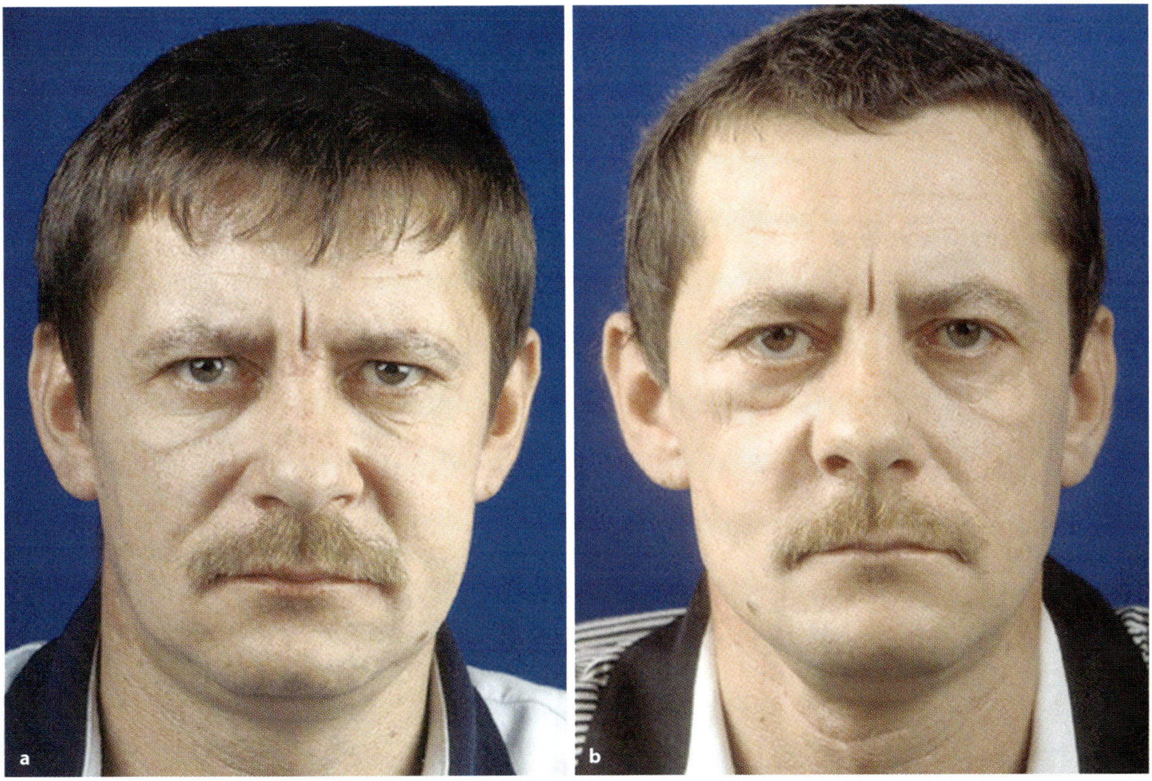

Fig. 79. Postoperative follow-up 2 years after a partial midfacial resection and primary reconstruction. Clinical appearance at presentation (a) and 2 years after operative treatment (b)

Fig. 80. Comparison of orbital volumes (in cm^3) before (*gray bars*) and after (*black bars*) the navigation-assisted primary reconstruction of a midfacial resection for a malignant tumor. Postoperative validation of the orbital reconstructions (n=10) showed an average postreconstruction decrease in orbital volume by 1.8 cm^3 (SD=0.3 cm^3), with preoperative values of 23.5–34.9 cm^3 and postoperative values of 22.3–33.5 cm^3

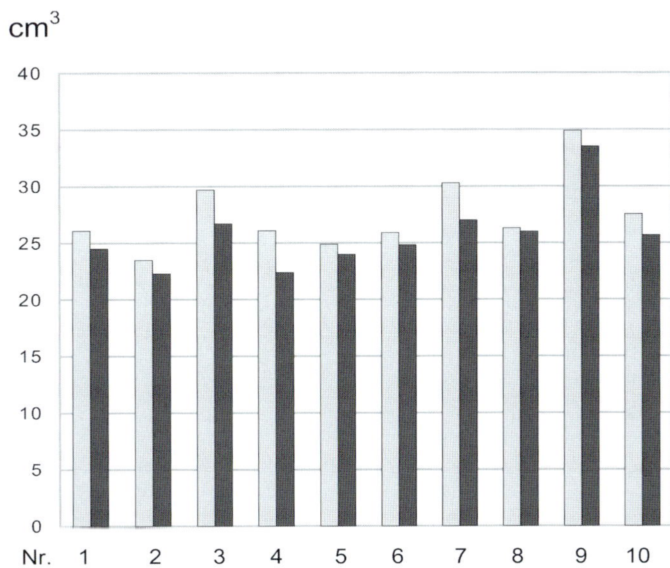

Intraoperative Radiotherapy

Pointer-based navigation can be used to plan the radiotherapy field in patients treated with intraoperative radiation (e.g., for intraoral carcinoma). This facilitates and expedites the complicated process of adjusting the X-ray tube (Fig. 81). However, the intraoperative soft tissue displacement caused by the resection limits this application to tumors that are situated near bone.

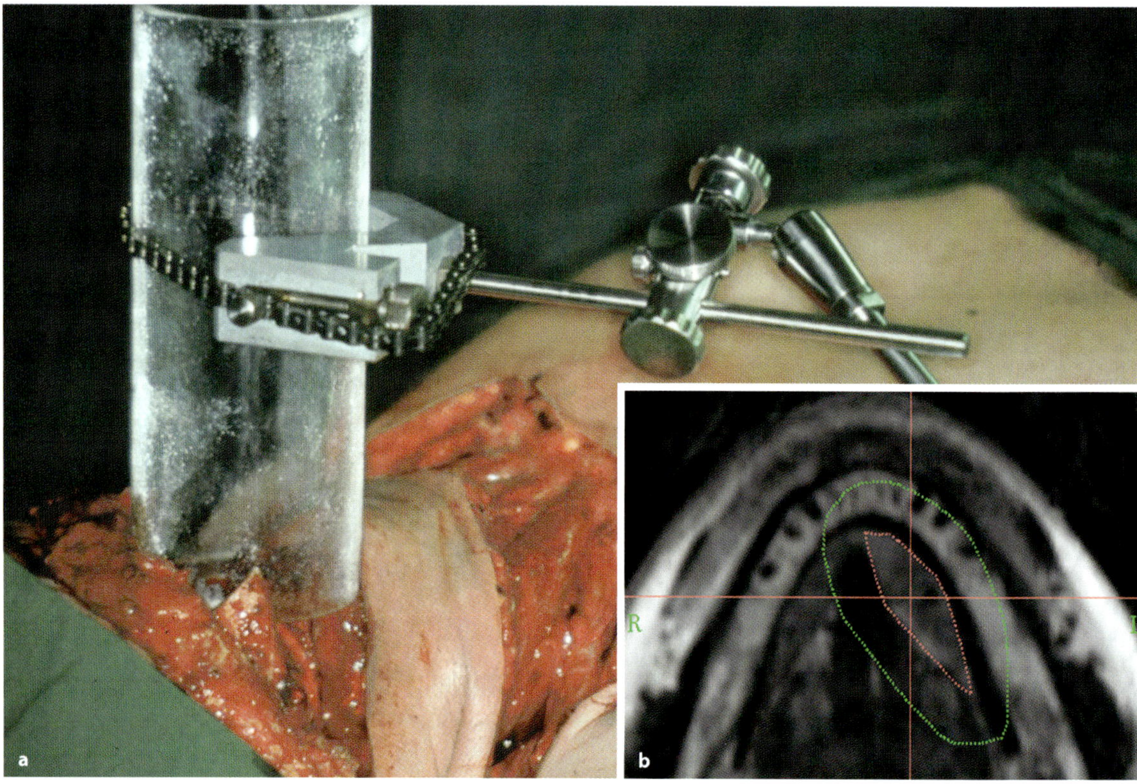

Fig. 81. Navigation-assisted alignment of the X-ray tube for intraoperative radiotherapy. a The resection of a malignant tumor is followed by the pointer-based alignment of the X-ray tube conforming to the preoperatively marked tumor boundaries. b MR image shows the outlines of the tumor (*red*) and resection margins (*green*)

Secondary Reconstructions after Tumor Resections

Secondary reconstructions of the midfacial region after tumor resections are challenging for the surgeon due to the soft tissue atrophy and scarring that take place after the initial operation. Often the original tumor site has also been subjected to radiotherapy, necessitating the transplantation and microvascular anastomosis of soft tissues and in some cases even hard tissue. Given the complex anatomy of the orbit and periorbital region, it is often difficult to achieve a functionally and esthetically sound reconstruction with autologous bone grafts. It is much easier to reconstruct the midface using a combination of titanium and soft tissue transfers with microvascular anastomosis. The bony reconstruction can be planned in detail with the aid of computer-assisted surgery, and the titanium reconstruction can be completed intraoperatively using mini- and microplates and mesh structures. The result of the reconstruction is evaluated postoperatively by fusing the image data sets or by superimposing the virtual template onto the postoperative data set (Figs. 82–87). The advantages of this method are a shorter operating time and fewer risks since composite grafts are considerably more likely to fail due to greater difficulties in handling. One disadvantage of using titanium combined with soft tissue in the presence of maxillary defects is the difficulty of prosthetic treatment with dental implants. Cases of this kind require the insertion of zygomatic implants without additional bony reconstructions of the maxilla.

Thus, the advantages for clinical therapeutic use are as follows:

1. By transforming pretherapeutic data into posttherapeutic data sets, we can measure the efficacy of chemotherapy based on the quantitative determination and localization of the tumor mass.
2. By transforming pretherapeutic data into posttherapeutic data sets, we can perform a navigation-guided resection that conforms to the original tumor boundaries.
3. By transferring the preoperative tumor boundaries into the postoperative data set, we can conduct a precise follow-up evaluation for tumor recurrence and refine the planning of postoperative adjuvant radiotherapy.
4. Through the use of virtual surgical templates during intraoperative navigation, primary and secondary reconstructions can be predictably carried out without the need for intraoperative imaging.
5. The correlation of pre- and postoperative image data sets permits an extremely accurate validation of the results of facial skeleton reconstructions. Measurement of the orbital volumes provides a particularly accurate measure of the quality of the reconstruction.

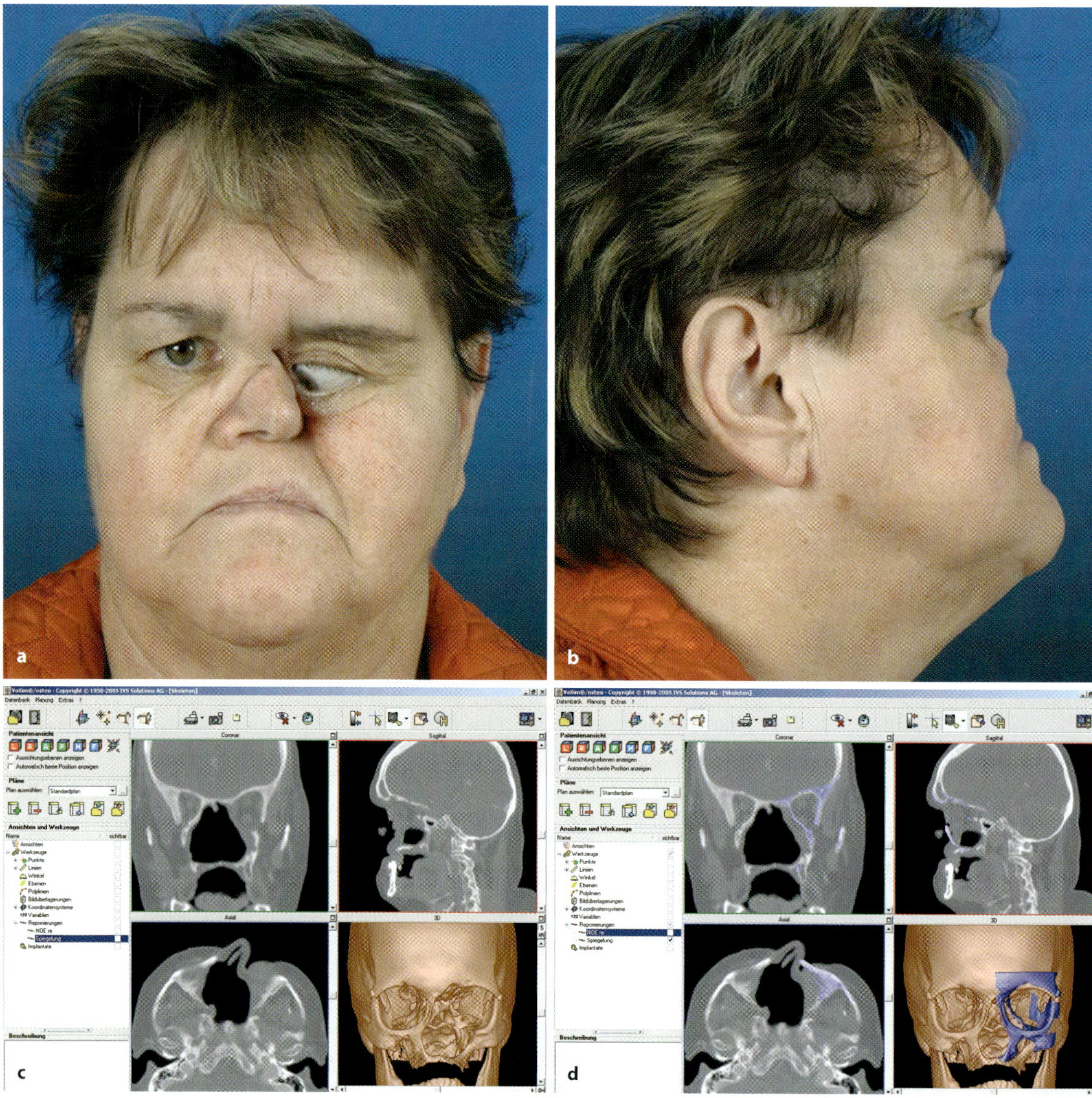

Fig. 82. Secondary reconstruction after a tumor resection – preoperative planning and simulation. This patient has an extensive left midfacial defect following a tumor resection (a,b). The CT images show the extent of the defect (c). Through segmentation and mirroring to the opposite side, a virtual surgical template is created that defines the contours of the ideal reconstruction (d)

Fig. 83. Secondary reconstruction after a tumor resection – intraoperative navigation. The titanium meshes and plates for midfacial and orbital reconstruction are provisionally inserted, and the surfaces of the implants are traced with the pointer and matched to the *blue outline* of the virtual surgical template in the CT data set. Reconstruction of the orbital walls with titanium mesh (a) and reconstruction of the paranasal pillar (b) and infraorbital margin (c) with titanium miniplates can be performed and controlled through an intraoral approach by this method

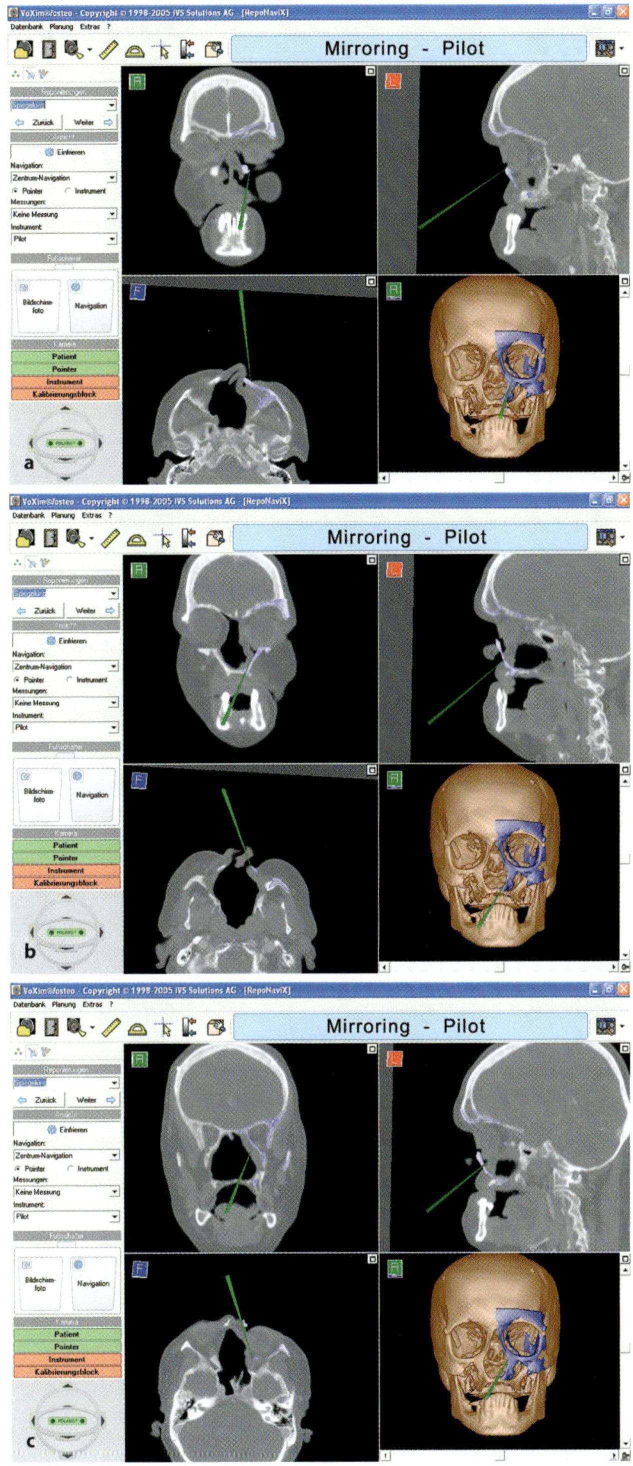

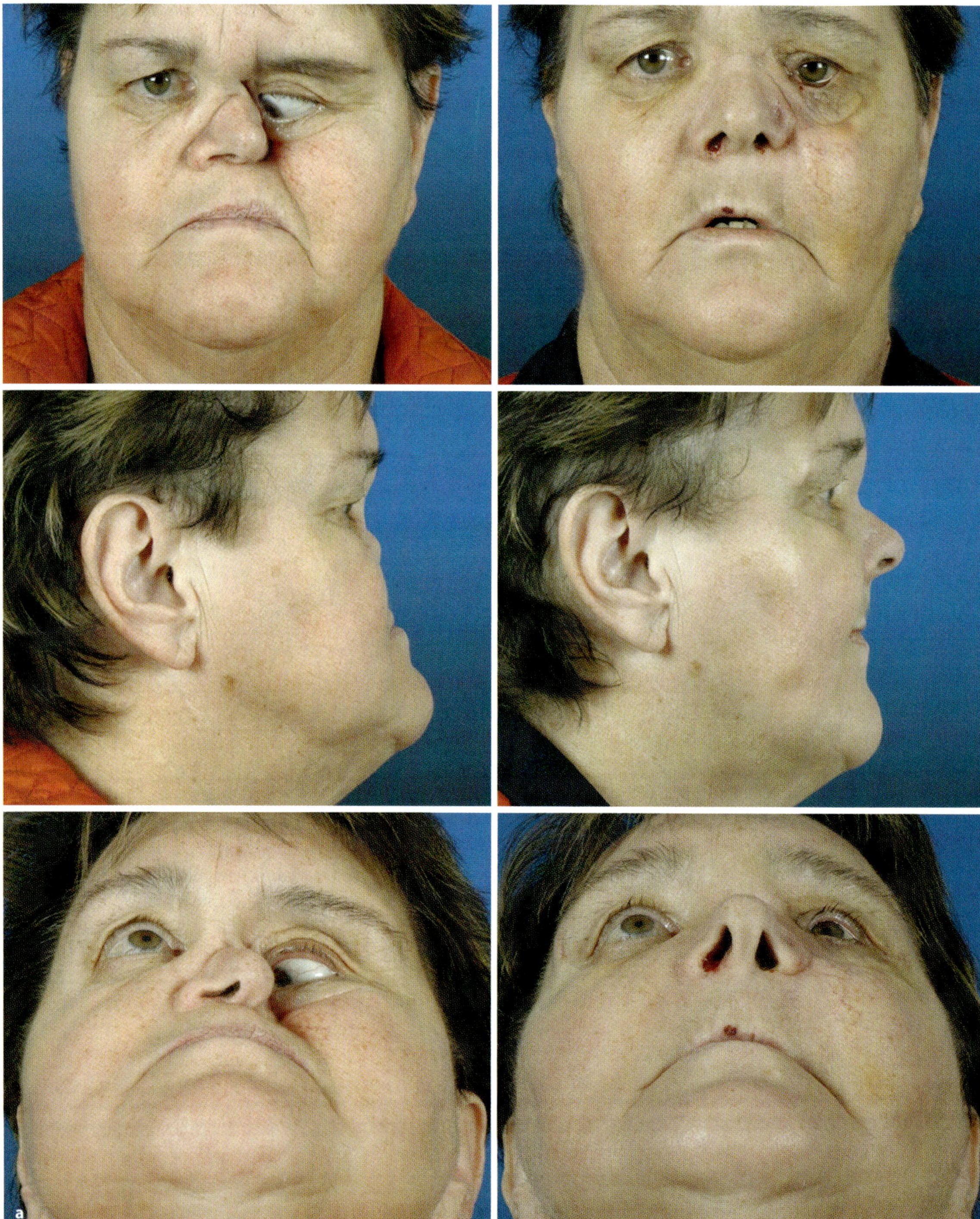

Fig. 84. a

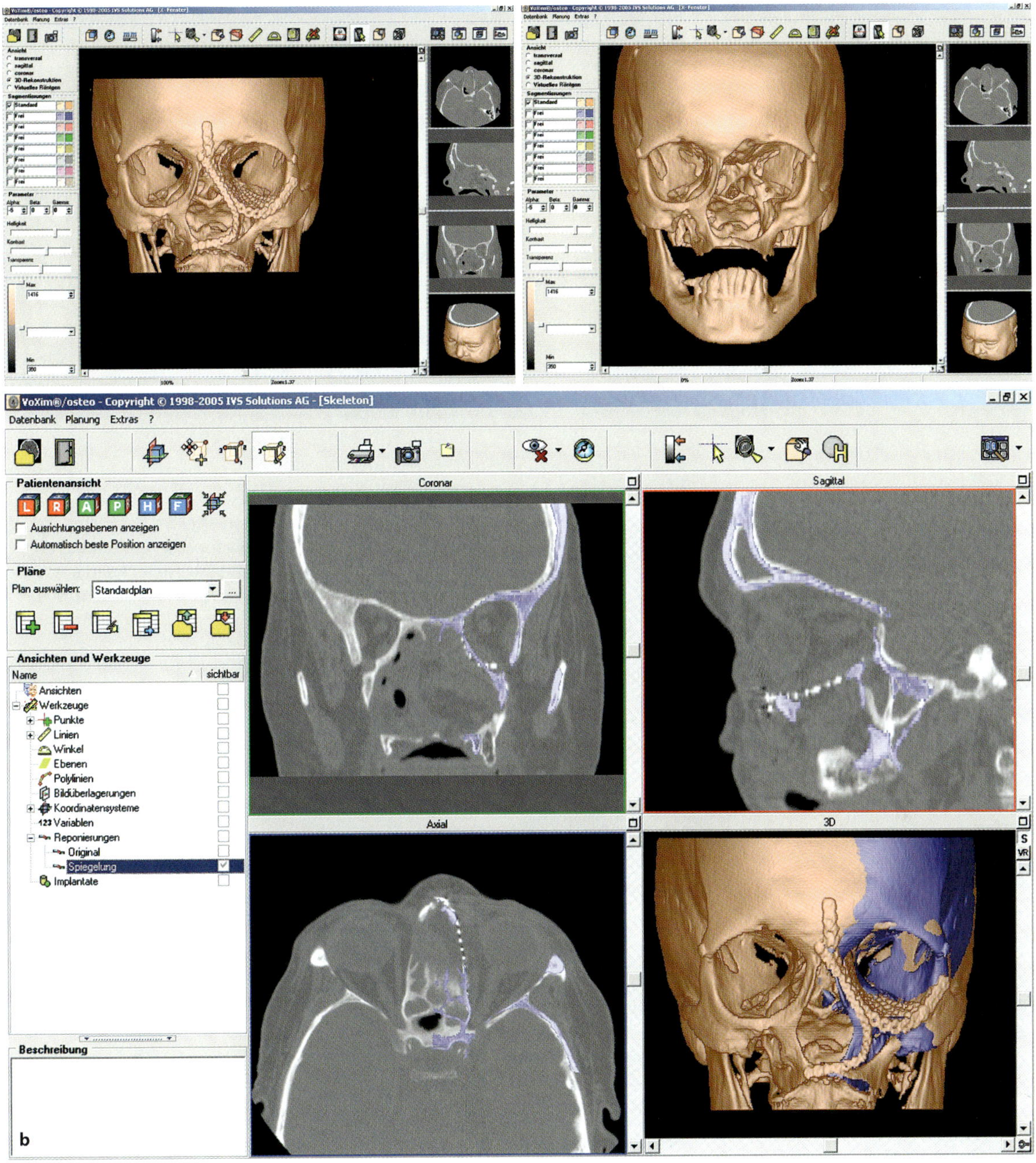

Fig. 84. (continued) Secondary reconstruction after a tumor resection – postoperative evaluation. **a** Clinical appearance before and after midfacial reconstruction with a navigation-assisted titanium reconstruction backed by a microvascular latissimus dorsi muscle transfer. Intraoral and transconjunctival approaches were used for the midfacial reconstruction. **b** Comparison of the pre- and postoperative 3D bone images shows the reconstruction of the osseous midfacial defect with titanium implants (*top*). The quality of the reconstruction can be checked qualitatively and quantitatively by superimposing the virtual surgical template onto the postoperative data set (*bottom*)

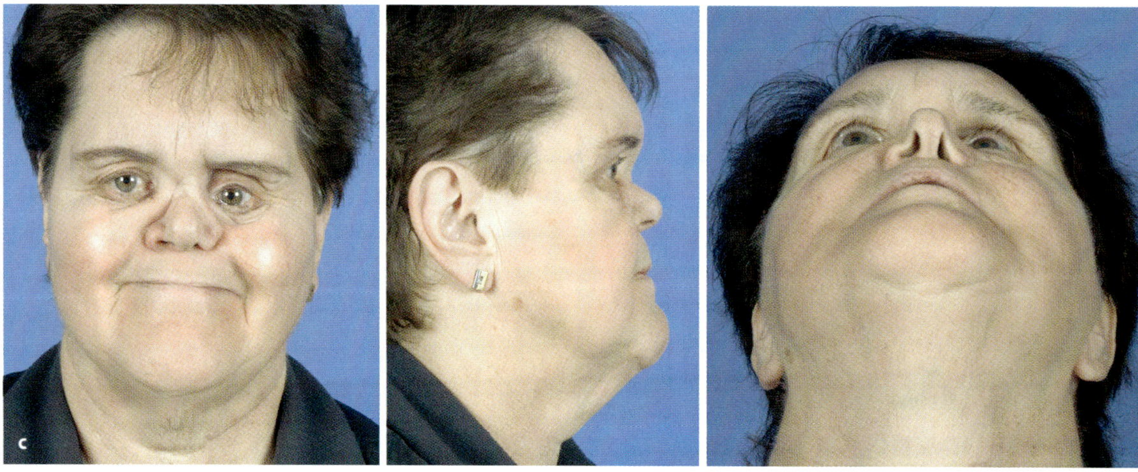

Fig. 84. (continued) c Clinical appearance one year after reconstructive surgery

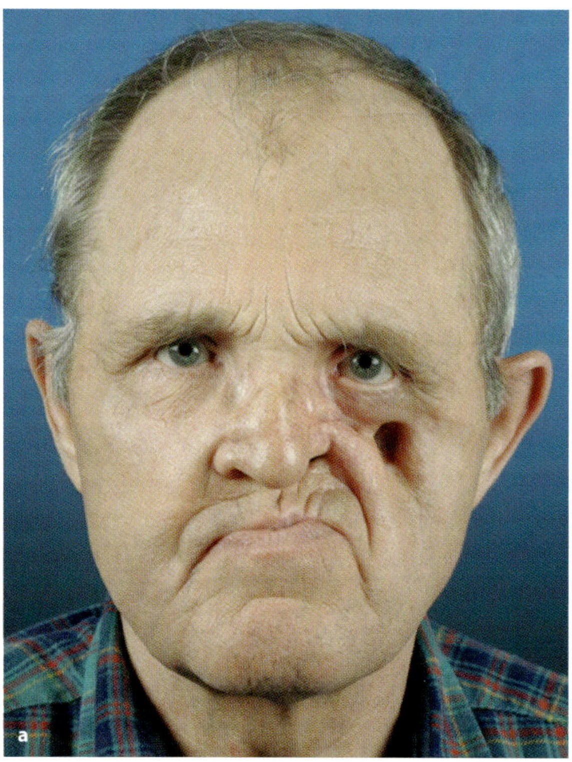

Fig. 85. Secondary reconstruction after a tumor resection – preoperative planning and simulation. This patient has an extensive intra- and extraoral soft tissue defect and a left midfacial bony defect following a tumor resection (a, b) (c, d see next page)

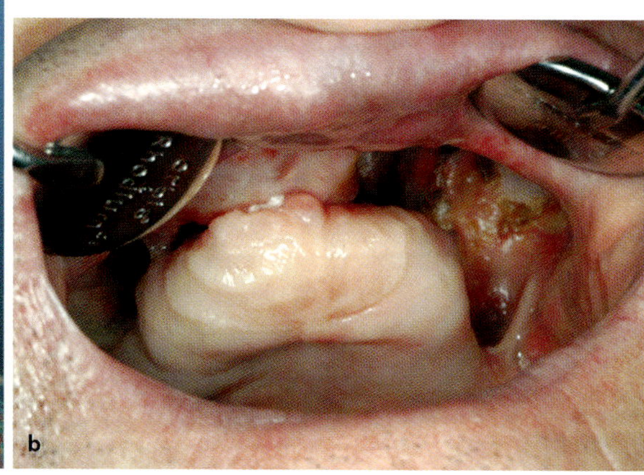

Fig. 86. Secondary reconstruction after a tumor resection – intraoperative navigation. The titanium meshes and plates for midfacial and orbital reconstruction are provisionally inserted, and the surfaces of the implants are traced with the pointer and matched to the *blue outline* of the virtual surgical template in the CT data set. The pointer tip is at the junction of the orbital floor and medial orbital wall, which is a critical site in determining the success of the reconstruction

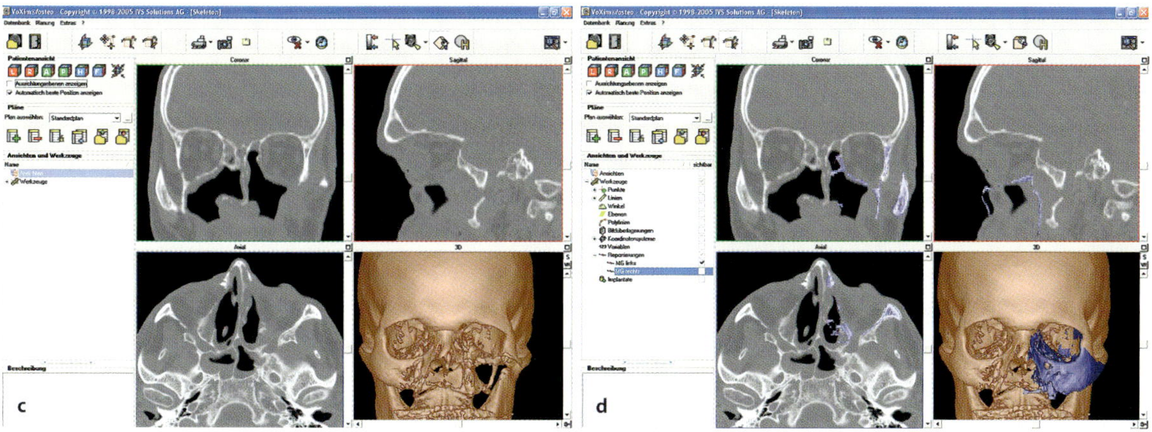

Fig. 85. (continued) The CT images show the extent of the defect (c). A virtual surgical template is created by segmentation and mirroring of the opposite side. This template predefines the contours of the ideal reconstruction (d)

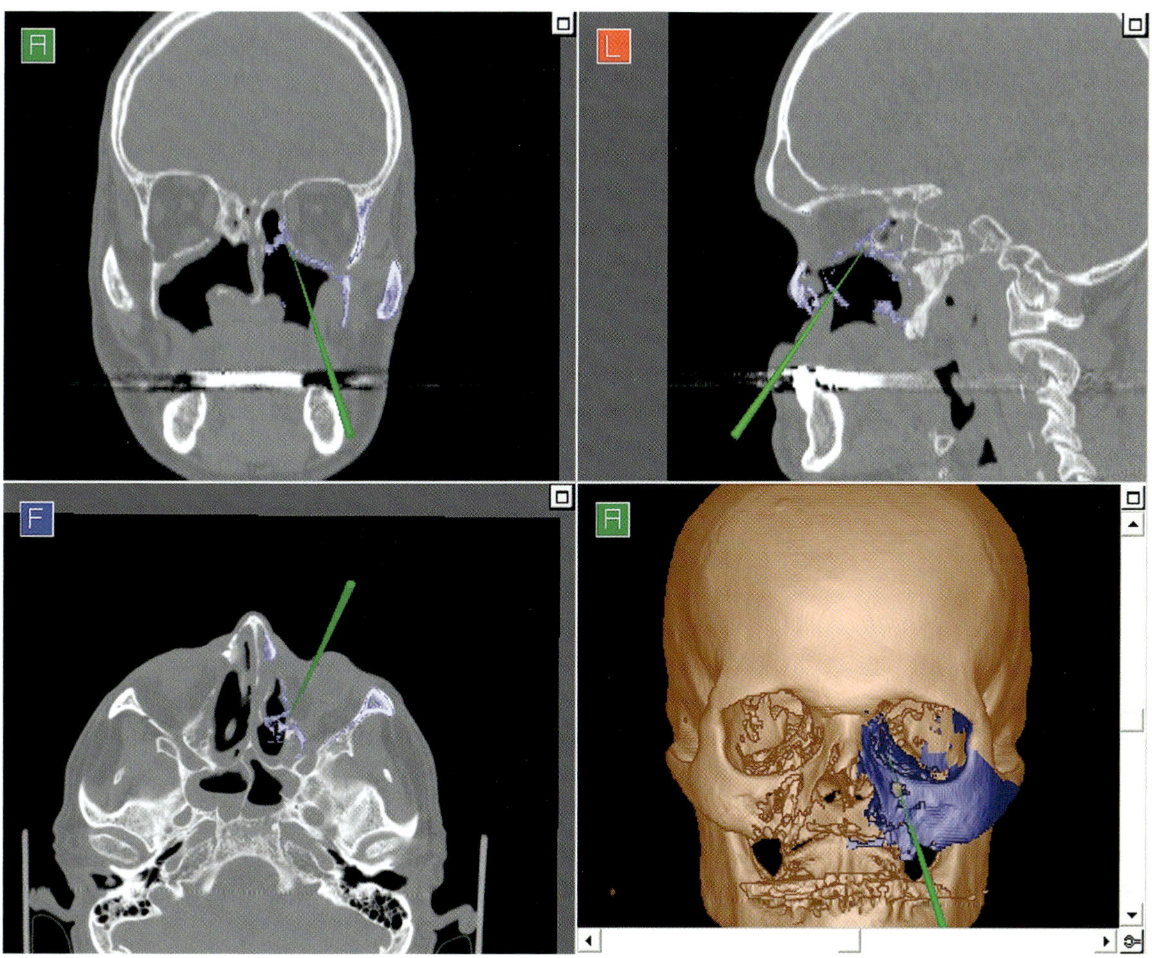

Fig. 86.

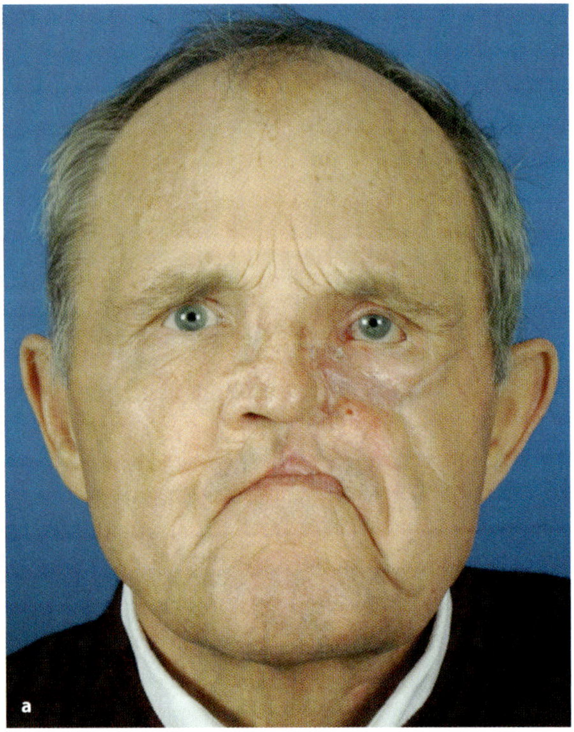

Fig. 87. Secondary reconstruction after a tumor resection – postoperative evaluation. **a** Clinical appearance after midfacial reconstruction with a navigation-assisted titanium reconstruction backed by a microvascular latissimus dorsi muscle transfer. **b** Comparison of the pre- and postoperative 3D bone images shows the reconstruction of the bony midfacial defect with titanium implants (*top*). The quality of the reconstruction is checked qualitatively and quantitatively by superimposing the virtual surgical template onto the postoperative data set (*bottom*)

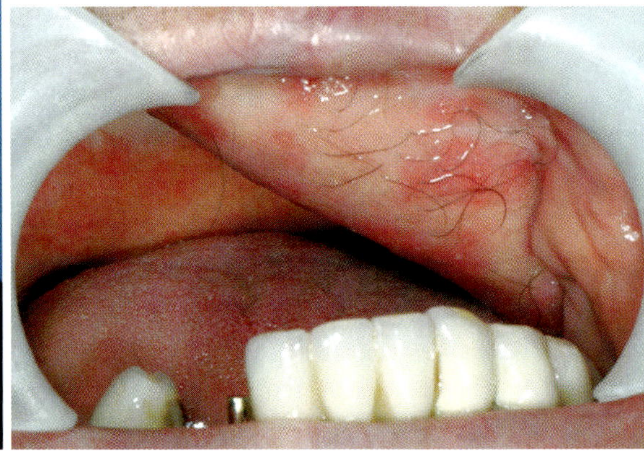

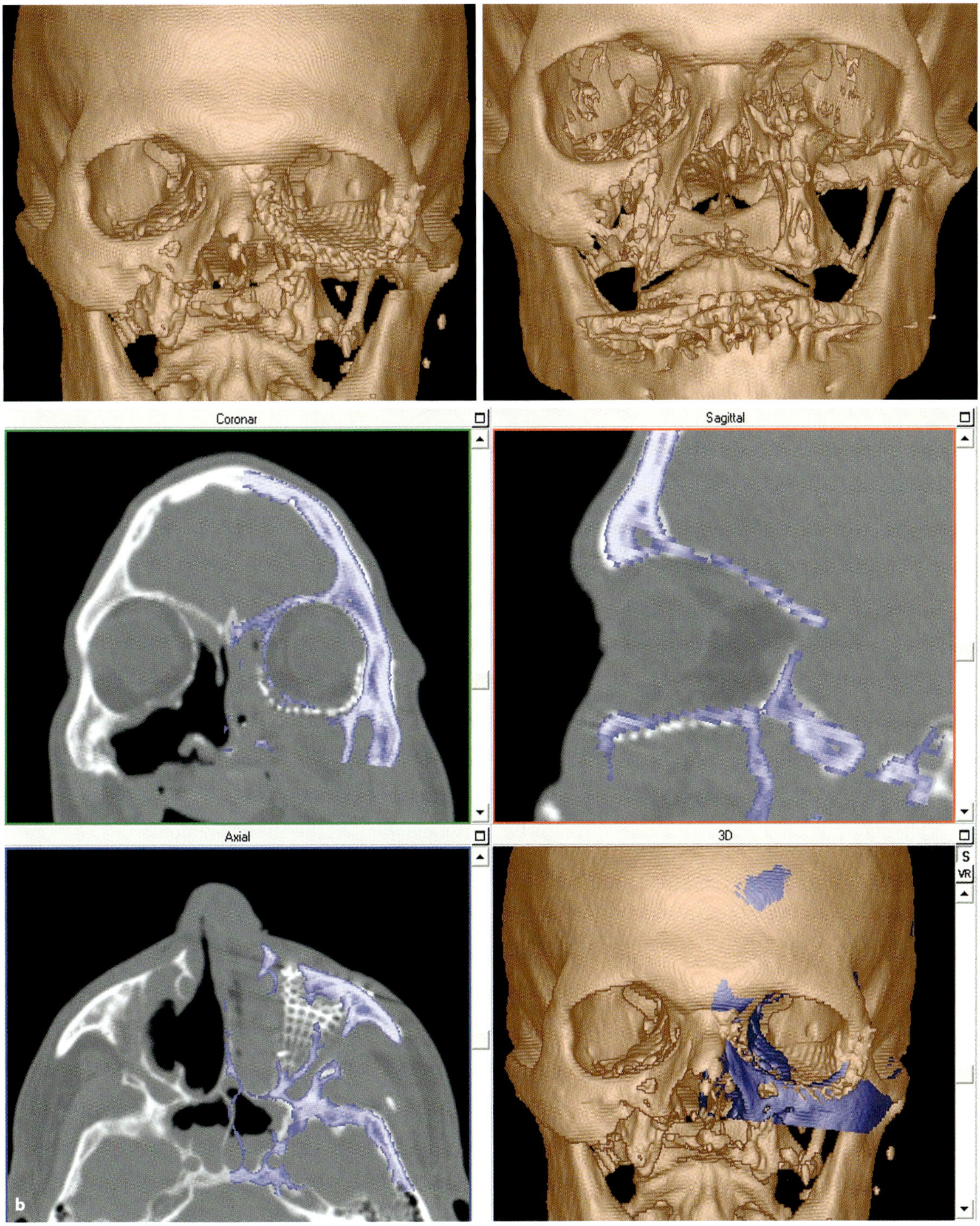

Fig. 87. (continued)

Traumatological Procedures

Primary Orbital and Midfacial Reconstructions

The primary treatment of facial fractures, especially those involving the naso-orbitoethmoid complex, is superior to secondary reconstruction in terms of functional recovery and should be the primary goal of treatment. The complex anatomy of the periorbital region requires an experienced surgeon with a detailed knowledge of functional anatomy who has access to 3D images for preoperative analysis and planning. CT is the imaging study of choice, and a 3D representation based on multiplanar algorithms (axial, coronal, and sagittal reconstructions) is essential. However, the limited access to the periorbital region makes intraoperative imaging desirable so that the surgeon can check the progress of the reconstruction at frequent intervals and ensure that the partial elements of the reconstruction are precisely coordinated and accurate in their details (Watzinger et al. 1997; Waldhart et al. 2000). Intraoperative CT is an option, but the need to check the various phases of the operation and the time-consuming process of data acquisition and processing the data sets have discouraged the clinical use of this method on a broad basis. Because imaging must be repeated after each corrective measure and a final postoperative check is still needed, the use of intraoperative CT leads to an unacceptable increase in radiation exposure, particularly to the sensitive lens of the eye. The progress of an orbital and midfacial reconstruction can also be checked by intraoperative navigation, which involves no radiation exposure and can be done without interrupting the surgical procedure. Intraoperative navigation permits the detailed direct or indirect visualization of the bony structures and, to a degree, of soft tissue structures during each phase of the operation. The use of this method is generally limited to secondary procedures, however, because of the long and often complicated preoperative preparations that are required. As a result, navigation-assisted primary reconstructions of the orbit have rarely been described in the literature. To date, invasive registration methods have been the only way to perform computer-assisted procedures with an acceptable degree of accuracy. But the registration markers should be inserted prior to initial imaging in order to avoid additional radiation exposure from a separate planning data set, and the prophylactic insertion of invasive markers prior to data acquisition cannot be recommended as a routine practice. Noninvasive registration methods such as headsets, adhesive skin markers, surface matching techniques, and anatomical landmarks cannot be used in patients with facial skeletal trauma for obvious reasons. Thus, besides the insertion of miniscrews, the use of an intraoral registration splint appears to be the only feasible option for conducting navigation-assisted procedures with high precision in the primary treatment of facial fractures. Most notably, the use of prefabricated silicone impression splints permits rapid preparation (10–15 minutes fabrication time at bedside) before data set acquisition, even in intubated patients. Prophylactic fabrications are justified and will eliminate treatment delays when computer-assisted surgery is indicated because the surgeon can conduct preoperative planning while the patient is being prepared and anesthetized. The preoperative planning of primary reconstructions includes analyzing the facial fractures and planning the surgical approach and mode of reconstruction (Figs. 88, 89). Moreover, the ideal result of the reconstruction can be simulated in unilateral orbital reconstructions by mirroring subvolumes of the data sets, i.e., reflecting portions of the unaffected side onto the affected side (Fig. 90). In patients with bilateral fracture patterns, the ideal reconstruction can be simulated by more complex segmentations of the affected regions.

The first step in the operation is registration with the intraoral splint. Afterward the splint is removed to avoid interference with the operating team and is reinserted only for intraoperative reregistration. Reregistrations should be done following all manipulations that may disturb the operative field, such as osteotomies or bone graft removal from the calvarium. The total duration of reregistration (1–3 per operation) averages 8–17 minutes in these procedures. Pointer-based navigation after registration includes checking the position of the zygomatic prominence and the surface of the zygoma after the fracture has been reduced and before the application of internal fixation material. Surface registration of the inserted titanium mesh and/or bone grafts in the orbit is done

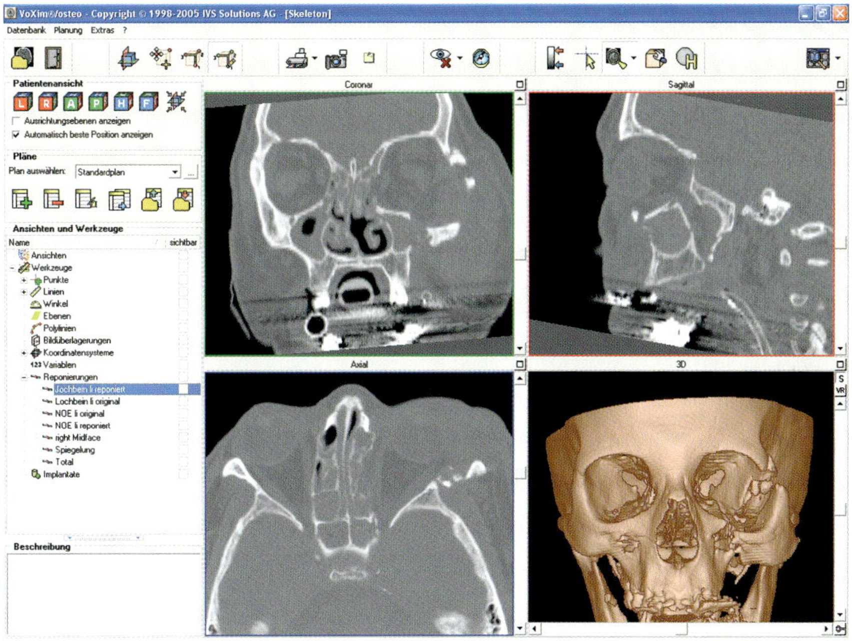

Fig. 88. Posttraumatic primary reconstruction of the midface – preoperative analysis. Multiplanar display (coronal, sagittal, axial, and 3D reconstruction) of a preoperative CT data set in a patient with comminuted midfacial and orbital fractures on the left side

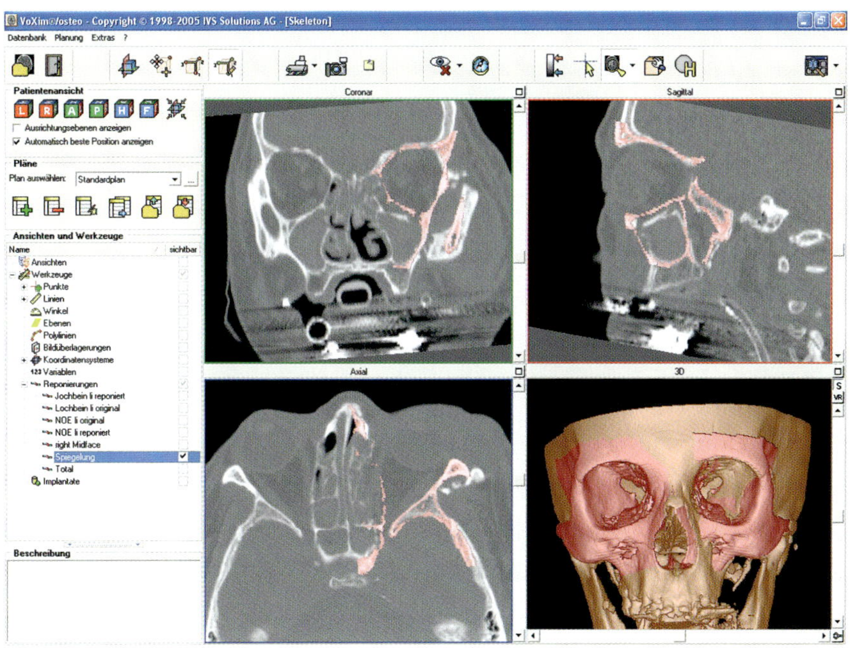

Fig. 89. Posttraumatic primary reconstruction of the midface – preoperative planning. The unaffected side is reflected onto the affected side, followed by segmentation and alignment to create a virtual surgical template for orbital reconstruction (*pink segments*)

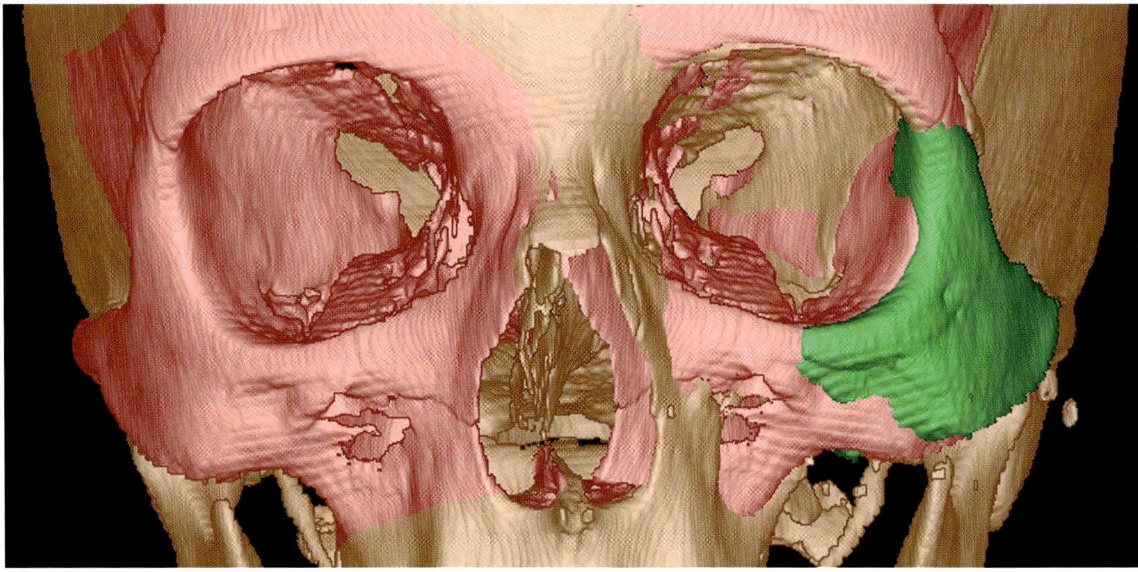

Fig. 90. Posttraumatic primary reconstruction of the midface – virtual reduction. The left zygoma (*green segment*) is virtually reduced based on the position of the mirrored segments (*pink*), creating a virtual template for reconstruction of the zygoma

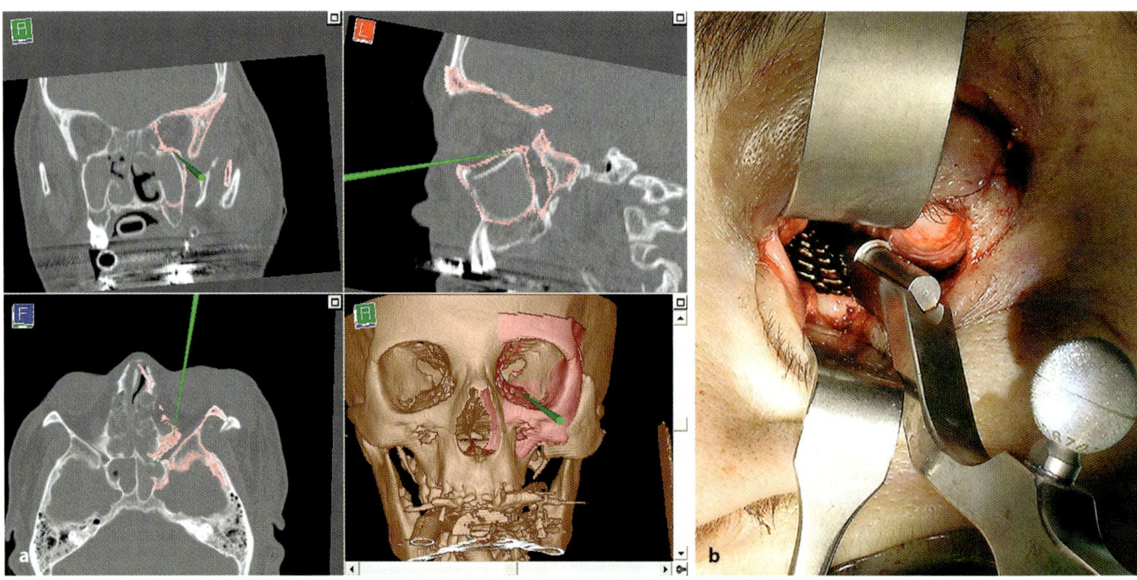

Fig. 91. Posttraumatic primary reconstruction of the midface – intraoperative navigation. Intraoperative multiplanar display shows pointer-based surface matching after titanium mesh insertion for left orbital reconstruction (**a**). The pointer tip has been touched to the inserted titanium mesh (**b** at *right*). The position of the pointer tip (*green line*) in relation to the virtual reconstruction template (*pink segmentation*) already shows an error in correction with no need for additional intraoperative imaging

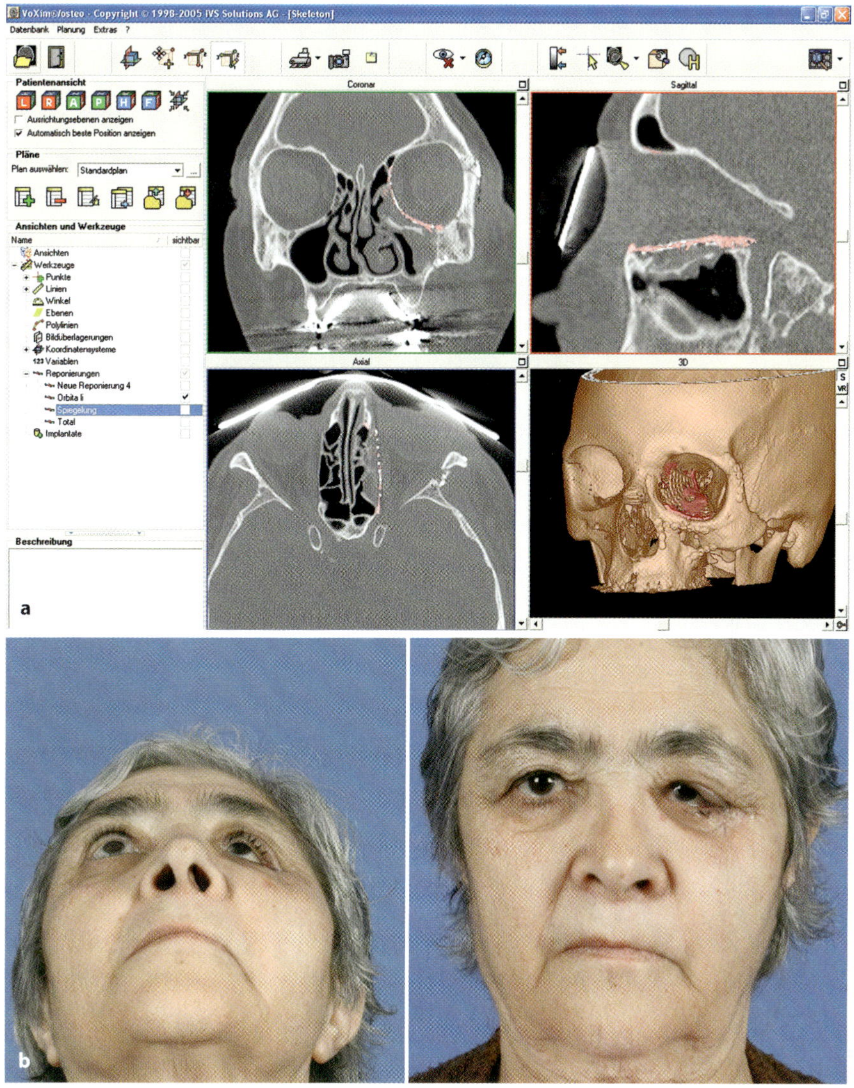

Fig. 92. Posttraumatic primary reconstruction of the midface – postoperative evaluation. Postoperative comparison of the result of the reconstruction with the virtual template (*pink segmentation*) confirms the accuracy of the titanium mesh orbital reconstruction with millimeter precision (a). Owing to the use of intraoperative navigation, this extensive reconstruction of the orbital floor and medial wall, plus the reduction and internal fixation of the zygoma, could be performed without a coronal incision. The laceration of the left lower lid is posttraumatic (b)

prior to the fixation (Ellis and Tan 2003; Fig. 91). Pointer-based navigation can also be used to determine the projection of the eyeball in order to evaluate swelling and determine the anticipated sagittal projection of the eye in relation to the opposite side. It is also possible to superimpose the virtual template onto the postoperative data set, enabling a detailed quantitative evaluation of the result (Fig. 92).

Isolated fractures of the orbital walls (medial wall or orbital floor) are generally an indication for delayed primary care, since these fractures are often missed on initial examination due to the absence of functional abnormalities (diplopia, sensory disturbances in the distribution of the infraorbital nerve) or are underestimated as a treatment priority. These fractures can be clearly visualized by digital volume

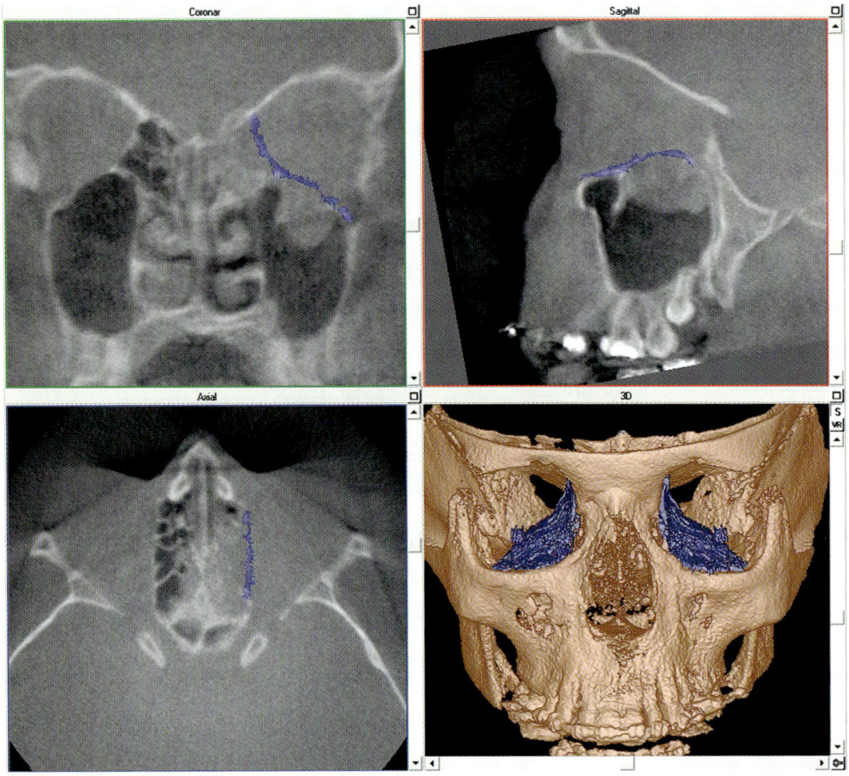

Fig. 93. Posttraumatic primary reconstruction of the orbit – creating the virtual template on the base of a Cone Beam CT scan. The unaffected side is reflected onto the affected side, followed by segmentation and alignment to create a virtual surgical template for the orbital reconstruction (*blue segmentation*)

tomography (DVT), which involves less radiation exposure than standard CT scanning. Because the volume of the image data set is limited, it is not always possible to image the entire skull, and soft tissue structures are imaged in relatively poor detail. Thus the application of this technique is limited to facial fractures and especially to preimplant workups. The resulting data set can be accessed in the DICOM format, making it suitable for intraoperative navigation (Fig. 93). With its rapid availability and low radiation exposure, it is reasonable to predict that DVT will increasingly replace conventional CT scans in patients with isolated midfacial fractures. When DVT data sets are used, the preoperative and intraoperative conduct of computer-assisted surgery are no different than when standard CT data sets are used.

Particularly in the case of orbital wall fractures that involve the junction of the orbital floor with the medial orbital wall or with a complete separation of the orbital floor, the difficult visual conditions associated with the standard transconjunctival approach often result in a faulty placement of the reconstruction materials. In many cases the junction of the orbital floor and medial wall is reconstructed at too sharp an angle, or the posterior part of the orbital floor is positioned too low. Both errors result in undercorrection of the bony orbit and may lead to persistent abnormalities of eye position. If a secondary correction is needed, it has significant disadvantages compared with an anatomically correct primary reconstruction because of the accompanying soft tissue changes and central compensatory processes (diplo-

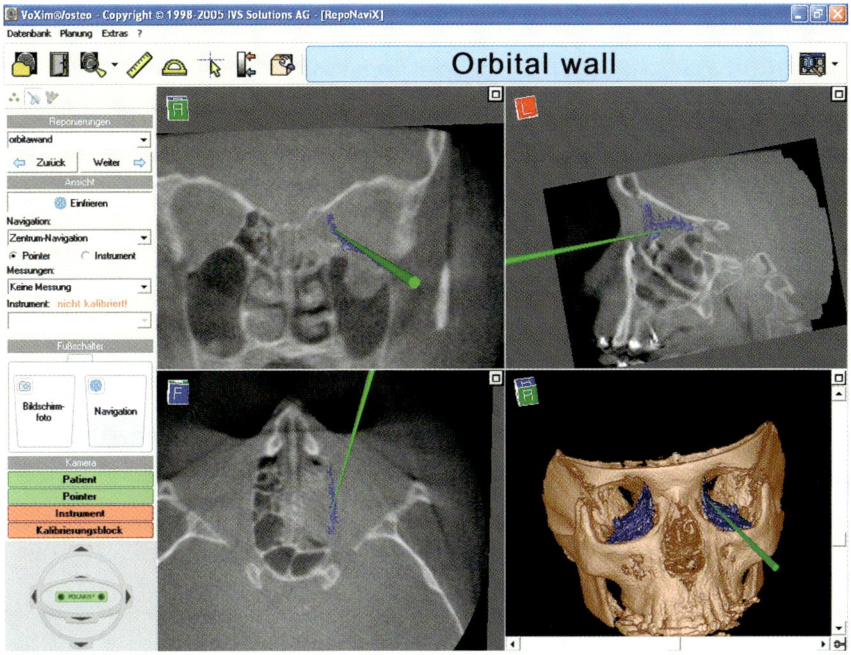

Fig. 94. Posttraumatic primary reconstruction of the orbit – intraoperative navigation. Intraoperative multiplanar display shows pointer-based surface matching after the transconjunctival insertion of titanium mesh for orbital reconstruction. The pointer tip has been touched to the inserted titanium mesh. The position of the pointer tip (*green line*) in relation to the virtual reconstruction template (*blue segmentation*) confirms the correct position of the titanium mesh at the very critical site between the orbital floor and medial orbital wall

pia is compensated in the visual cortex and may persist after secondary corrections). In the primary treatment of these fracture patterns, then, intraoperative visualization is necessary in order to avoid these positioning errors and reduce the need for secondary reconstructions (Fig. 94). The operative technique of navigation-assisted orbital wall reconstructions differs from conventional protocols only in the use of a head restraint (Mayfield clamp). The length of the operation is increased by approximately 30 minutes. In complex periorbital reconstructions, the ideal reconstruction is simulated preoperatively by mirroring the unaffected side onto the affected side (Zizelmann et al. 2005a,b). Synthetic materials such as titanium mesh will increasingly supersede the use of autologous bone grafts owing to their better predictability and absence of donor site morbidity (Fig. 95).

With the aid of voxel-based planning and intraoperative navigation, a coronal incision can be omitted even in patients with extensive orbital wall fractures and panfacial fractures, provided there are no multiple fractures of the naso-orbitoethmoid complex and the medial canthus does not require reattachment (Fig. 96). Even in these extensive orbital reconstructions, we were able to eliminate the need for a coronal incision by means of intraoperative navigation. The titanium implants were inserted through a transconjunctival approach and checked by pointer-based navigation. The zygoma and maxilla were accessed through the upper lid on each side and through the maxillary vestibule. A fracture in the

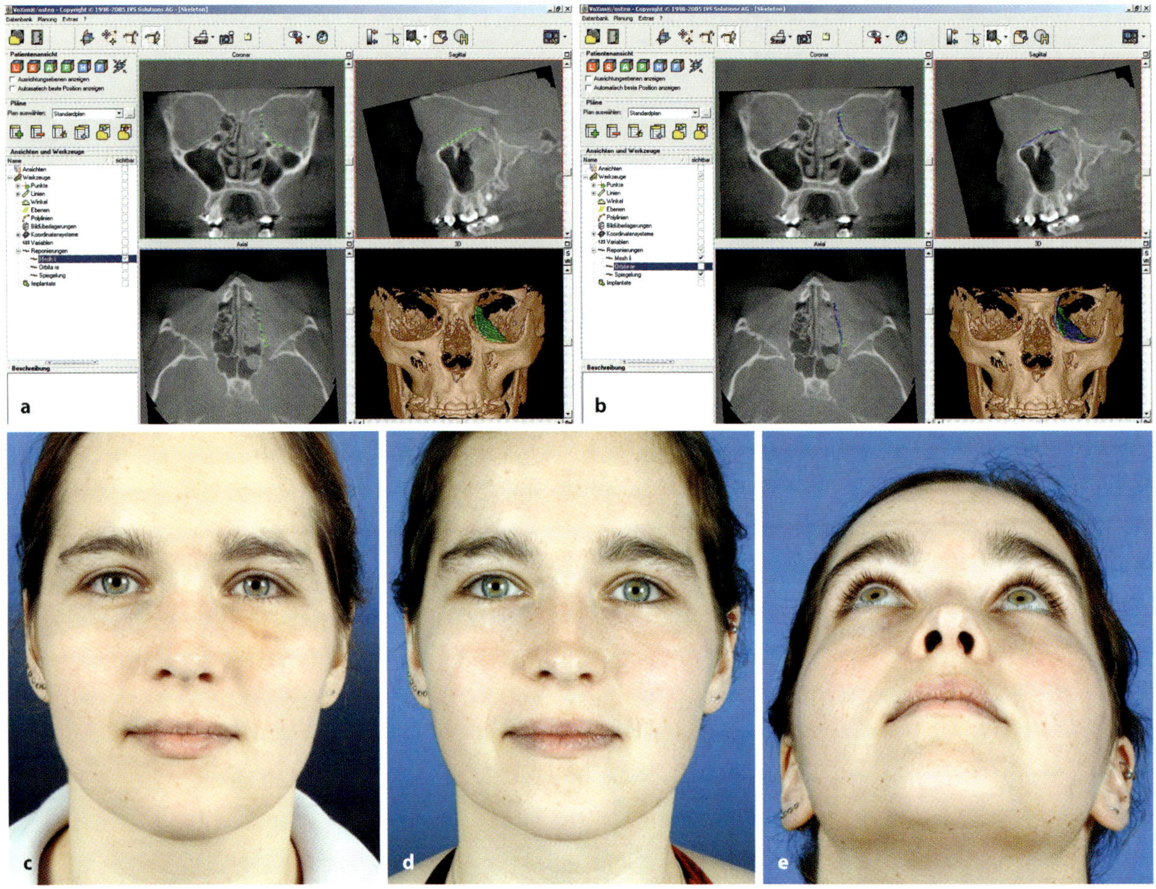

Fig. 95 a, b. Posttraumatic primary reconstruction of the orbit – postoperative evaluation. Postoperative comparison of the result of the reconstruction (*green segmentation*) with the virtual template (*blue segmentation*) confirms the accuracy of the titanium mesh orbital reconstruction with millimeter precision. Owing to the use of intraoperative navigation, this extensive reconstruction of the orbital floor and medial wall could be performed entirely through a transconjunctival approach. Clinical appearance 10 days (**c**) and 2 years (**d, e**) after primary reconstruction of the left orbit

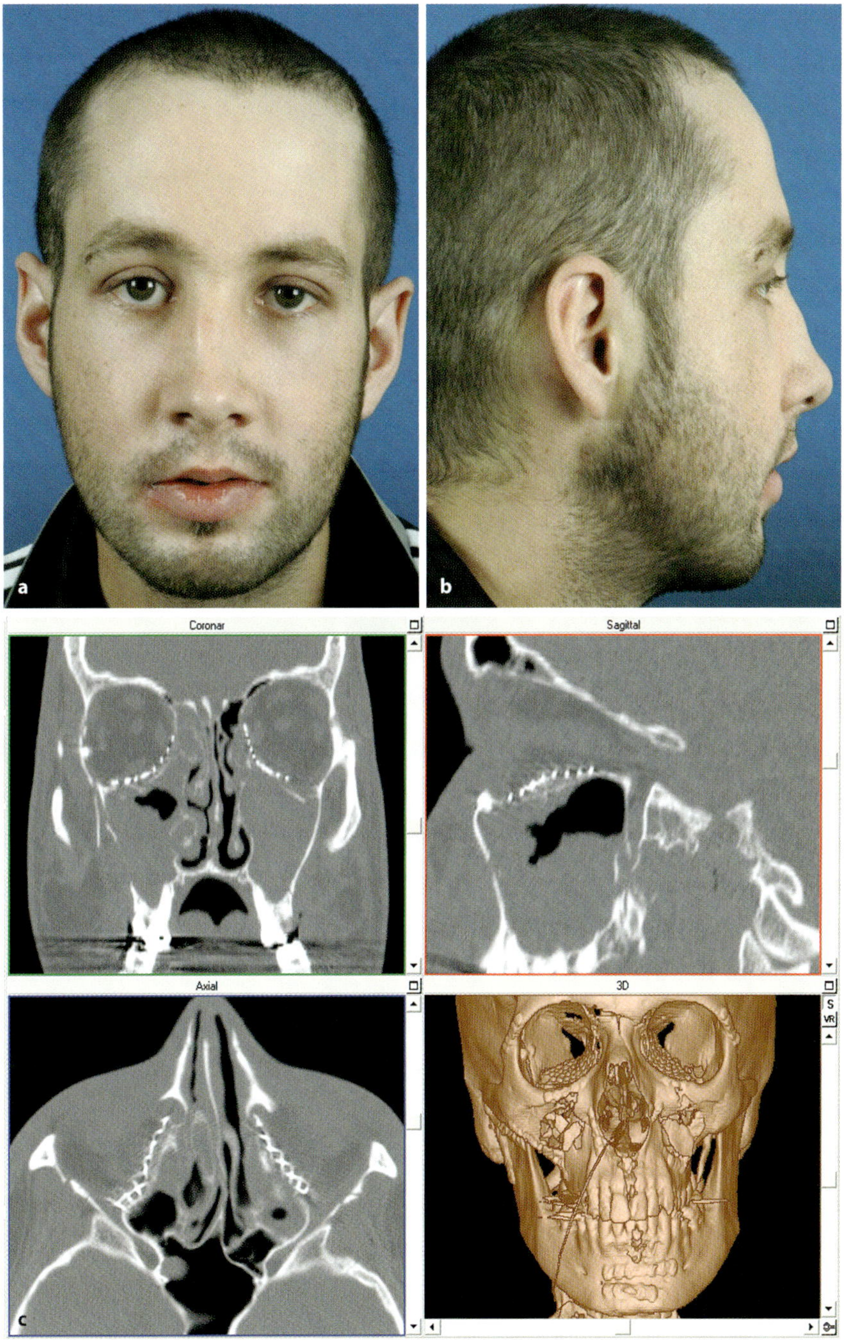

Fig. 96 a–c. Posttraumatic primary reconstruction of a panfacial fracture – postoperative status with no visible surgical scars

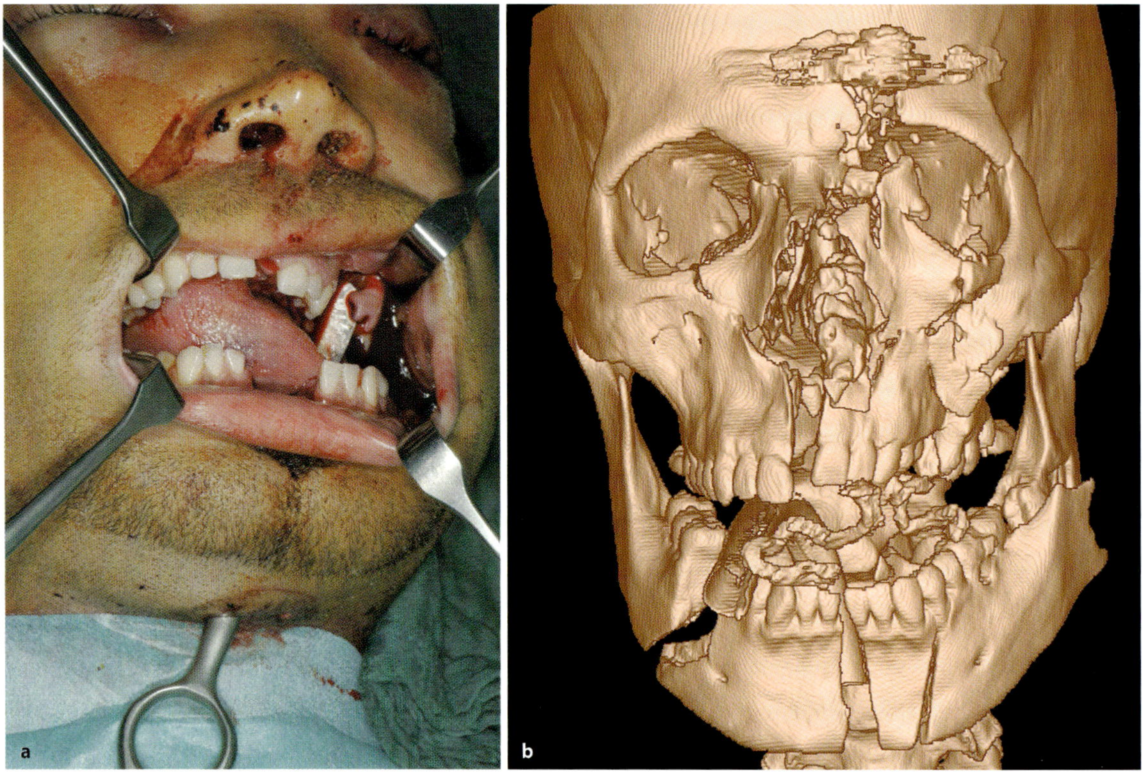

Fig. 97. Panfacial fracture after a gunshot injury. a A surgical instrument placed in the bullet track following a submental pistol shot in a suicide attempt. b The 3D reconstruction shows an overview of the fracture pattern. The projectile exited the bone and lodged in the supraorbital soft tissue

right condylar process was treated through an intraoral approach using an endoscopically assisted technique. When seen 10 days postoperatively, the patient had no visible surgical scars.

In cases with extensive comminution of the facial skeleton, voxel-based data processing can supply a detailed view of the fracture patterns in two and three dimensions. In cases with bilateral or central comminution or bone defects, free segmentations are necessary in order to simulate the ideal reconstruction. These segmentations are considerably more difficult and time-consuming than mirroring and aligning segments from the unaffected side. Checking the anatomical reconstruction of the junction of the orbital floor and medial wall is a particularly useful intraoperative aid in achieving an optimum reconstruction of the comminuted orbit (Figs. 97–100).

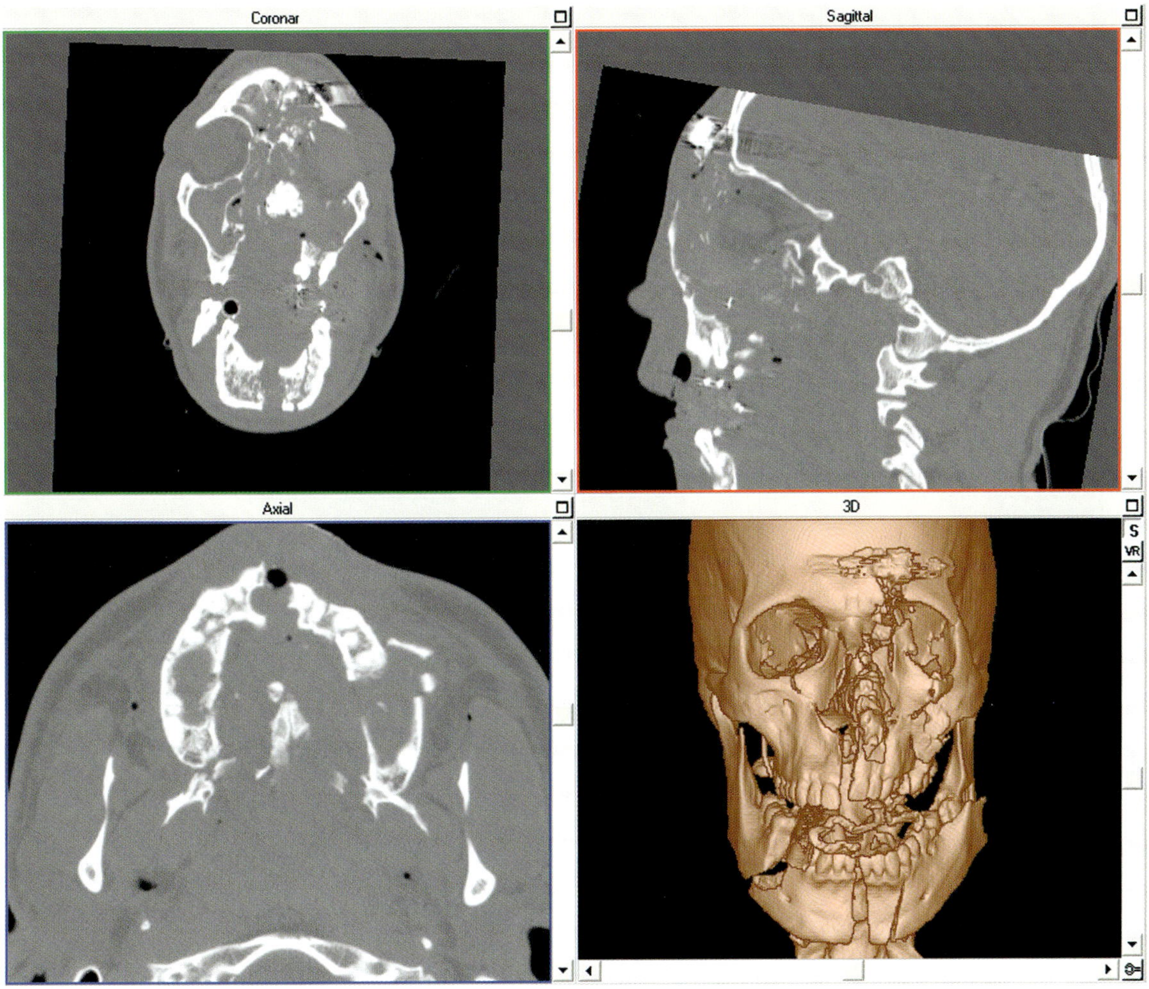

Fig. 98. Panfacial fracture after a gunshot injury – preoperative analysis. The multiplanar display of the preoperative CT data set (corona, sagittal, axial, and 3D reconstruction) reveals the extent of the destruction

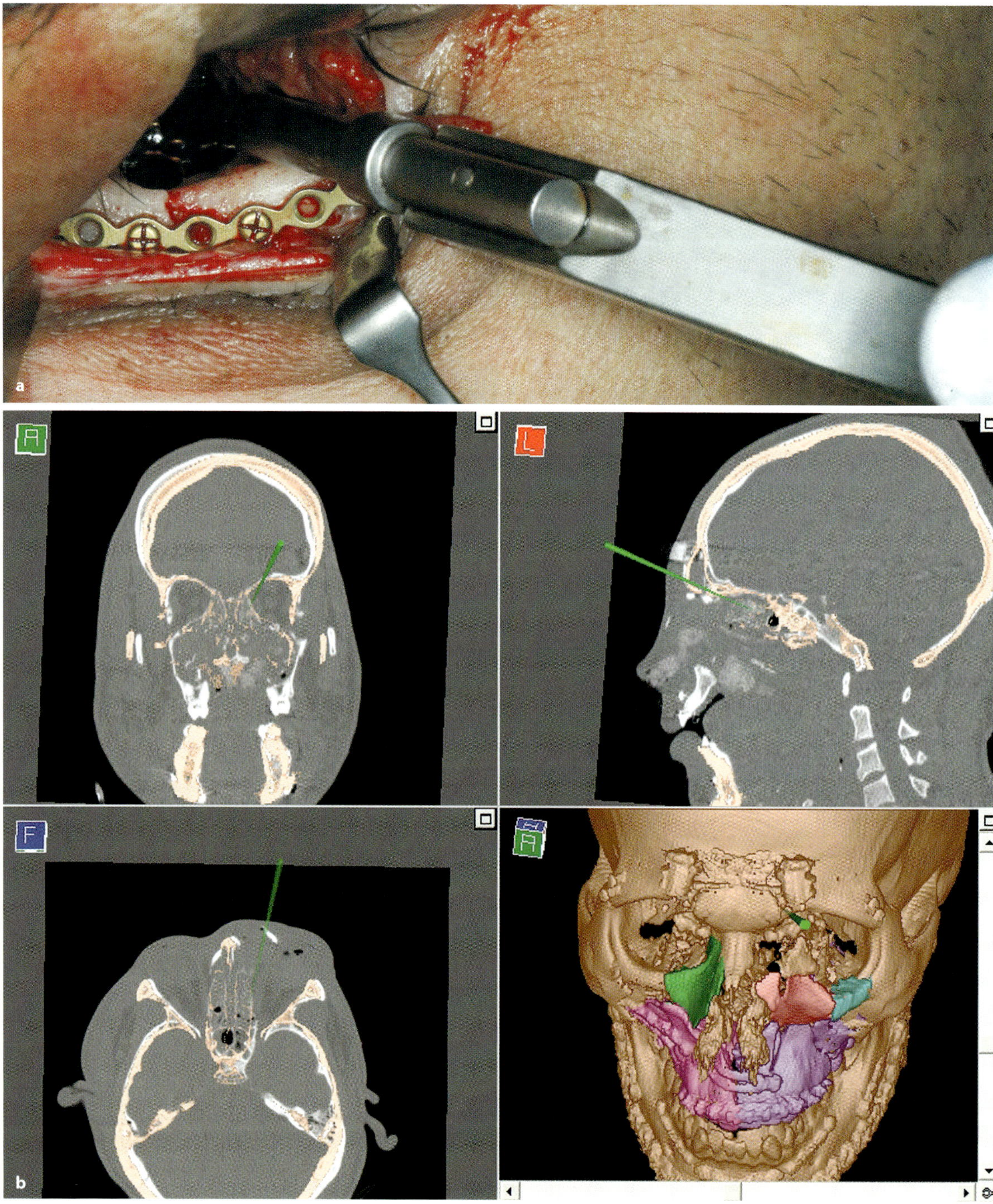

Fig. 99. Panfacial fracture after a gunshot injury – intraoperative navigation. Pointer-based position check following orbital reconstruction with titanium mesh (a). The surface of the titanium implant is traced with the pointer, which is introduced through a transconjunctival approach (b), and is compared intraoperatively with the contour of the virtual surgical template displayed on the screen (*light brown contour*)

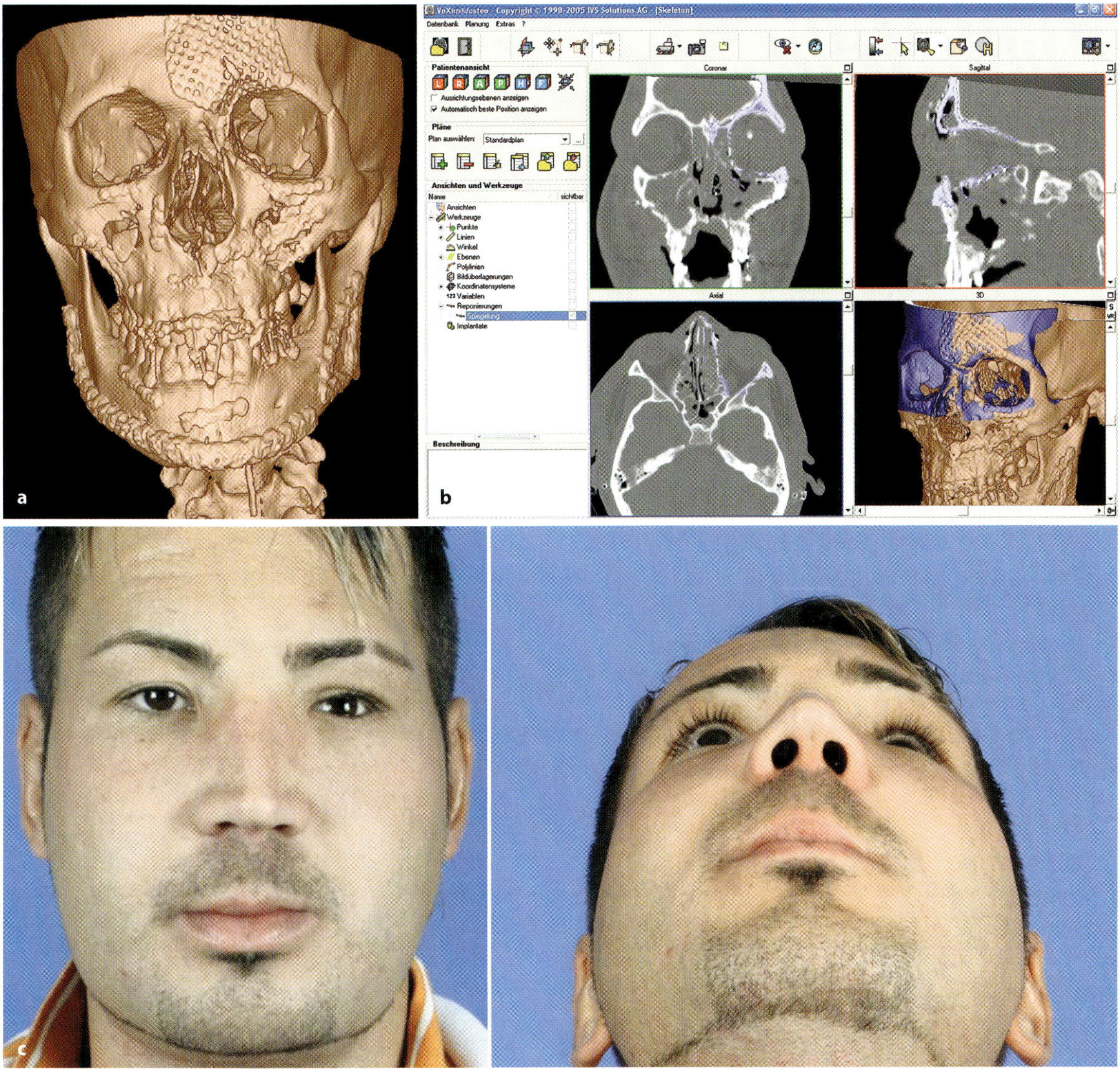

Fig. 100. Panfacial fracture after a gunshot injury – postoperative evaluation. Postoperative 3D reconstruction (**a**) shows the overall result of the reconstruction. Postoperative comparison of the result of the reconstruction with the virtual template (*blue segmentation*) confirms the accuracy of the titanium mesh orbital reconstruction (**b**). The clinical appearance after 1 year with eye prosthesis (**c**)

Secondary Orbital and Midfacial Reconstructions

The interval between patient selection and surgery is highly variable in these elective procedures. It may range from 1 to 100 days. Because a CT data set acquisition is already necessary for patient selection, there are many cases in which invasive registration methods cannot be used. The only way to proceed with high accuracy is by using registration splints (Gellrich and Schramm 2002).

Besides analyzing the deformity and the defect, preoperative planning should include a preoperative simulation of the desired result of the reconstruction (Fig. 101). In unilateral reconstructions, the desired result can be simulated with a mirroring program that reflects a subvolume of the CT data set from the unaffected side to the affected side. The simulation begins with correct 3D positioning of the plane of symmetry. This process is the most time-consuming planning step because the result must be checked several times and the plane of symmetry must be adjusted. Thus, software programs have been developed that position the plane of symmetry semiautomatically on the basis of congruent surfaces. These programs are still in the experimental stage, however.

After the plane of symmetry has been correctly positioned, the subvolume of the data set to be reconstructed is defined, or, in a surface-based simulation, the surfaces to be reconstructed are marked and segmented. This is followed by the mirroring process. In volume-based simulations, the subvolume to be reconstructed is overwritten by the corresponding subvolume on the unaffected side. In surface-based simulations, the marked surface segment on the opposite side is reflected onto the side to be reconstructed while preserving the surface segments located there. The advantage of the volume-based simulation is that soft tissue structures can also be mirrored. This makes it possible, for example, to check the predicted position of the eye following the reconstruction. One disadvantage of overwriting the original structures by the mirror image is that intraoperative visualization of the anatomical structures can be done only indirectly based on outlines of the original contours that were made preoperatively. Another option is "image fusion" of the mirrored data set and original data set. This can also be done by intraoperative navigation. The disadvantage of surface-based simulations is that either bony or soft tissue segments can be mirrored. Again, however, this problem can be solved by image fusion and data set correlation (Gellrich et al. 1999b).

When the mirroring steps have been completed, a virtual template is obtained in the form of a new data set (Figs. 102, 103). This template must be compared with the original data set of the patient by data set correlation and checked for plausibility. If the simulated result of the reconstruction is satisfactory, the reconstruction parameters can be calculated. These parameters include the sagittal, axial, and vertical correction heights of the orbital walls, the size of the grafts, and the possible necessary graft volumes (Rojas et al. 2001).

In the reconstruction of bilateral facial deformities, the simulation and creation of the virtual surgical template consists of boundary lines and line segments that are positioned based on measurements of orbital and midfacial parameters and on anatomical landmarks that are still intact. With this method, the bony contours of the ideal reconstruction and reference lines for shifting bony or soft tissue structures can be imported into the data set. This new CT data set has been used intraoperatively as a reconstruction template to check the position of the zygoma and the reconstruction of the bony orbit.

The results have been qualitatively and quantitatively validated by comparison of the CT data sets (Gellrich et al. 2002a). In 20 unilateral isolated orbital reconstructions, the quality of the reconstruction was evaluated based on comparative measurements of pre- and postoperative orbital volumes (Fig. 104). The comparative measurements of the preoperative CT data sets indicated a mean volume of 26.5 cm^3 for the unaffected orbit, with a standard deviation of 2.8 cm^3. As expected, the volumes of the deformed orbits were considerably greater (mean volume = 30.7 cm^3, SD = 3.4 cm^3). Analysis of the postoperative data sets indicated an average 4.0 cm^3 reduction of orbital volume on the operated side (SD = 1.8 cm^3). Comparison of the symmetry of the operated side with the control side showed a volume disparity of 0.2 cm^3 (SD = 1.2 cm^3). Our analysis is summarized in Table 1.

Table 1. Orbital volumes before and after navigation-assisted unilateral secondary reconstructions. The mean values and standard deviations are shown at the bottom of the table

Number of patients	Control side (cm^3)	Affected side: preoperative (cm^3)	Affected side: postoperative (cm^3)	Volume reduction (cm^3)	Difference between the sides (cm^3)
1	25.5	27.5	26.2	1.3	0.7
2	28.2	32.1	28.1	4.0	–0.1
3	29.0	33.8	30.1	3.7	1.1
4	30.9	33.3	30.2	3.1	–0.7
5	30.3	34.9	30.5	4.4	0.2
6	23.1	26.5	22.4	4.1	–0.7
7	31.0	36.3	32.6	3.7	1.6
8	24.2	29.6	22.5	7.1	–1.7
9	22.6	29.1	23.9	5.2	1.3
10	24.5	26.5	20.8	5.7	–3.7
11	25.9	27.6	27.4	0.2	1.5
12	29.2	36.5	29.8	6.7	0.6
13	29.4	34.8	29.9	4.9	0.5
14	27.8	32.5	27.3	5.2	–0.5
15	23.2	27.0	24.0	3.0	0.8
16	23.9	30.3	24.2	6.1	0.3
17	23.1	26.4	24.1	2.3	1.0
18	26.4	28.6	27.2	1.4	0.6
19	25.9	29.4	25.8	3.7	–0.1
20	26.2	30.9	27.3	4.3	0.9
Mean	26.5	30.7	26.7	4.0	0.2
SD	2.8	3.4	3.2	1.8	1.2

Virtual reconstruction is more difficult in cases with preexisting defects, and changes must be made in the virtual patient model. The virtual reconstruction of unilateral defects is relatively simple. In this case either the intact side or a subvolume of the intact side can be used for mirroring (Perry et al. 1998). The mirroring is done on a freely definable plane of symmetry (Schramm et al. 1999b, 2001a,b; Gellrich et al. 2002c). It may prove difficult to define the plane of symmetry in the midline because the skull does not have precise mirror-image symmetry and this leads to inaccuracies. Thus, the result of the mirroring requires a visual evaluation and should be repeated as required.

The capabilities of preoperative planning are significantly improved by the use of voxel-based simulations (VoXim, IVS Solutions, Chemnitz). This method is illustrated below for the planning and simulation of a posttraumatic secondary reconstruction of the orbit and periorbital region.

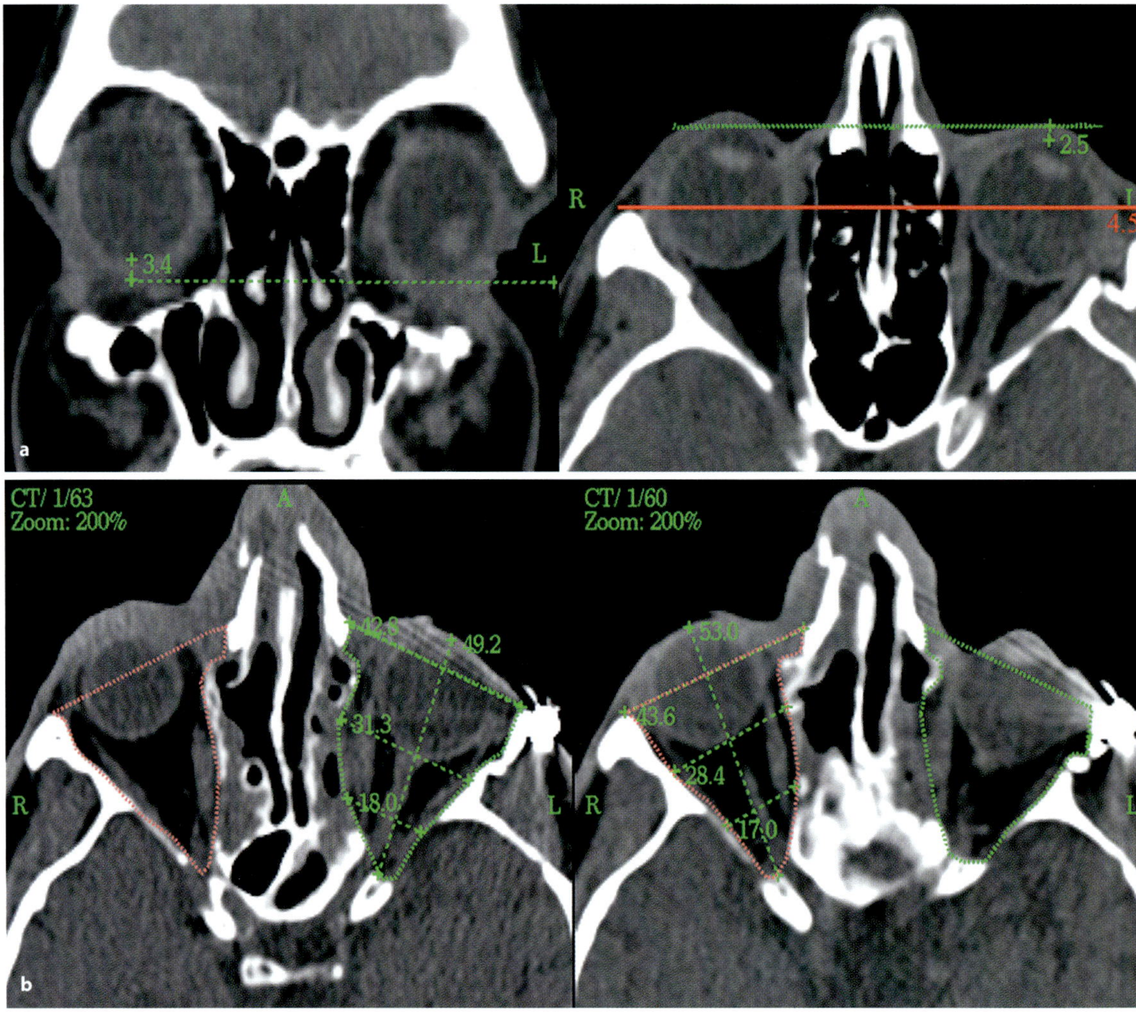

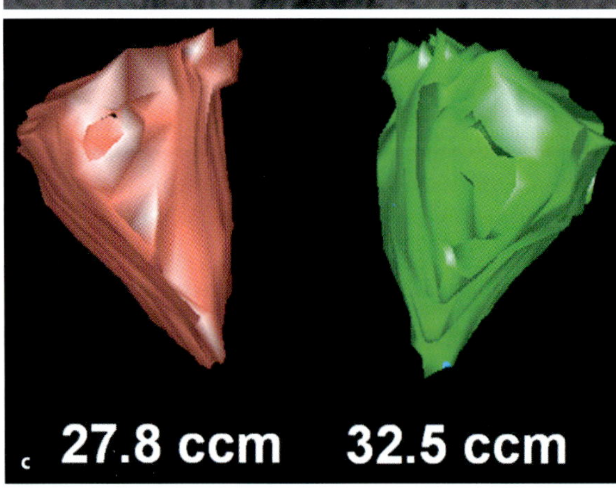

Fig. 101. Preoperative analysis of an orbital deformity. **a** Measurements of the vertical and sagittal malalignment of the left eye. The Hertel measurement of ocular prominence (*right*) is faulty in cases where the lateral orbital margins are deformed. **b** Orbital dimensions (longitudinal diameter plus anterior, middle, and posterior transverse diameters). **c** 3D surface-rendered images permit a quantitative and qualitative comparison of the orbital volumes on each side

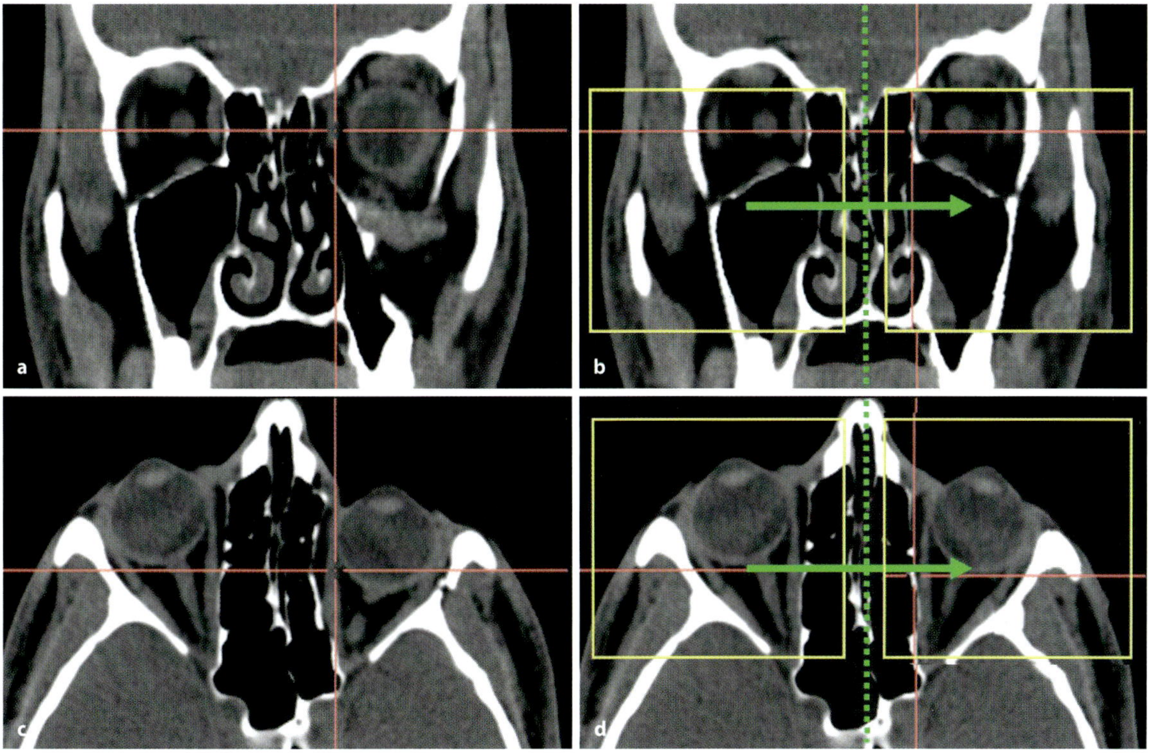

Fig. 102. Simulation of the ideal reconstruction of a left-sided orbital deformity by mirroring the unaffected side. **a, c** The biplanar display (coronal and axial slices) shows pronounced left-sided enophthalmos caused by the deformity of the orbital floor and medial wall. **b, d** The reflected (mirrored) data set. The subvolumes on the right side (*yellow frames*) have been reflected onto the affected left side

After the data set has been entered, it is first aligned with respect to the plane of symmetry (Fig. 105). This results in a new patient-specific coordinate system. Next the bony elements of the facial skeleton are segmented according to surgical and anatomical requirements (Fig. 106). The next step in planning is to copy and reflect (mirror) the unaffected side onto the affected side. Fine adjustments are then made in the anatomical position of the segments, resulting in a virtual reconstruction template. The template can be used to simulate the ideal placement of grafts or implants for reconstructing defects, or it may be used to align the displaced bone segments of the facial skeleton. In addition, areas that are to be resected can be virtually removed (Fig. 107). When the virtual reconstruction is completed, a metric analysis of the deformities can be carried out (Fig. 108). In this way the bone-based surgical procedure can be accurately simulated, and this can provide a more comprehensive understanding of individual patient anatomy during the planning stage. The reference points (splint-based markers or screw markers) are marked after the virtual template has been created.

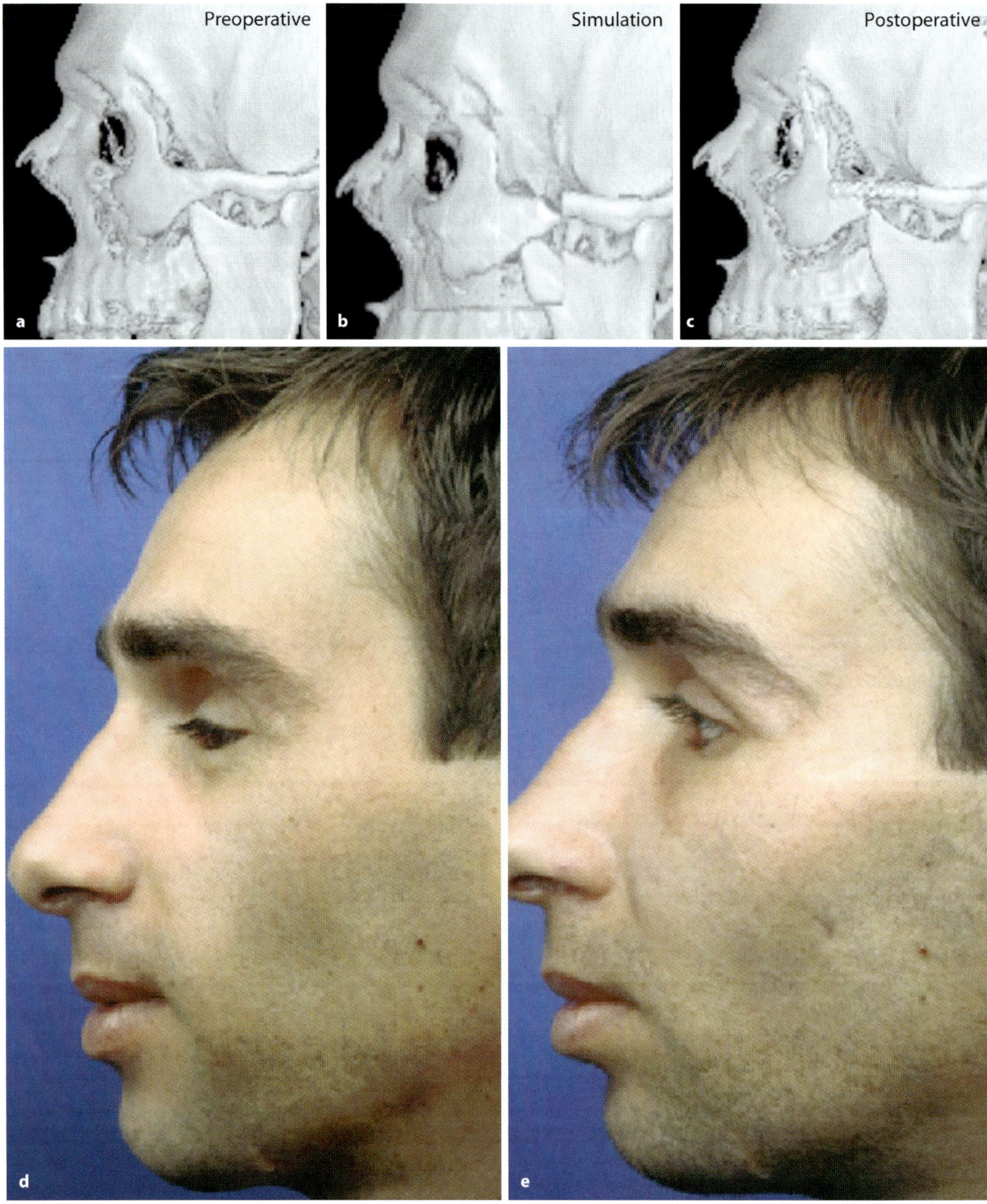

Fig. 103. Computer-assisted orbital and midfacial reconstruction. The 3D reconstructions show the preoperative right zygoma (a), the computer simulation after mirroring the subvolume (b), and the postoperative result (c). The clinical photographs show the appearance of the profile before (d) and after (e) the reconstruction

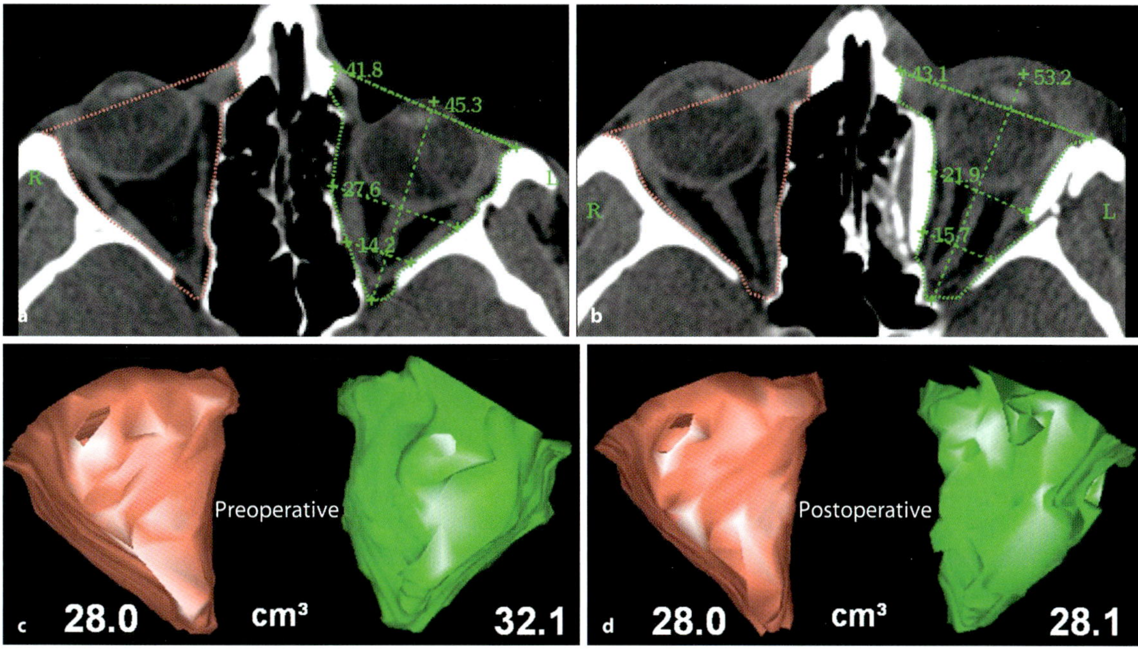

Fig. 104. Postoperative validation of the reconstruction. The orbital volumes were measured to compare the unaffected side with the operated side before and after navigation-assisted reconstruction based on the preoperative (**a, c**) and postoperative (**b, d**) CT data sets

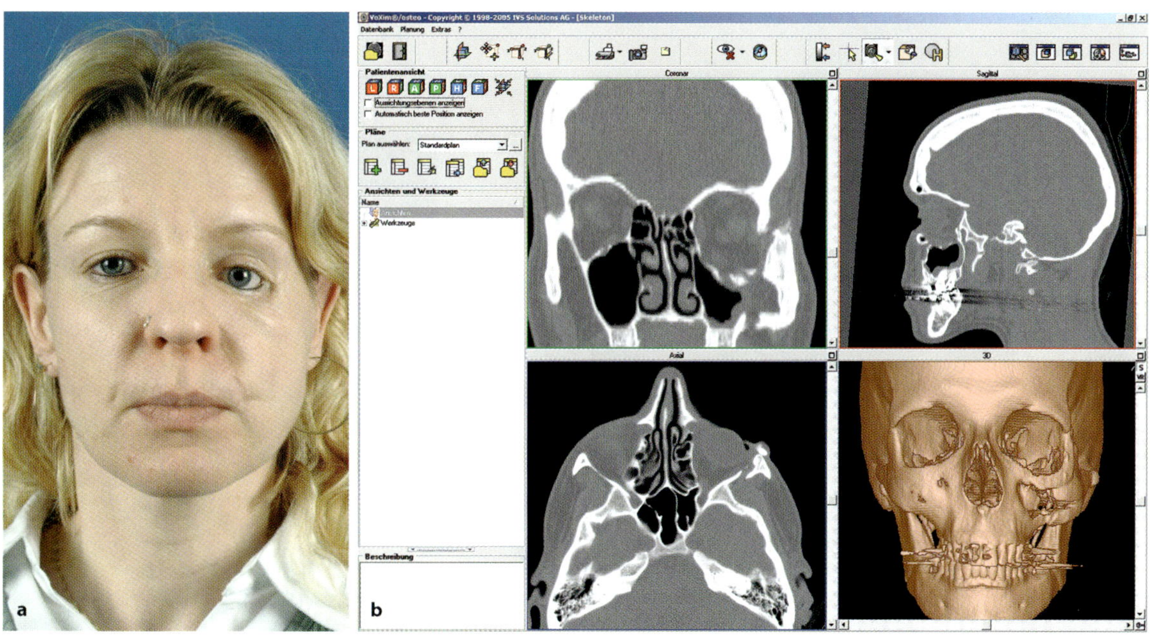

Fig. 105. Posttraumatic orbital deformity (**a**). The multiplanar display shows a periorbital deformity on the left side following multiple attempts at reconstruction and augmentation of the left zygoma (**b**)

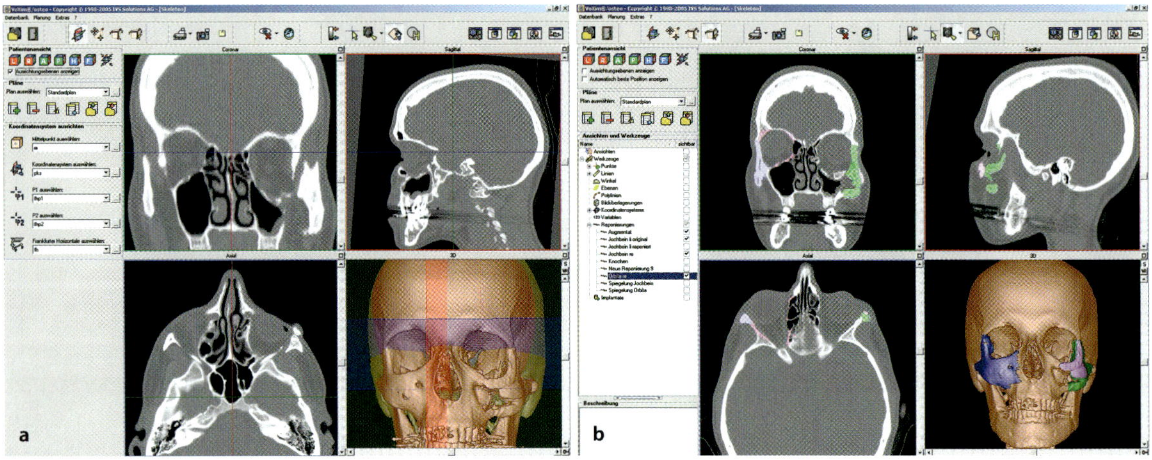

Fig. 106. Computer-assisted simulation of orbital reconstruction – part I. After alignment of the data set in the patient-oriented coordinate system (**a**), segmentation of the anatomical regions is performed (**b**)

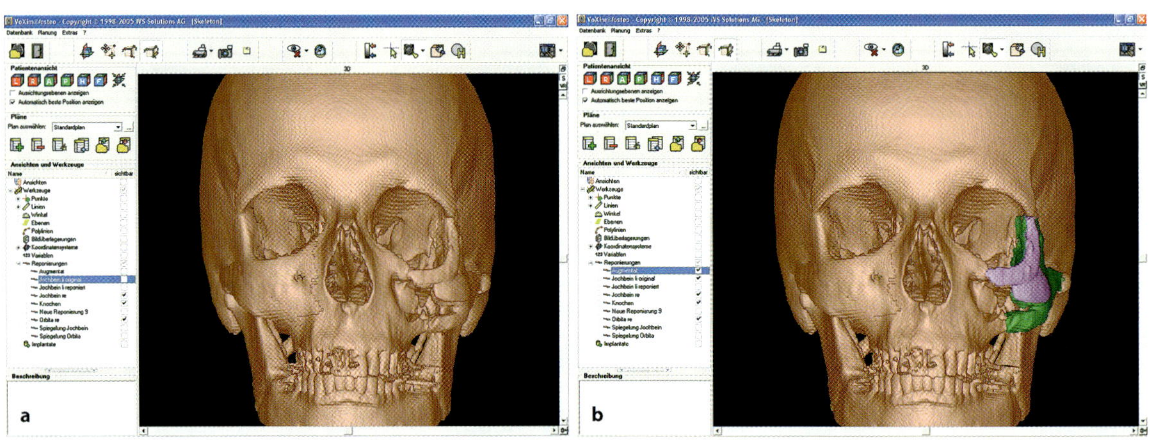

Fig. 107. Computer-assisted simulation of orbital reconstruction – part II. The original data set (**a**) is segmented to extract anatomically relevant structures such as augmentation material (*purple* in **b**) and the zygoma (*green* in **b**). This permit a virtual resection of the augmentation (**c**). After the contralateral zygoma has been segmented (*blue* in **d**), it is reflected onto the opposite side to create a positioning template for the displaced left zygoma (**e**). The displaced zygoma can now be aligned to conform with the mirrored zygomatic contour (**f**). After this alignment is completed, the mirroring can be removed to obtain a virtual surgical template for repositioning the left zygoma (**g**). Mirroring of the opposite side is adequate for reconstruction of the bony orbital walls (**h**)

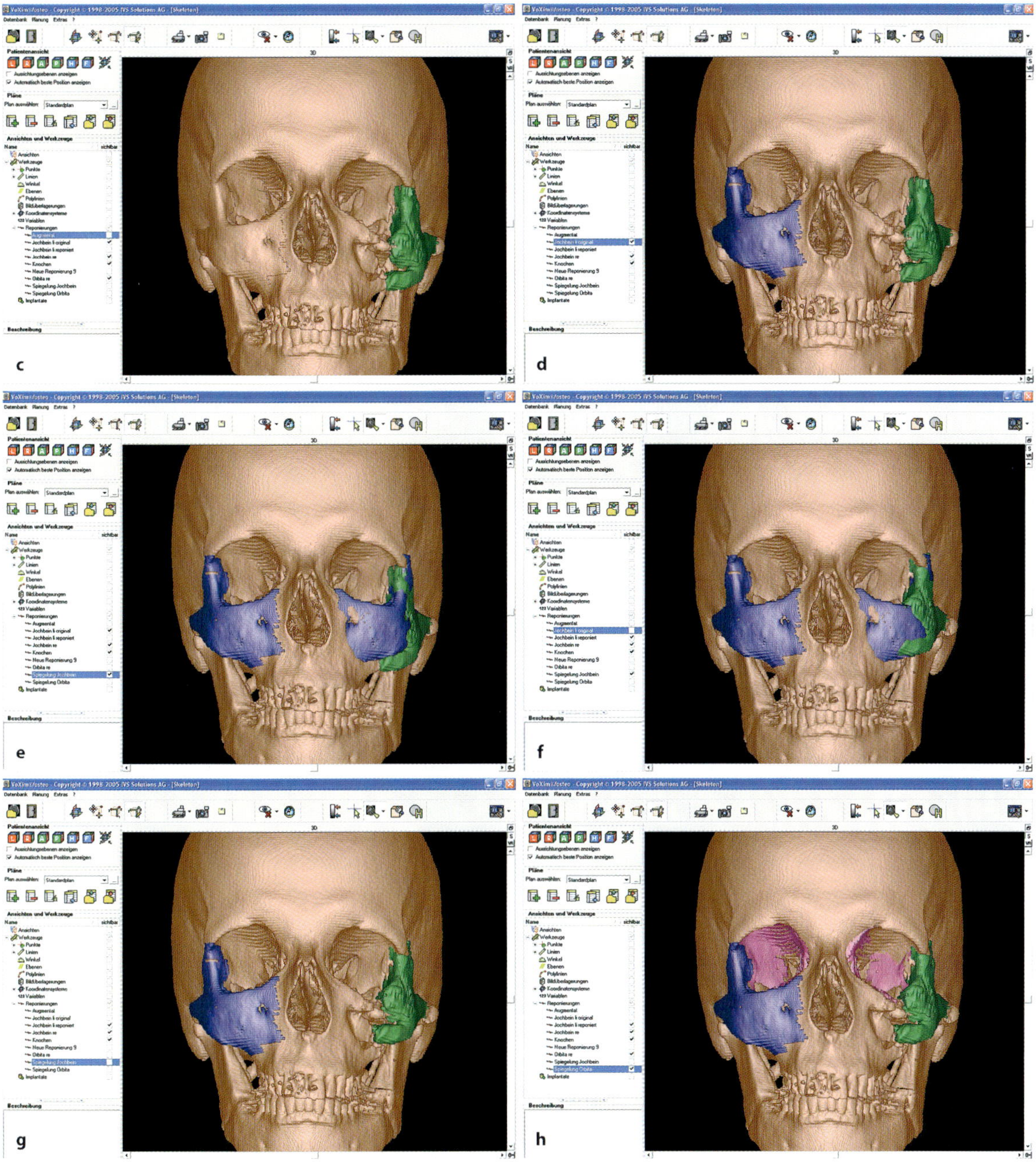

Fig. 107. (continued)

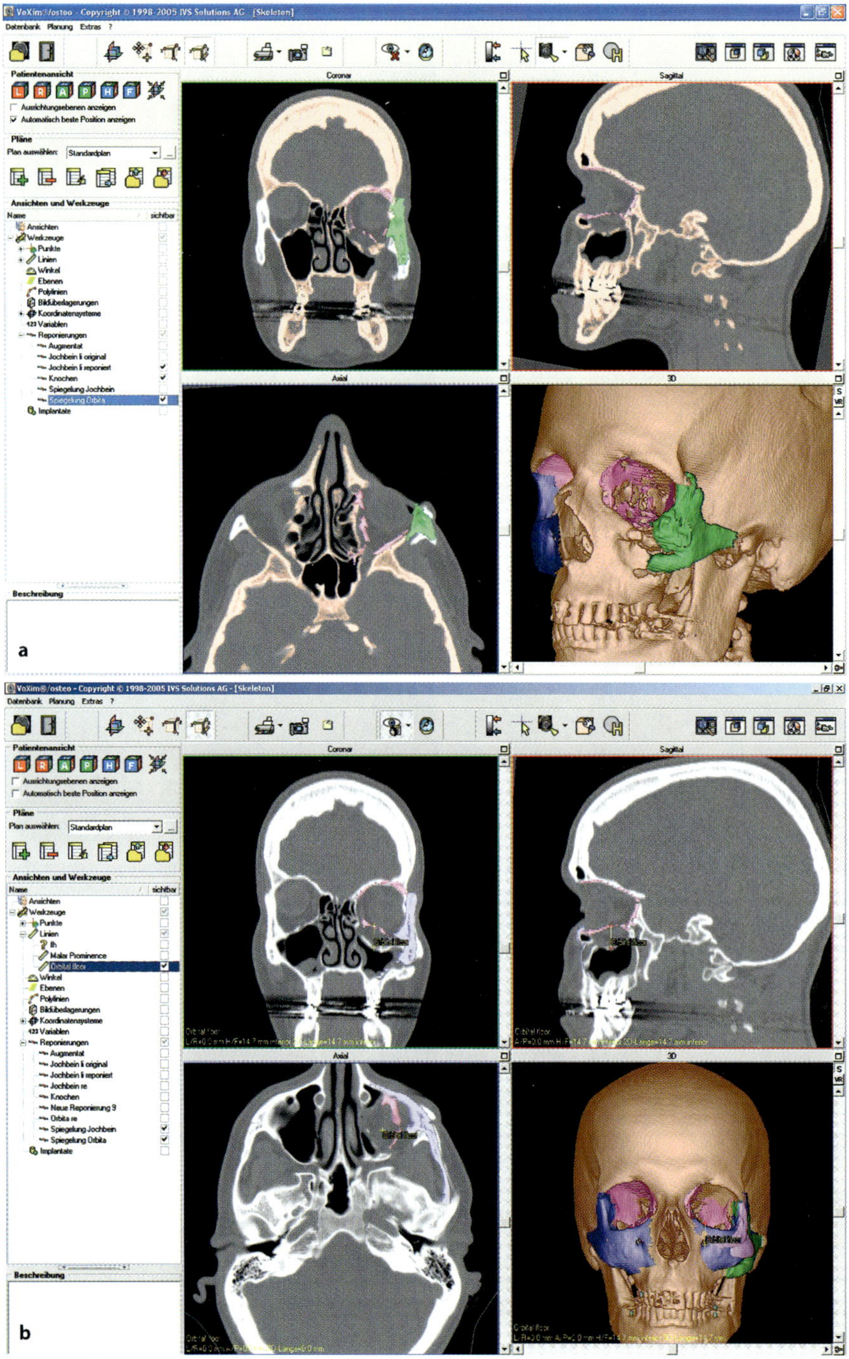

Fig. 108. Computer-assisted simulation of orbital reconstruction – part III. Virtual resection of the augmentation material, repositioning the displaced left zygoma, and mirroring the right orbit have yielded a 3D surgical template that is available through intraoperative navigation (a). Comparison of the virtual reconstruction and original structure permits a detailed metric analysis of the deformity (b)

Guided by intraoperative navigation, the surgeon can check the reconstruction repeatedly during the operation and adjust it to match the desired ideal. After the zygomatic contour has been corrected, it is probed with the pointer and its position is adjusted until the virtual pointer tip matches the key points on the virtual template. This can avoid unwelcome "surprises" during subsequent analysis of the postoperative CT data set (Figs. 109–112). Intraoperative imaging (CT, DVT, C-arm) could be used as an alternative, but multiple position corrections would significantly increase the radiation exposure to the patient. It would certainly be desired in these cases to use intraoperative navigation followed by a single intraoperative imaging check. The latest generation of C-arm fluoroscopes are especially promising in this regard. In contrast to primary reconstructions, posttraumatic soft tissue changes are of major importance in secondary corrections of the orbit. As a result, the reconstruction of the bony orbit cannot always be based on anatomical criteria alone (Ramieri et al. 2000). Often it is necessary to make overcorrections, which are difficult to predict preoperatively. But even in these cases, intraoperative navigation is an essential aid to carrying out the planned reconstruction at operation. Graft and implant positions can be checked as often as desired by probing them with the pointer and adjusting them to match the virtual template. This significantly increases the predictive value of these difficult procedures.

Reconstruction with CAD-CAM Implants

The planning and fabrication of titanium implants for the reconstruction of deficient facial and calvarial bones is based on the preoperative CT data set (Vougioukas et al. 2004). The figure illustrates the primary reconstruction of a postresection defect in the parietal bone. After virtual resection in the CT data set, the titanium implant was fabricated (CranioConstruct, Bochum, Germany) and pointer-guided resection of the cranial bone was carried out intraoperatively to accommodate the implant (Eufinger et al. 2001; Weihe et al. 2002; Fig. 113).

CAD-CAM reconstructions can be combined with midfacial revision osteotomies and orbital reconstructions (Gellrich et al. 2001). Pointer-based navigation can then be used intraoperatively to direct the revision osteotomy of the zygoma and also reconstruct the adjacent calvarium with a CAD-CAM implant (Fig. 114).

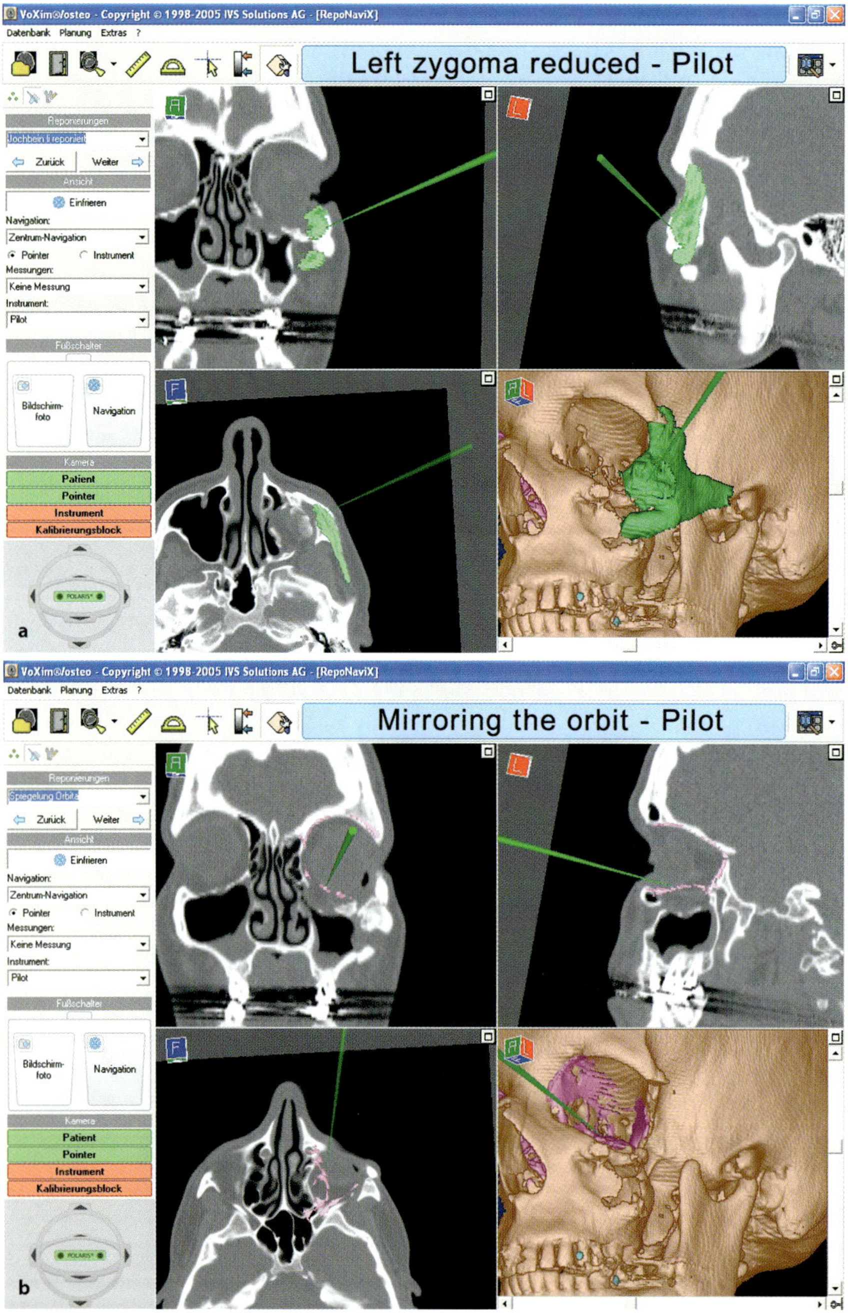

Fig. 109. Secondary reconstruction – intraoperative navigation. After repositioning and provisional fixation of the left zygoma, the surface of the zygoma is touched with the pointer and its position is adjusted until it conforms to the contour of the virtual template (*green segmentation* in **a**). The same method is used in positioning the orbital mesh (**b**)

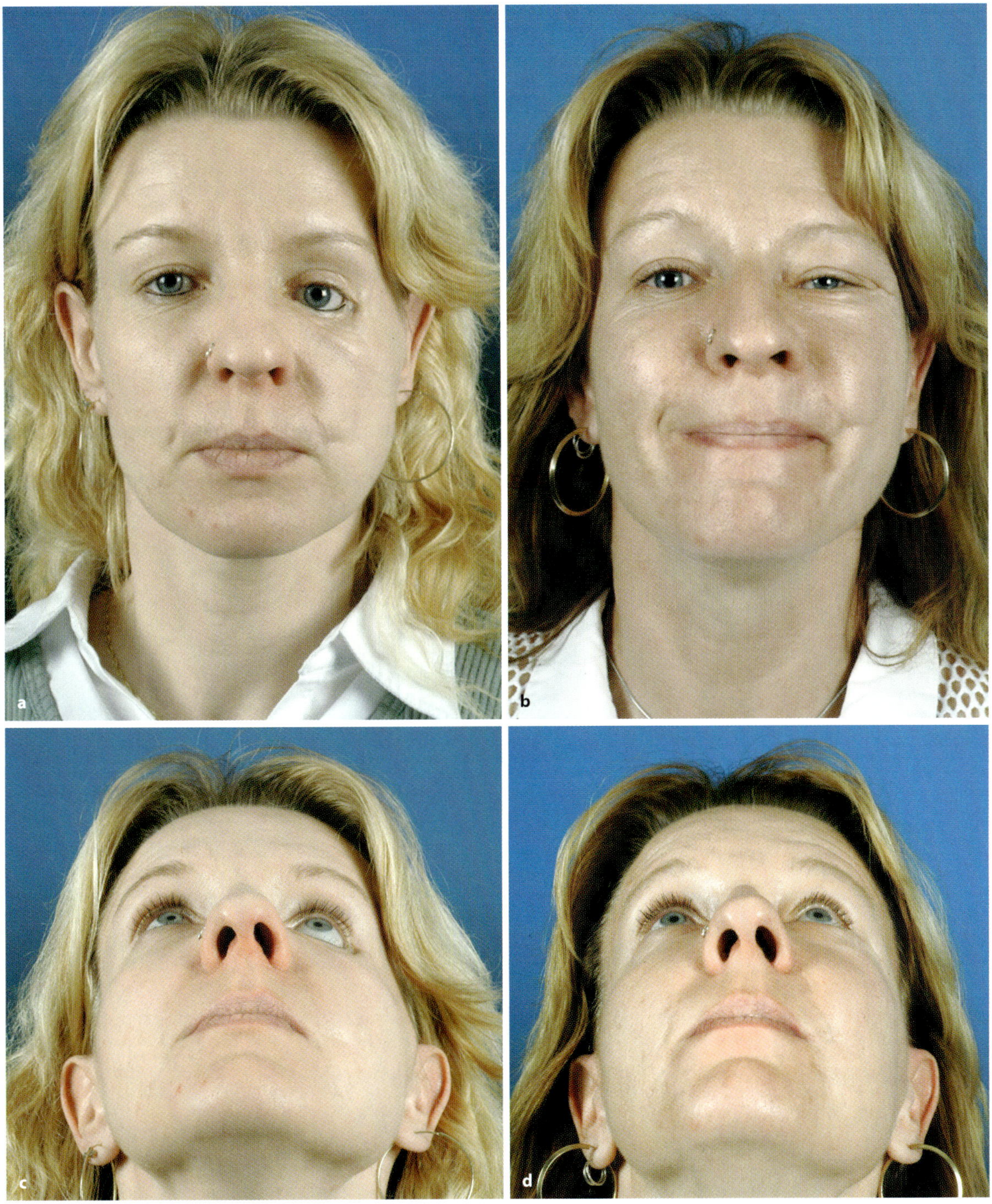

Fig. 110. Secondary reconstruction – postoperative follow-up. Clinical appearance before (**a, b**) and 1 year after (**c, d**) the navigation-assisted secondary correction. The operation has restored ocular symmetry and the symmetry of the zygomatic prominences

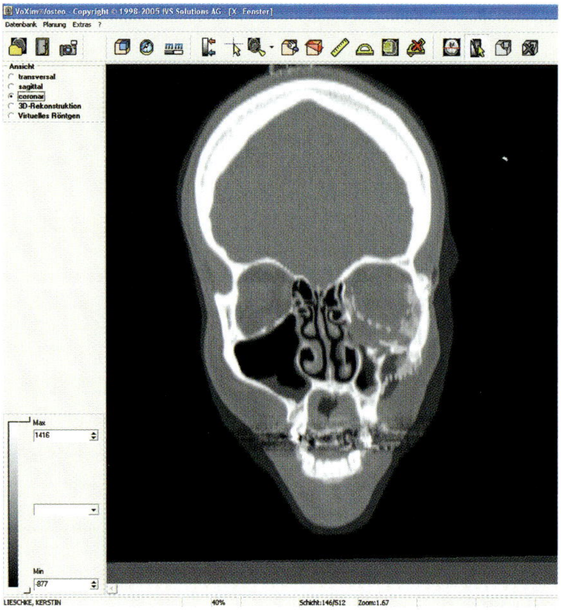

Fig. 111. Secondary reconstruction – postoperative evaluation by image fusion. Superimposing the two CT data sets before and after the reconstruction allows better visualization and quantitative evaluation of the postoperative result

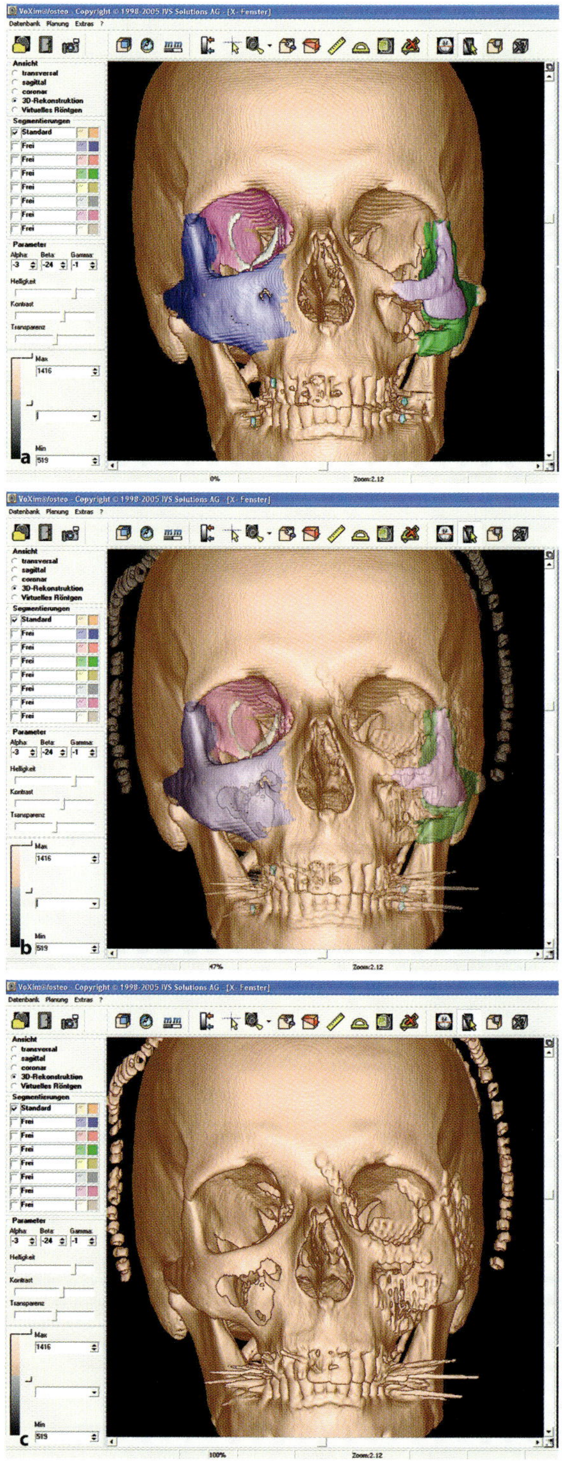

Fig. 112. Secondary reconstruction – postoperative evaluation by image fusion. The result of the reconstruction is vividly portrayed by successively superimposing the pre- and postoperative CT data sets (from a to c)

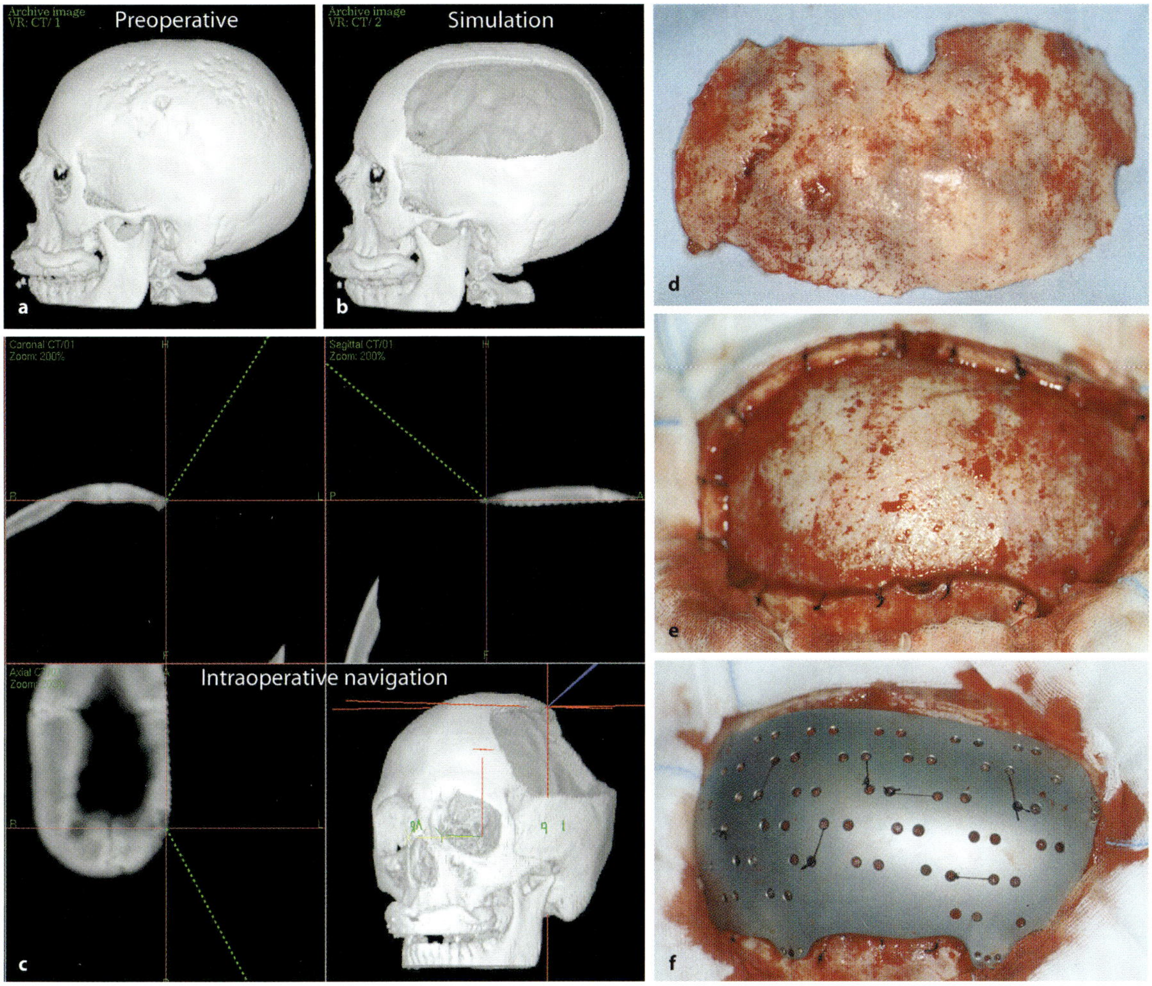

Fig. 113. Navigation-assisted resection of the left temporoparietal calvarium for chronic osteomyelitis. After virtual planning of the resection (3D reconstruction, a, b), the titanium implant was fabricated (d). Intraoperatively the resection was guided by pointer-based navigation (c), followed by insertion of the titanium implant (e, f)

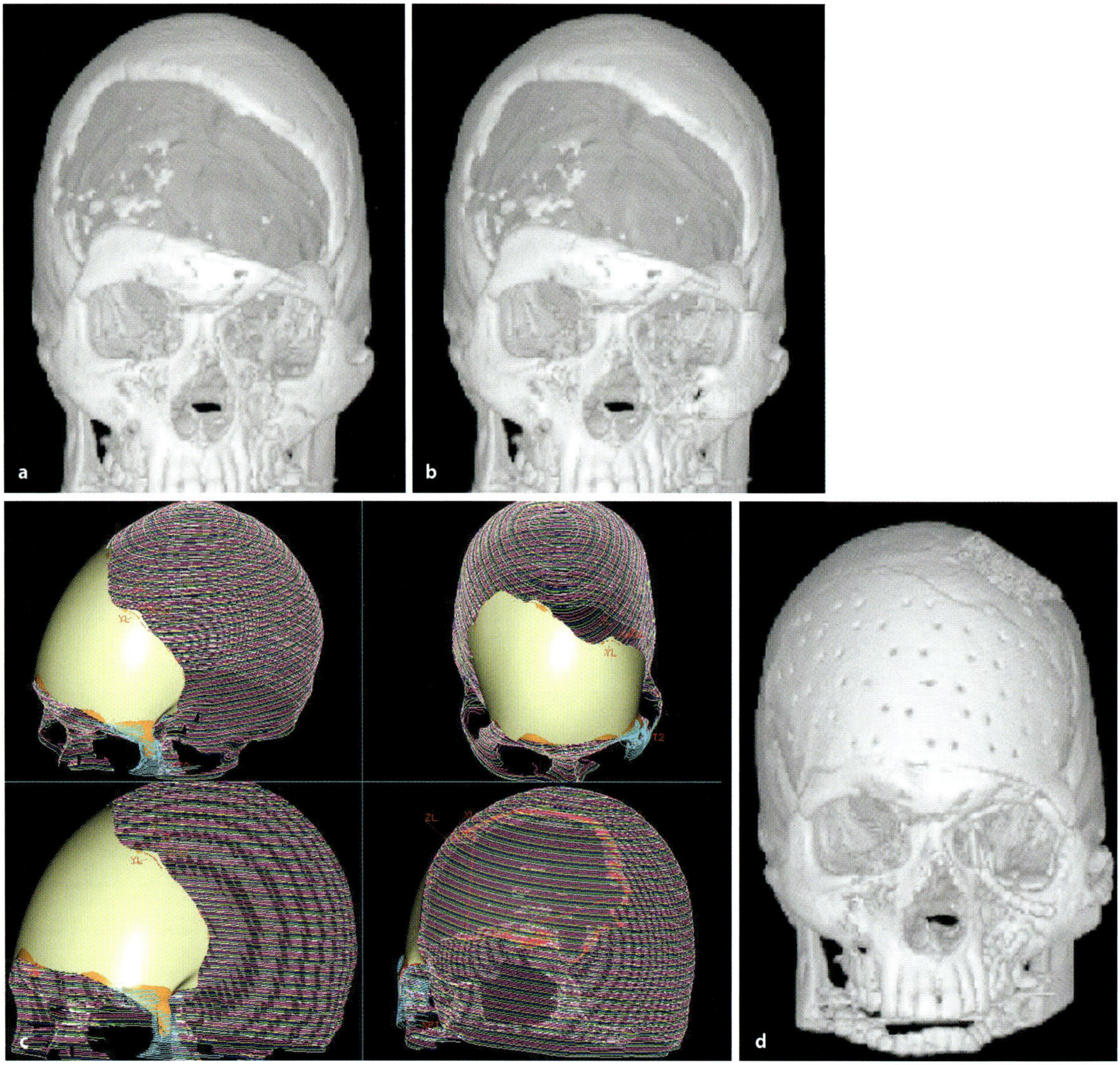

Fig. 114. **a** Three-dimensional CT data set of a trauma patient with an extensive frontal bone defect and a displaced centrolateral midfacial fracture on the left side. **b** First the reconstruction of the left zygoma and left orbit was simulated by mirroring the data set. **c** This formed the basis for planning and fabricating a custom-made titanium implant for reconstructing the frontal bone. Intraoperatively, the titanium reconstruction and midfacial reconstruction were performed simultaneously with navigational assistance. **d** Postoperative CT scan. **e, f** Clinical appearance before and after combined frontal bone reconstruction with a custom-made titanium implant (CAD-CAM) and navigation-assisted midfacial and orbital reconstruction on the left side

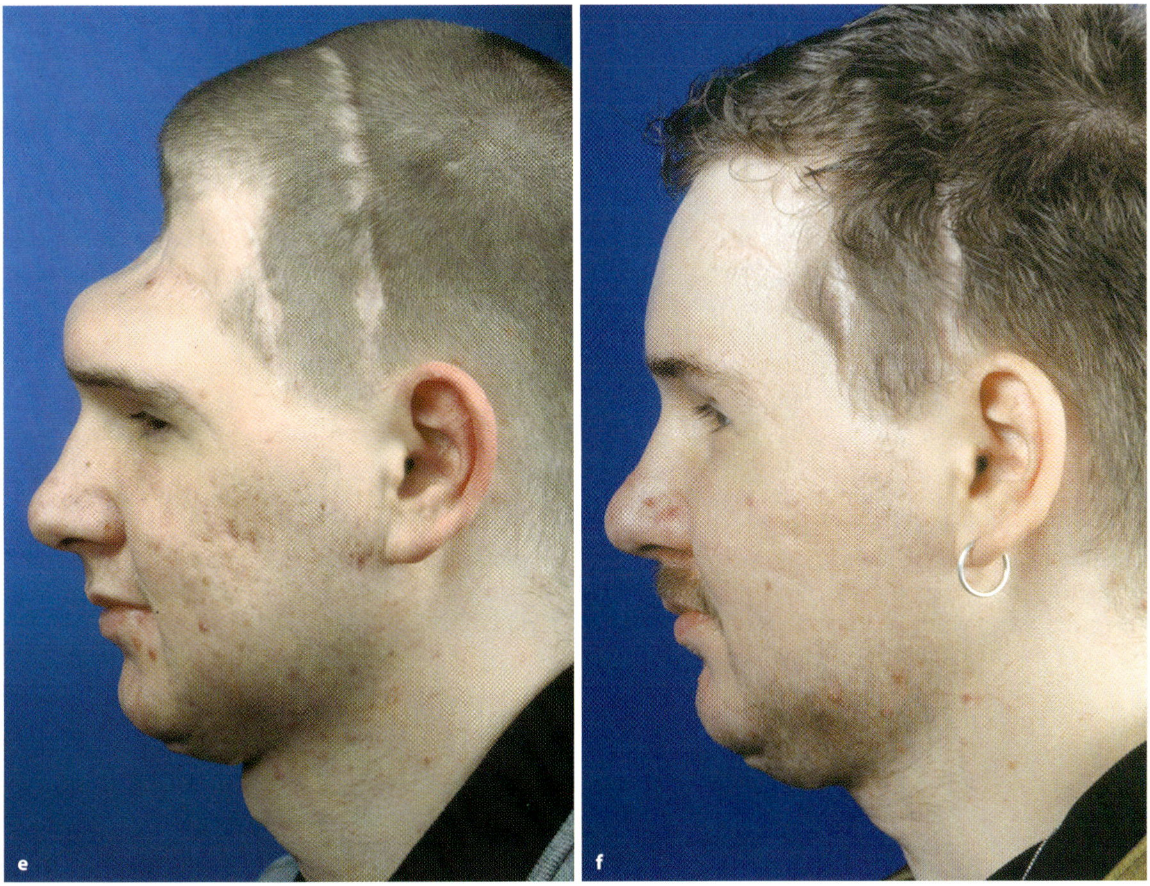

Fig. 114. (continued)

Procedures for Midfacial Correction

Syndromic anomalies and complex dysgnathias require 3D planning to evaluate the asymmetries and define the appropriate treatment concept (Mommaerts et al. 2001). Two-dimensional imaging must often be supplemented in these cases by CT-based evaluation. With modern planning systems, the necessary corrections of individual cranial regions can be simulated prior to distraction therapy or corrective midfacial osteotomies to test the efficacy of the proposed treatment strategy (Wagner et al. 1997; Zeilhofer et al. 1997; Watzinger et al. 1999a; Santler 2000; Schramm et al. 2001a). Intraoperatively, osteotomies can be navigationally guided in anatomically hard-to-reach areas, and correction distances and the positioning of bone segments can be directed in accordance with preoperative planning. Le Fort III midfacial osteotomies are particularly challenging in terms of planning and execution (Schmelzeisen and Schramm 2002). The necessary surgical treatment can be accurately determined preoperatively by segmentation and virtual repositioning of the midface and mandible. The simulation enables the surgeon to perform the osteotomies and reposition the bone segments with very high precision. Because the clinical use of intraoperative navigation cannot and should not replace the use of surgical splints, it is still necessary to produce these splints in a conventional way. In order to transfer the virtual planning to the conventional model operation using plaster models, it is necessary to fabricate a registration splint on the articulated jaw models. This splint bears the registration markers that are necessary for intraoperative registration and which also allow the virtual correction distances to be displayed separately for each marker. So with synchronous alignment of the CT data set and plaster models based on the hinge axis-orbital plane, the conventional model operation can be performed using the virtually determined correction distances for the upper jaw. The surgical splint for the mandible can still be produced in the conventional way (Schwestka-Polly et al. 1993). Intraoperatively, the osteotomy is performed under navigational guidance to protect vital structures. After placing the maxillary surgical splint, the surgeon can check and make fine adjustments of midfacial position in the region of the zygomatic prominences and nasal skeleton. The position of the maxilla can also be checked by pointer-based navigation using the reference markers (Schramm 2001; Figs. 115–119).

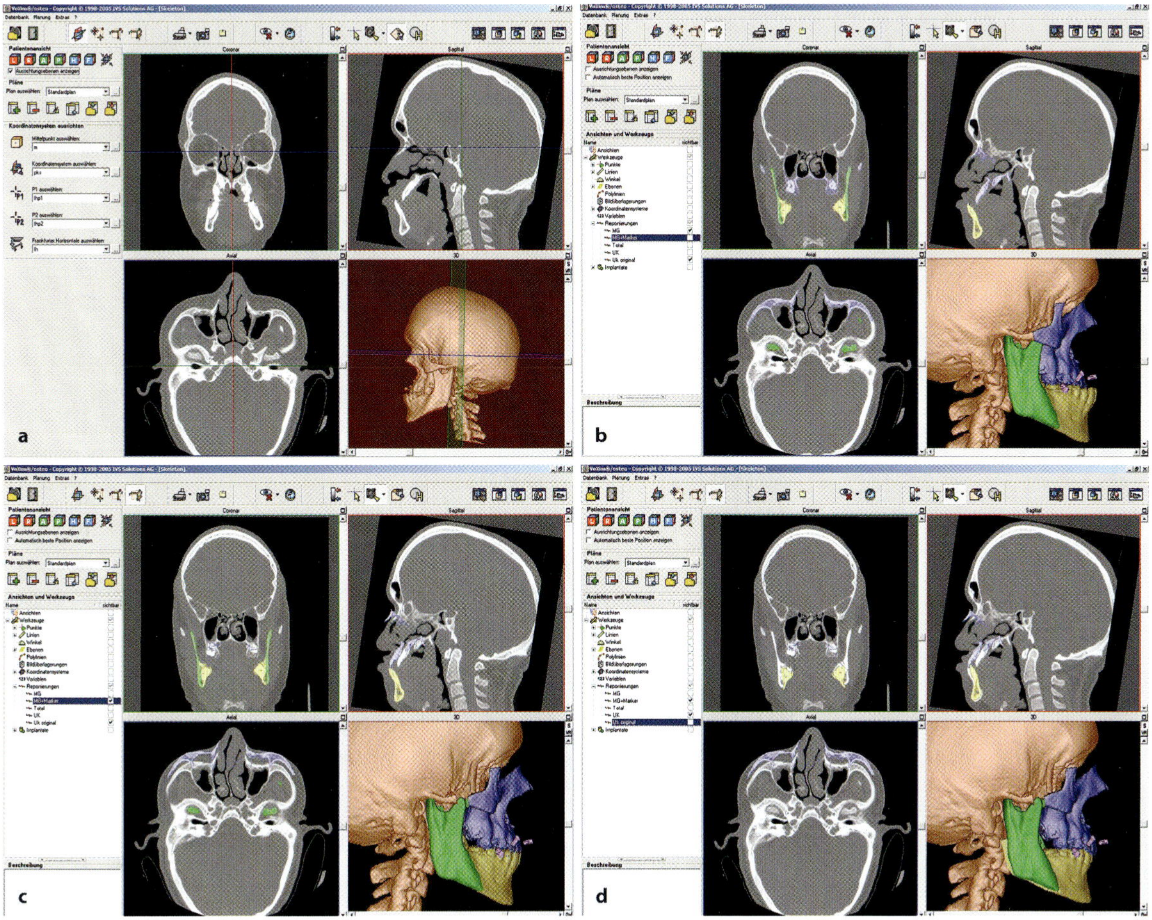

Fig. 115. Facial correction in Crouzon's disease – preoperative planning and simulation. When the data set has been symmetrically aligned in the individual patient coordinate system and positioned parallel to the hinge axis-orbital plane, it can be correlated with the articulated plaster models (**a**). Segmentation of the data set based on the osteotomy lines forms the basis for simulating the correction (**b**). The midfacial advancement at the level of the Le Fort III plane is planned and simulated based on anatomical criteria (**c**). The mandibular ramus osteotomy is planned last (**d**)

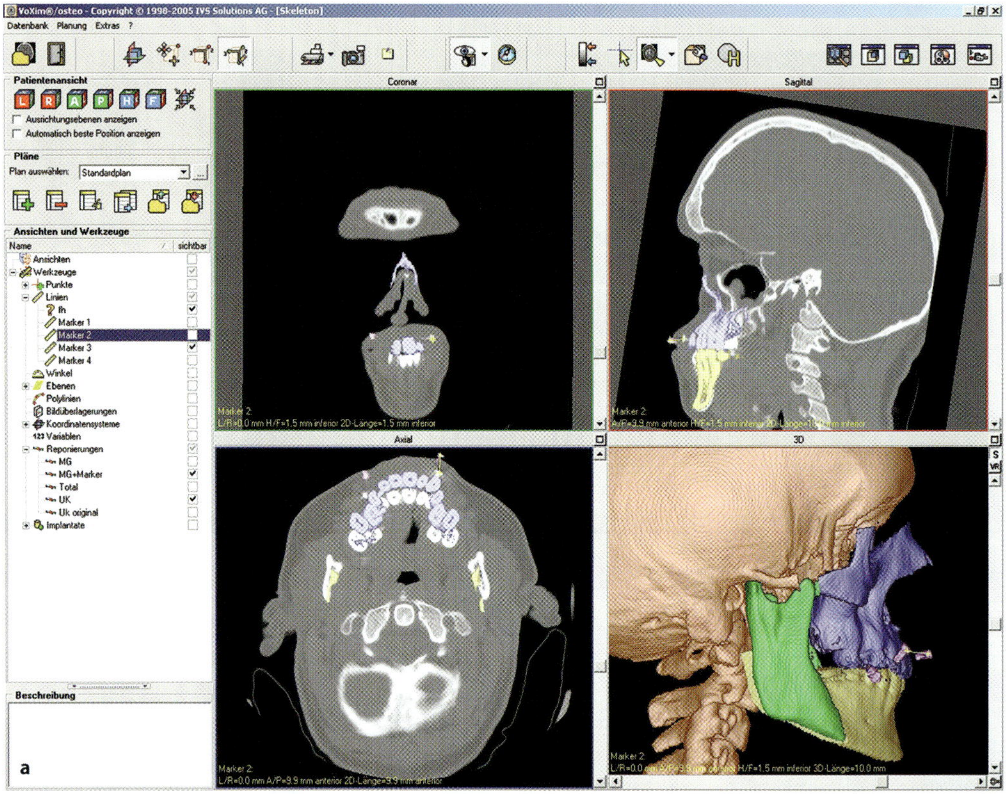

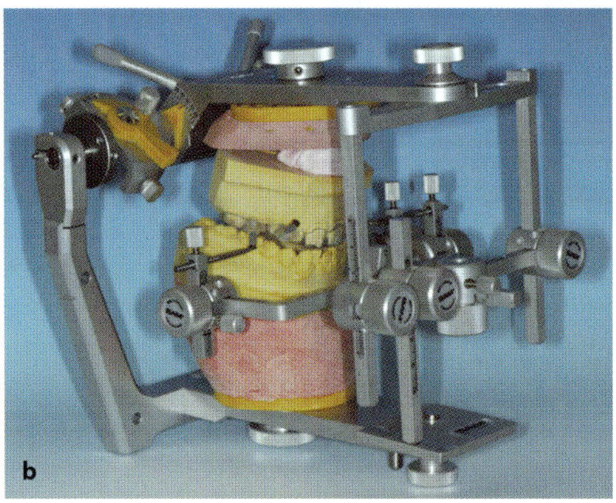

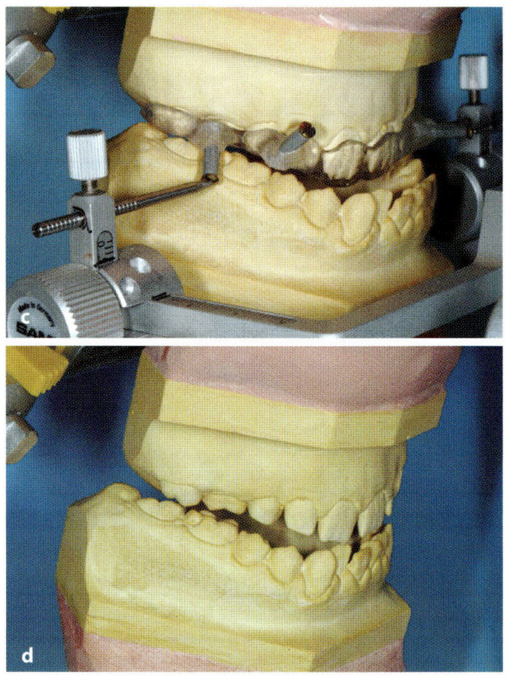

Fig. 116. Facial correction in Crouzon's disease – transferring the CT plan to plaster models. Since the data set has been aligned on the hinge axis-orbital plane, it can be correlated with the articulated plaster models. The virtual advancement of the splint-based markers is determined by CT planning (a), and the desired mandibular correction is transferred to the plaster jaw model with the aid of a fully adjustable articulator (b). After the maxilla has been articulated in i ts new position, a surgical splint can be fabricated for midfacial advancement (c). A second surgical splint for the mandibular correction is made conventionally by moving the plaster models to the desired interocclusal relation (d)

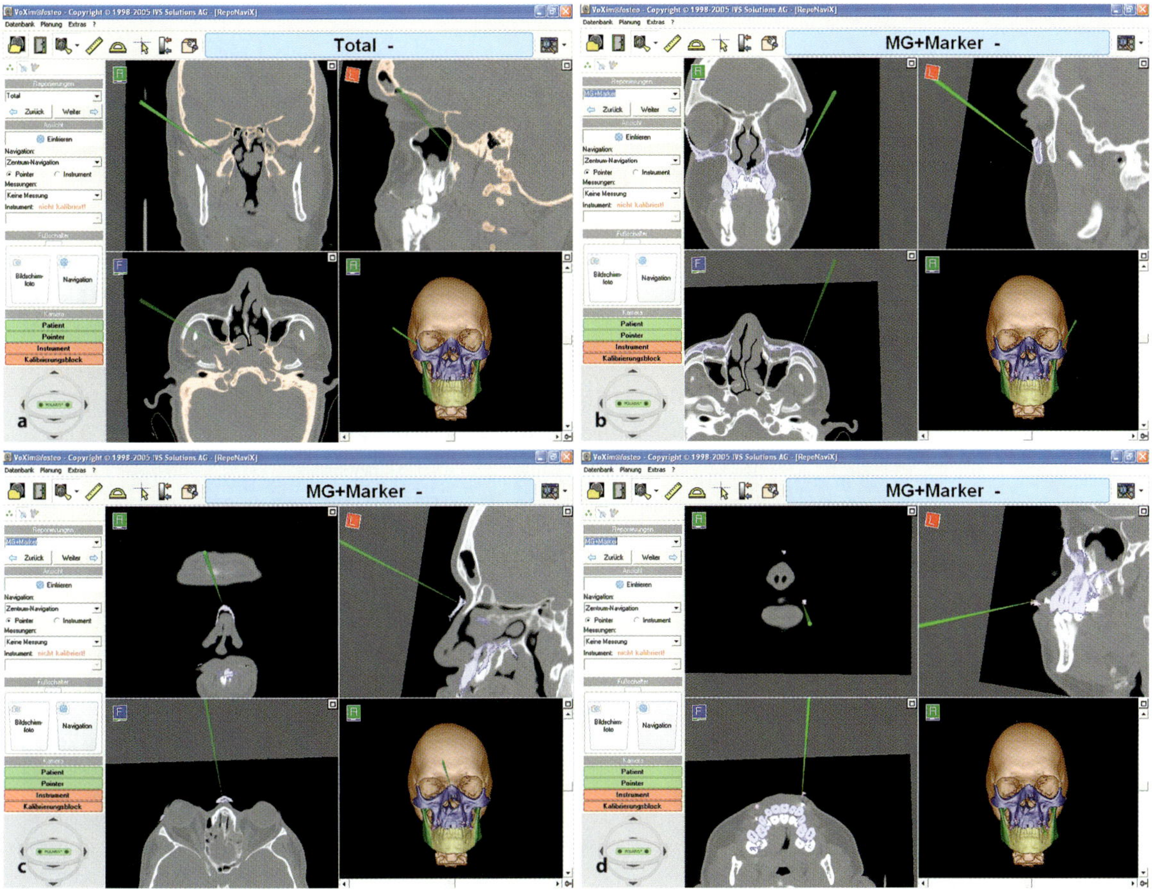

Fig. 117. Facial correction in Crouzon's disease – intraoperative navigation. Following a navigation-assisted osteotomy to avoid injury to vital structures during the skull base osteotomy (a), the midface is positioned using pointer-based surface control. The most critical landmarks for checking midfacial position are the zygomatic prominences (b) and the nasal skeleton (c). The position of the occlusal plane is predetermined by the surgical splint. Additionally, the displacement of the splint-based markers can be checked by intraoperative navigation so that fine adjustments can be made (d)

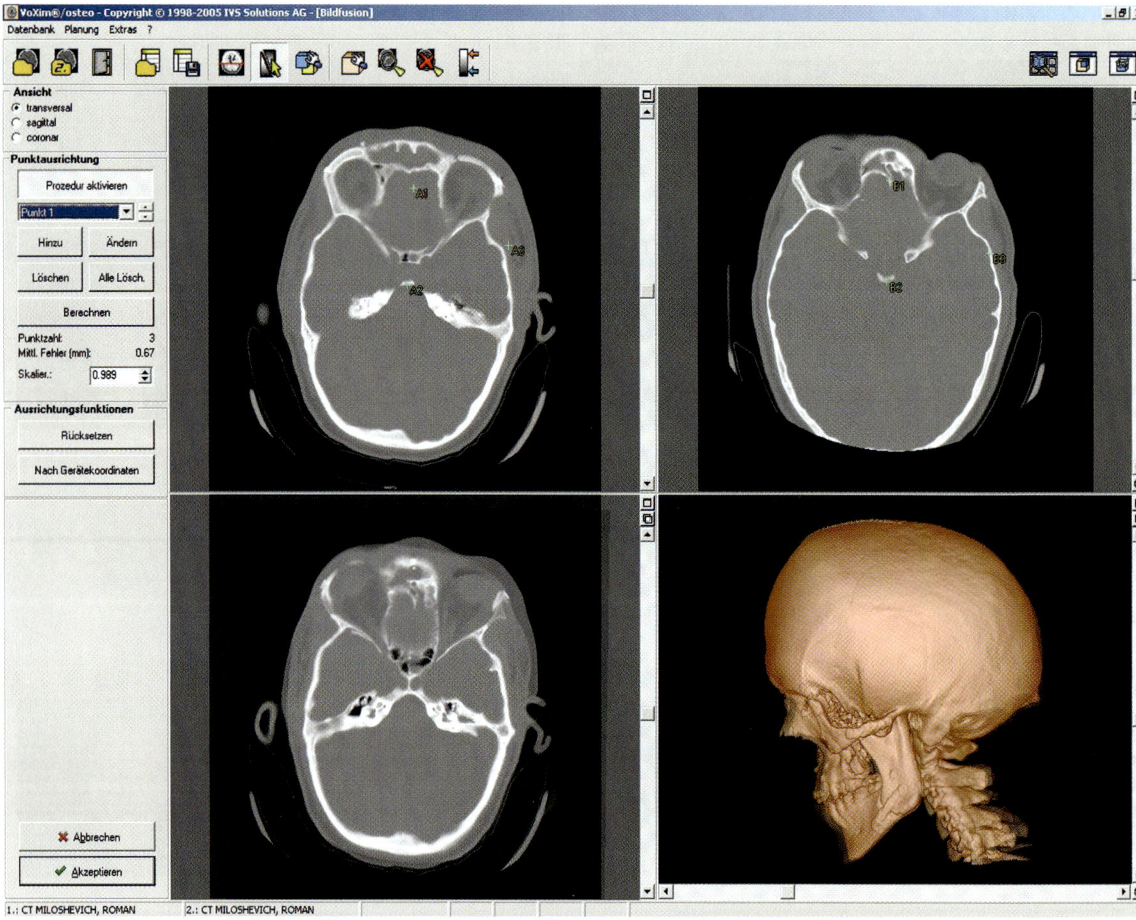

Fig. 118. Facial correction in Crouzon's disease – image fusion. Superimposing the pre- and postoperative data sets is accomplished by a point-based correlation of anatomical landmarks that have remained unchanged. The preoperative (*left*) and postoperative (*right*) data sets are shown at the *top* of the figure. Point-to-point correlation yields a 3D overlay of the data sets, shown in two and three dimensions at the *bottom* of the figure

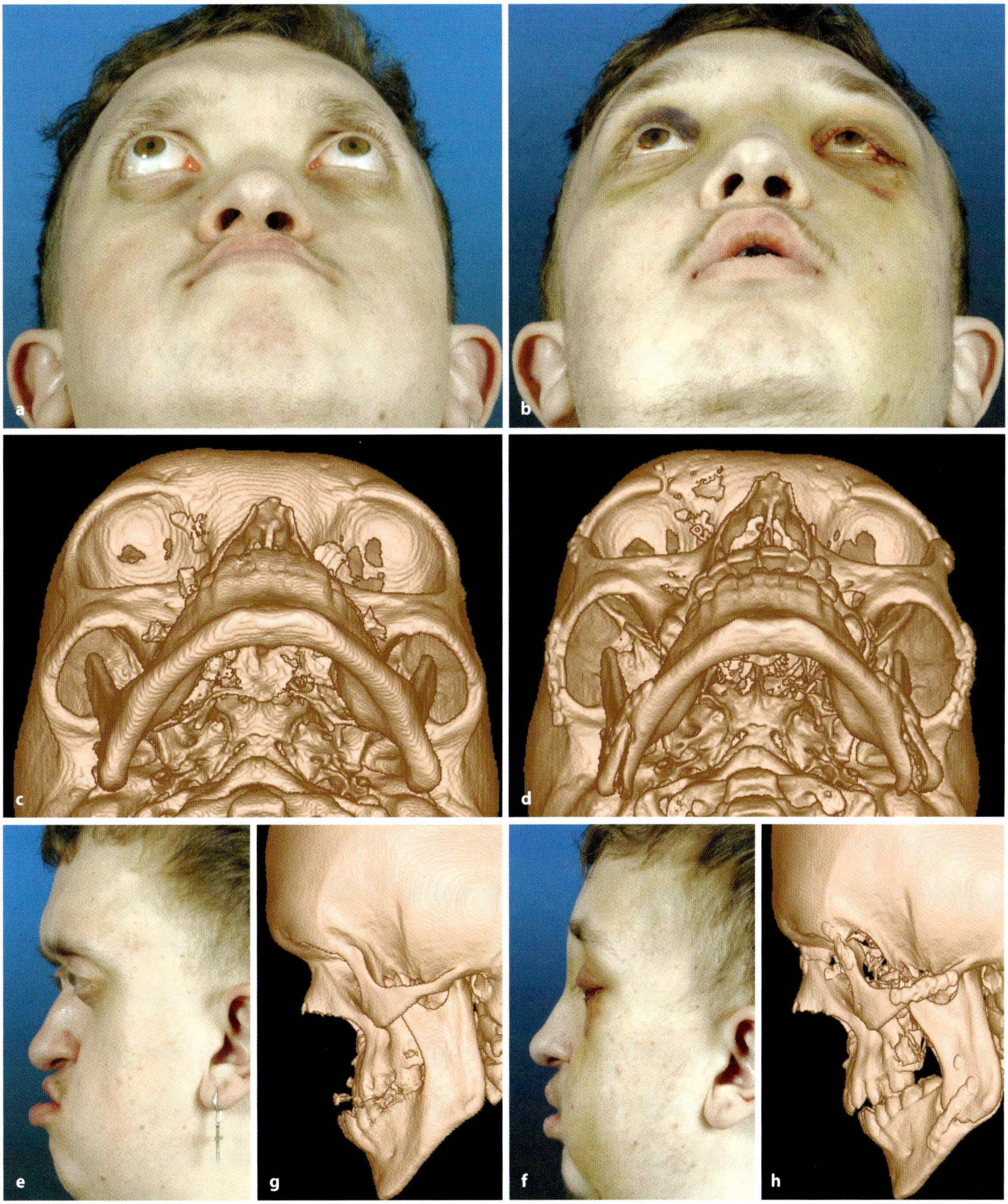

Fig. 119. Facial correction in Crouzon's disease – postoperative evaluation. Comparison of the clinical photographs with 3D reconstructions of the bony skull before (**a, c, e, g**) and after (**b, d, f, h**) midfacial advancement reflects the relationship of the soft tissue and bony corrections

Complex dysgnathias, especially those involving rotation and angulation of the maxillary occlusal plane, are challenging in terms of preoperative planning and intraoperative execution (Hohoff et al. 2002). Virtual planning software is available that allows the surgeon to plan all the osteotomies down to the smallest detail and simulate the corrective displacements of the jaw segments. The following points and problems should be noted. Surgical splints should still be used at operation, as they allow 3D positioning of the osteotomized jaw segments to be carried out more easily and accurately than would be possible with navigational assistance alone. The fabrication of the surgical splints, however, is often based on approximate model operations that do not always conform to actual anatomy, especially in cases where maxillary rotation is proposed. But even in complex dysgnathias, the positioning of the mandible is usually determined by occlusion. This can easily be simulated in a conventional model operation by the tactile control of plaster models. The visualization and adjustment of occlusion with imaging procedures is definitely too cumbersome and is even unnecessary as the following planning method will show.

A combination of conventional articulator planning and virtual CT data set-based planning can be used for the simulation of complex bignathic corrective osteotomies. It is necessary to have an articulator with a freely movable upper part that can be locked in any desired position. The upper and lower parts of the articulator are connected to a registration array that can register the movements of the plaster jaw models in relation to each other. The initial position of the models is taken from an intermaxillary splint that is made conventionally on the patient with the jaws in centric relation. Registration markers are attached to the splint, and the patient undergoes a CT examination with the navigation splint in place. This uniquely defines the position of the mandible relative to the maxilla, and the registration markers can also be used to correlate the CT data set to the plaster models made from the patient. When computer-assisted planning is used, this makes it possible to transfer all simulated jaw movements directly to the articulator. The rest of the procedure is described below and is analogous to pointer-based navigation in the patient.

Initially, registration is performed on the "model patient," which consists of the articulator and the attached registration array. The centric splint is inserted to align the upper part of the articulator with the upper jaw model to the lower part of the articulator with the lower jaw model, and then registration is performed using the markers on the centric splint. This process correlates the CT data set of the patient to the plaster models of the patient's jaws. A navigation-assisted model operation can now be carried out. The upper part of the articulator can be moved and repositioned in accordance with the previously performed simulation and virtual correction of the maxilla in the CT data set. This is done until the position of the upper part of the articulator coincides with the virtual plan (Chapuis et al. 2005). The upper part is then fixed in that position, and the surgical splint for positioning the maxilla can be fabricated in a conventional way.

This procedure can be reversed for positioning the lower jaw. The lower part of the articulator is positioned in optimal interocclusal relation to the upper part and is locked in place. It does not matter which part of the articulator is moved, since both parts are tracked separately from each other by the infrared tracking system. The surgical splint for positioning the mandible can now be fabricated. This part of the procedure is the same as in a conventional model operation, except that the corrections are carried out simultaneously in the planning data set. This permits an accurate simulation of the optimum positional relation between the upper and lower jaws, and it may contribute to the decision of whether a bony advancement of the chin is also necessary. This simulation may also be done as a prelude to virtually manipulating and repositioning a bimaxillary block consisting of the maxilla and mandible in ideal occlusal relation. This can greatly facilitate operative planning in some forms of dysgnathia.

Intraoperative navigation is necessary to determine the vertical dimension and for fine adjustments, since the surgical splint for the maxilla represents an exact reproduction of the preoperative simulation in all other dimensions. This method provides a clinically useful improvement over the conventional model operation, combining the advantages of tactile control on plaster models with 3D patient-based planning (Figs. 120–124).

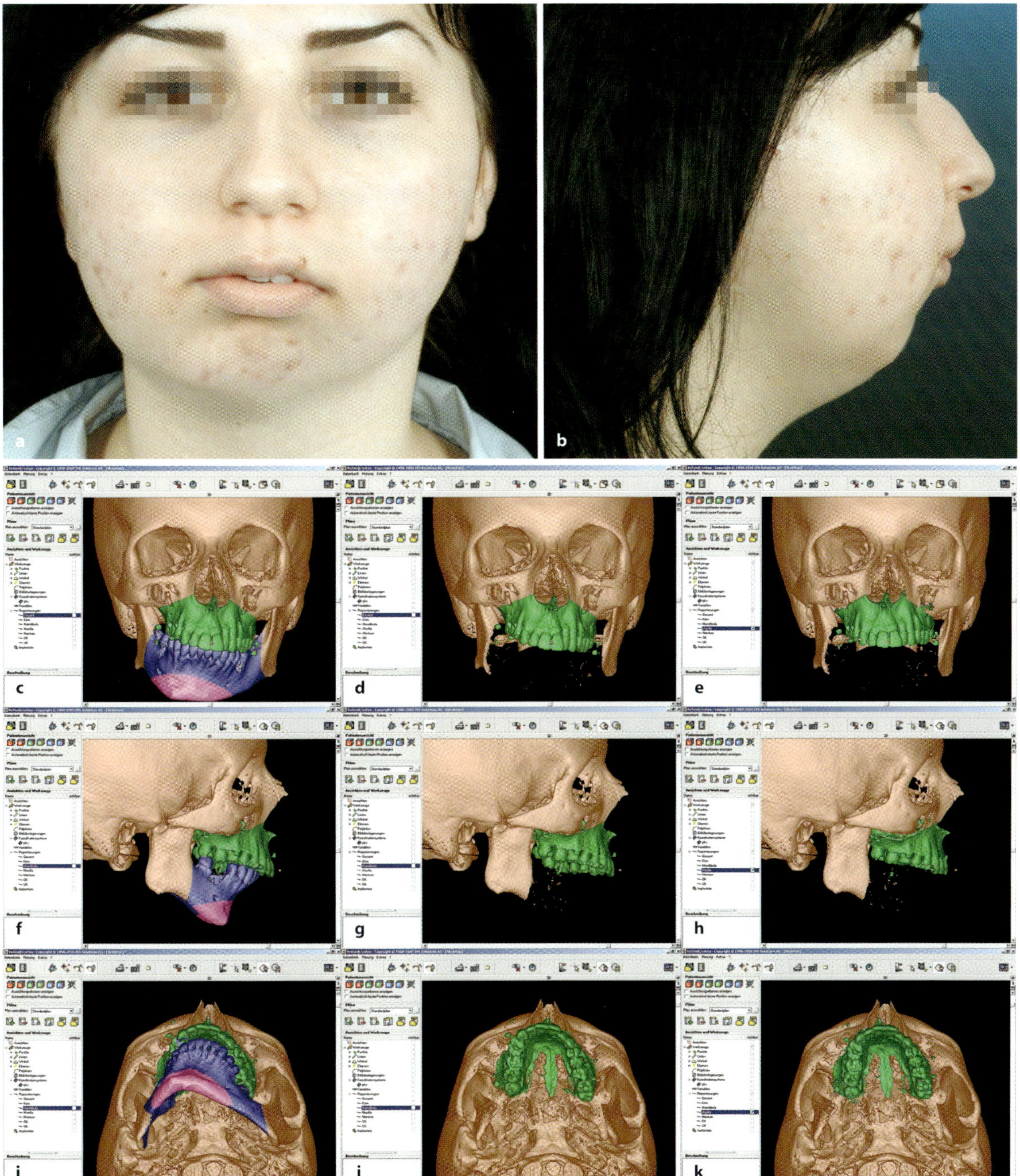

Fig. 120. Complex dysgnathia (a, b) – preoperative planning of the maxillary correction. First the data set is segmented based on the osteotomy lines for the midfacial, lower facial and chin corrections (c). To plan the maxillary correction, the mandible is virtually resected (d) and the maxilla is realigned based on anatomical relationships (e). These should include the findings of the clinical examination (level of the nasolabial fold, center of the maxilla). The planning steps are evaluated in various views (f–k)

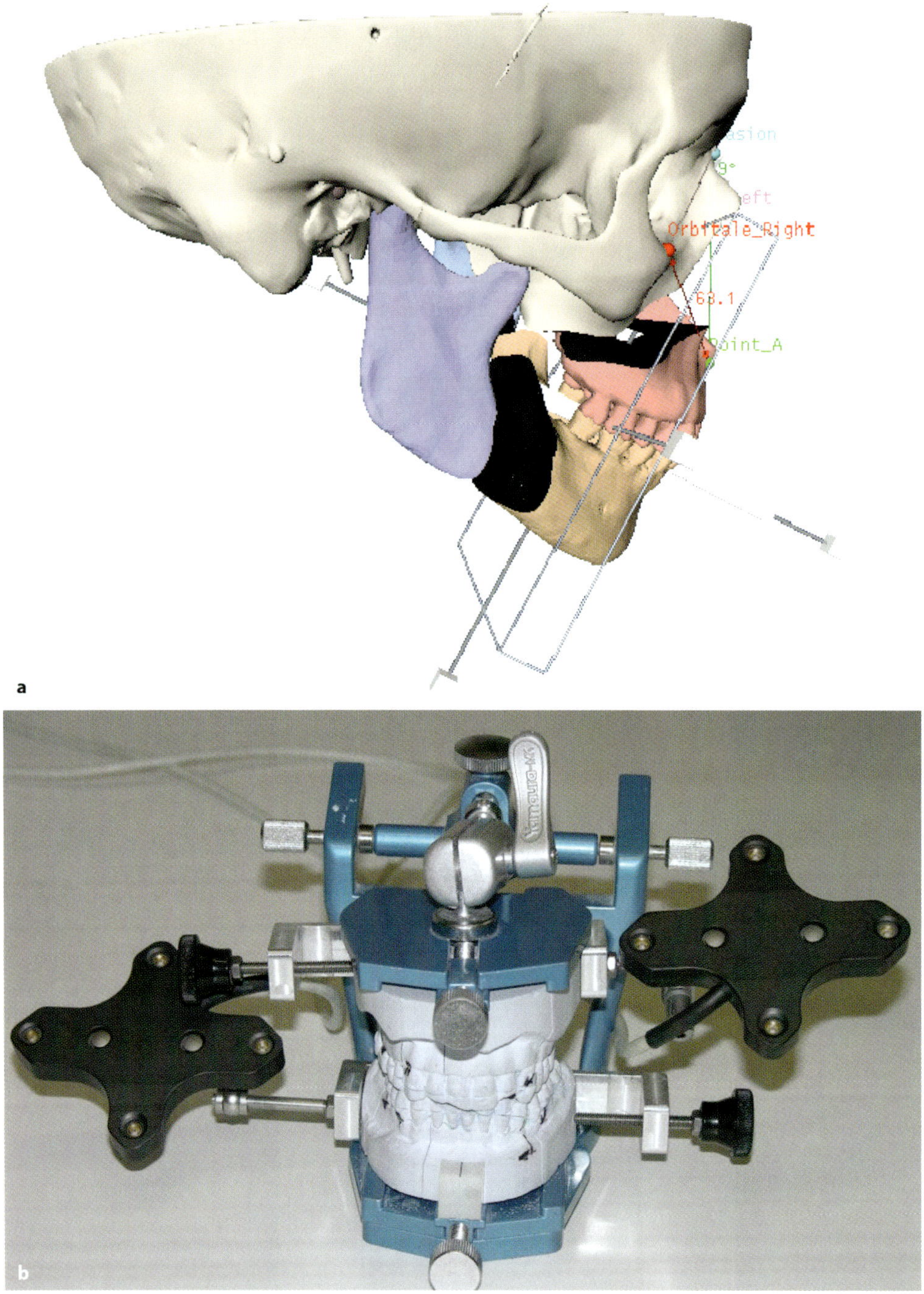

Fig. 121. Complex dysgnathia – transferring the CT plan to the articulator. By segmental navigation of the upper and lower parts of the articulator, a correlation can be established between the plaster models and the CT data set by registering the models with the registration splint. Movements of the upper part of the articulator can now be visualized in the CT data set by segmental navigation, and the position of the maxillary model can be adjusted to match the virtual plan (**a**). The articulator is fixed in that position, and the surgical splint for the maxilla is produced (**b**)

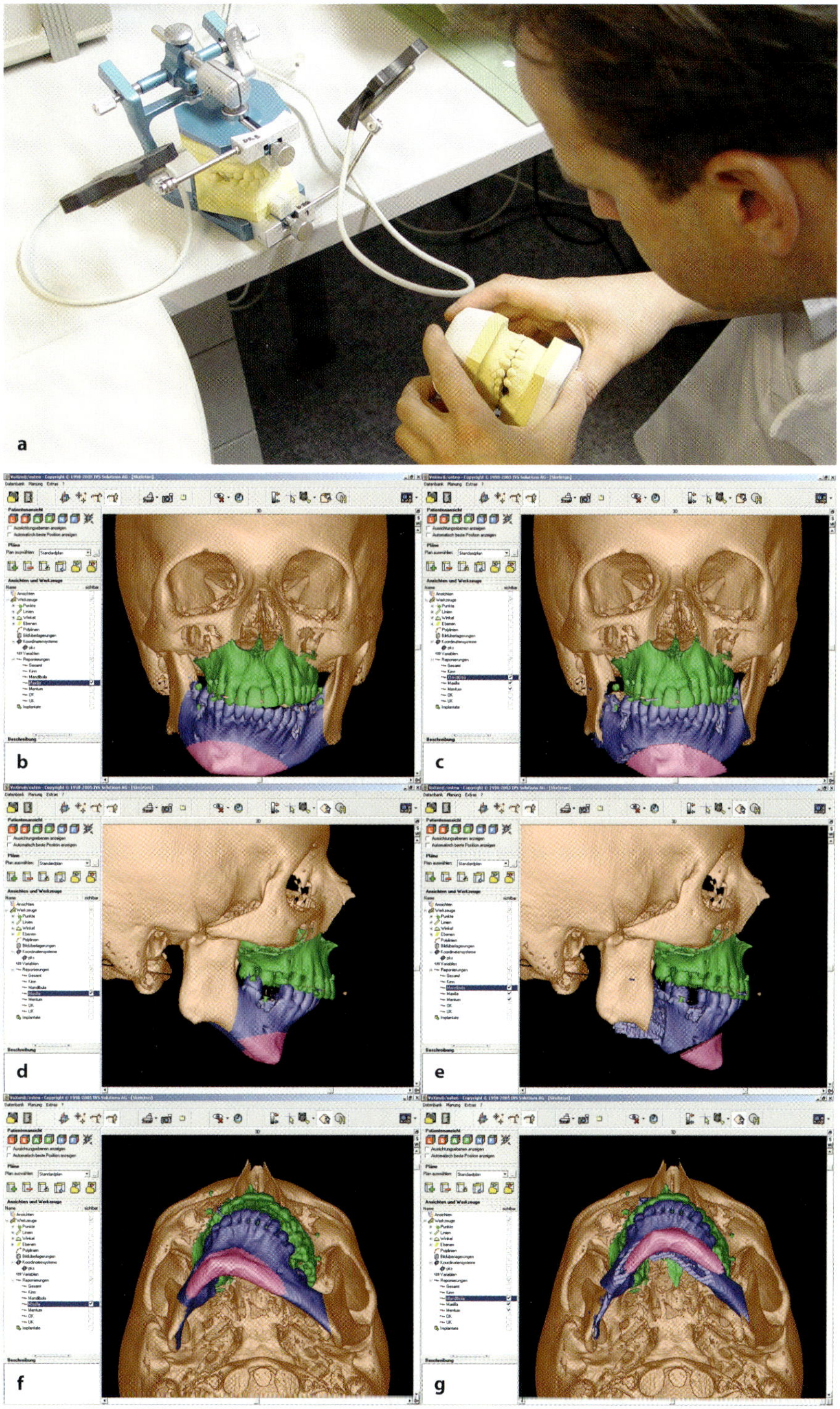

Fig. 122. Complex dysgnathia – planning the mandibular correction and mentoplasty. After the maxilla has been positioned, the mandible is placed in the desired occlusal relationship to the maxilla in the articulator (**a**). This correction is registered and simulated in the planning data set. Next a mentoplasty can also be simulated (**b–g**)

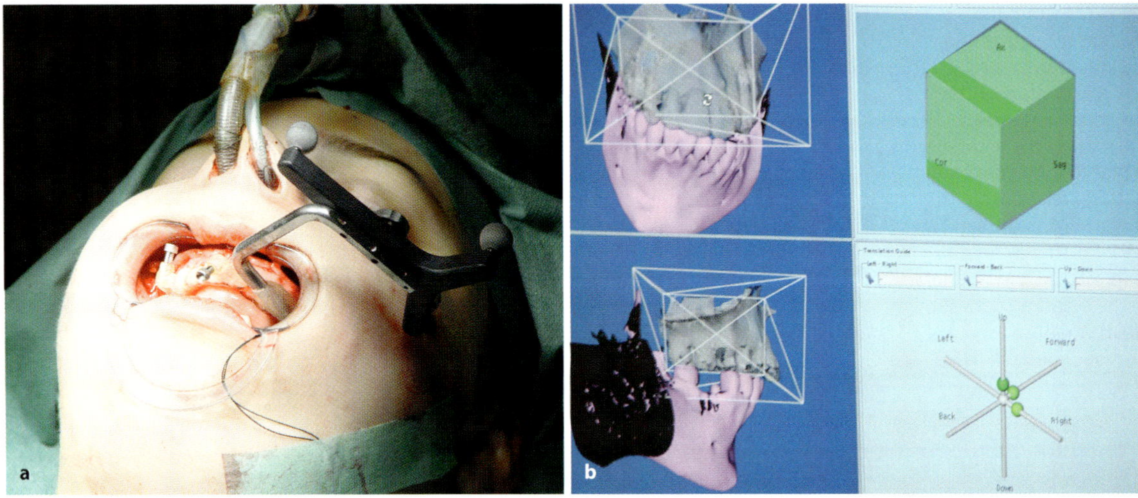

Fig. 123. Complex dysgnathia – intraoperative navigation. After the maxilla has been positioned with the surgical splint, its new position is checked on the monitor by segmental navigation and fine adjustments are made (**a**). The movements of the maxilla at this stage are tracked by a registration array that is attached to the registration splint (**b**)

When reliable surgical splints are available for intraoperative use, it is likely that intraoperative navigation can be dispensed with altogether. CAD/CAM-based fabrication of the surgical splint should be mentioned as a possible future trend in preoperative planning. However, this requires computer scanning of the plaster models and the use of cutting or polymerizing machines, which would substantially increase the costs. It seems doubtful that this technology would achieve more accurate results than the method described here.

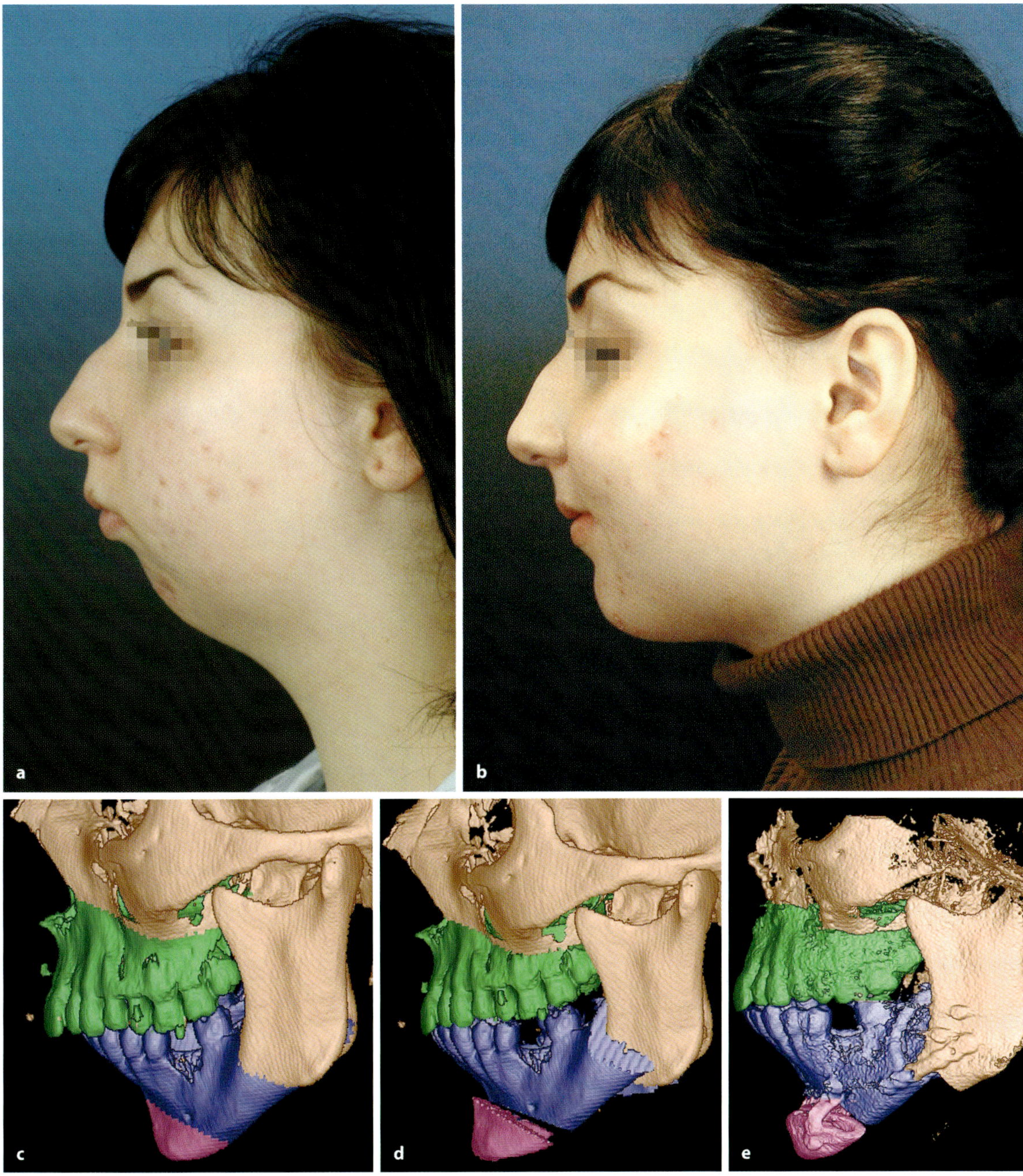

Fig. 124. Complex dysgnathia – postoperative evaluation. Comparison of clinical appearance before (a) and after (b) corrective osteotomy, and comparison of the preoperative CT data set (c) with the simulation (d) and postoperative DVT data set (e). Image fusion permits a metric comparison of the simulation and postoperative result

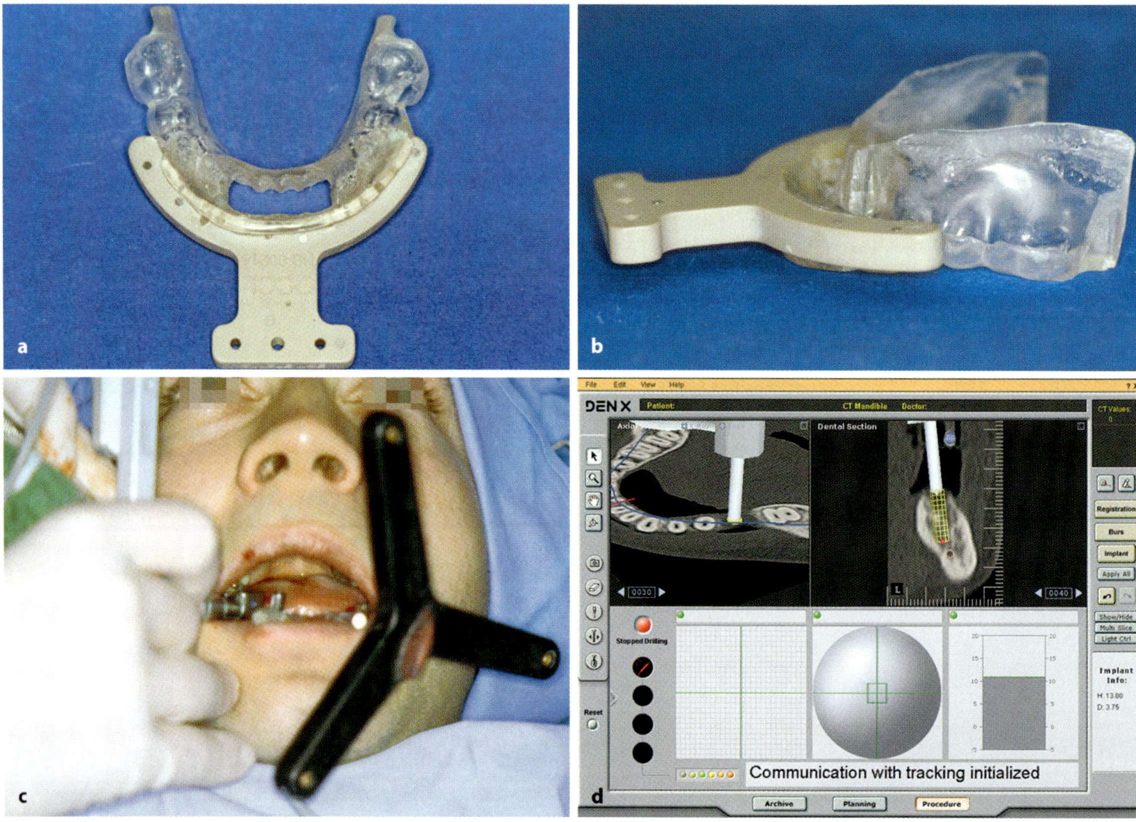

Fig. 125. Navigation-assisted insertion of dental implants. By attaching the registration array to a mandibular splint, it was possible even in 1997 to perform navigation-assisted predrilling for dental implants in the conscious patient (a, b). Using commercially available systems (Robodent), a ready-made frame is polymerized to a dental arch splint. The frame bears the registration markers, and a registration array can be attached to it intraoperatively (c). The intraoperative navigational interface (d) varies in different systems; the track-ball system (Confident, DenX) is very easy to handle

Implant Insertions

Despite initial euphoric reports on the use of intraoperative navigation in the insertion of dental implants, broad clinical application has failed to materialize. There are several reasons for this, including the fact that the equipment and logistical costs are disproportionately high in relation to the intraoperative gain. For example, registration in edentulous patients may be possible only after the preliminary insertion of temporary implants, because splint-based registration can be successful only in at least partially dentulous patients (Fig. 125).

The navigation errors that are measured in phantom models cannot be applied to the clinical situation; they usually show considerably greater values (Watzinger et al. 1999b; Meyer et al. 2003; Wagner et al. 2003). Because of these issues as well as problems of nonreimbursement, intraoperative navigation cannot be recommended for routine implantations. The main challenges in implantology relate to patient selection, planning, and soft tissue management. With adequate bone stock and careful preoperative planning, an experienced surgeon should be able to position dental implants with acceptable accuracy. More difficult are implantations in cases with borderline-deficient bone, where a few tenths of a millime-

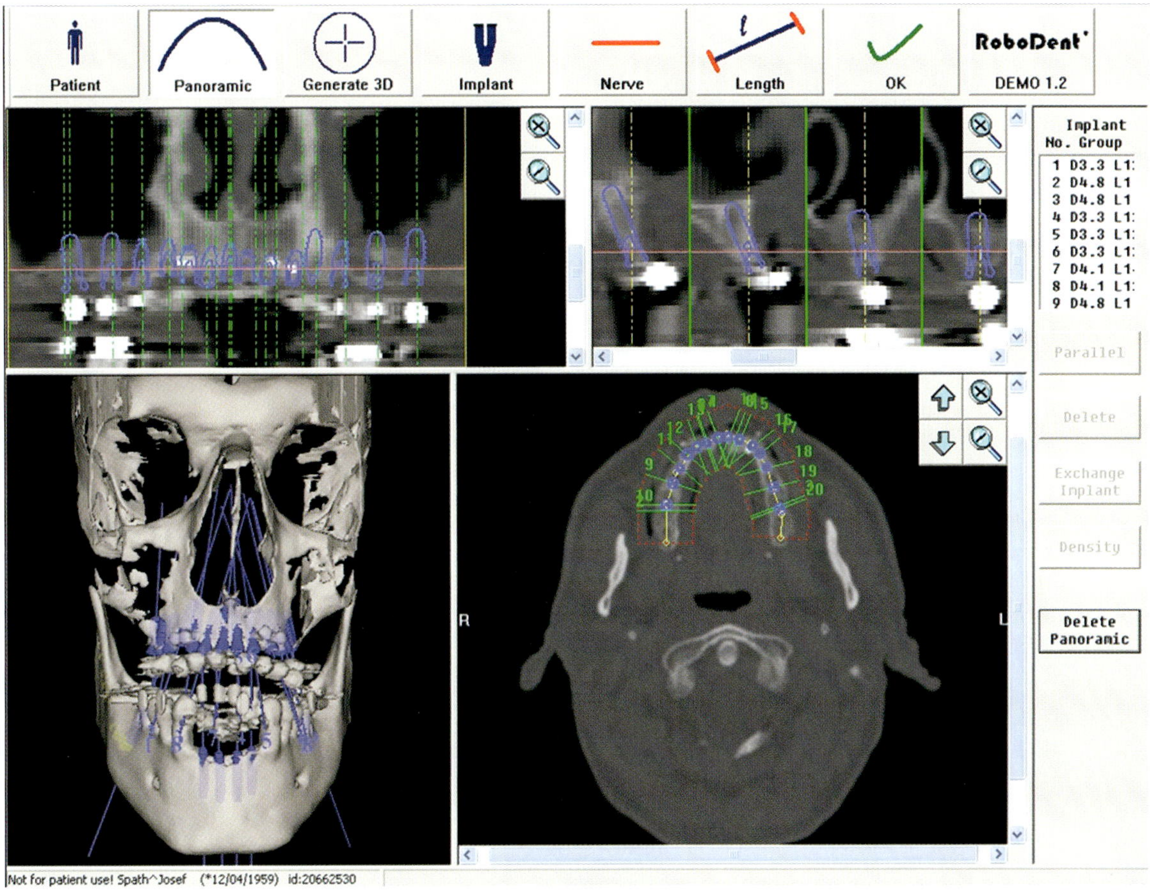

Fig. 126. Planning and simulation of dental implants. For complex issues in implantology, the need for augmentation or bone splitting can be determined preoperatively by a CT- or DVT-based analysis and simulation of the implant insertion. Intraoperative navigation was used only for the transgingival insertion of the two posterior mandibular implants

ter may prove critical. But even in these situations, the use of intraoperative navigation may not be helpful due to the problems noted above. By contrast, there is no question as to the advantage of 3D analysis and planning in complex cases based on CT imaging or DVT, which involves less radiation exposure. Three-dimensional planning can simulate the prosthetically correct positioning of the implants and can also help direct the preoperative decision for or against additional bone augmentation. Especially in the anterior part of the maxilla, it is difficult to make an accurate prediction based on conventional two-dimensional radiographs (Fig. 126).

Conversely, a rationale may exist for using intraoperative navigation for the transgingival insertion of implants, especially in the posterior part of the lower jaw (Randelzhofer et al. 2001). The ability to check the intraoperative position and especially the depth of implant insertions is helpful in avoiding injury to the inferior alveolar nerve (Fig. 127). But these cases are also indications for the use of CAD/CAM-fabricated drilling templates, which surpass the accuracy of intraoperative navigation (Fig. 128). One drawback of drilling template systems is that the presurgical plan cannot be modified during the operation. To summarize, it may be said that

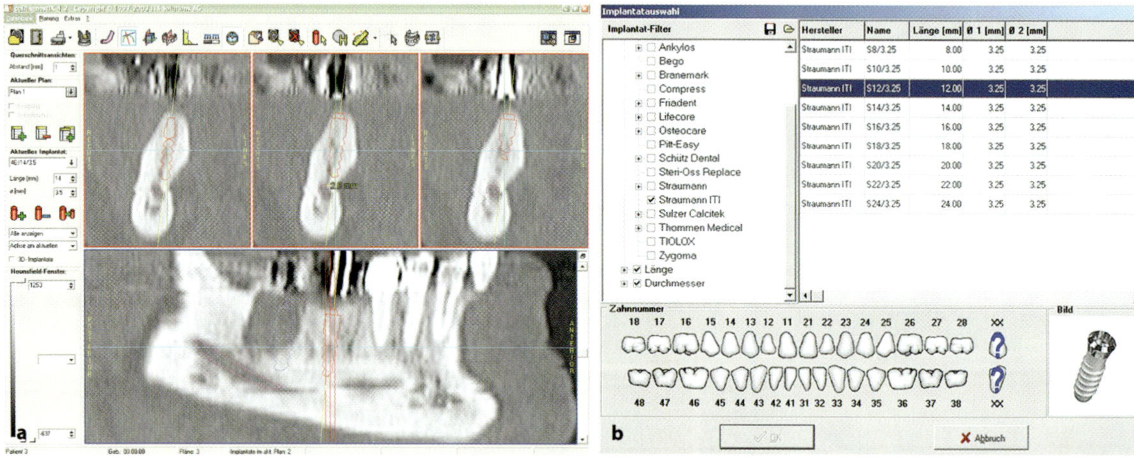

Fig. 127 a, b. Planning and simulation of dental implants. With modern software (CoDiagnostiX, IVS Solutions, Chemnitz), the planning of implant insertions in the posterior mandible can be done for any implant for which CAD data are available from the manufacturer

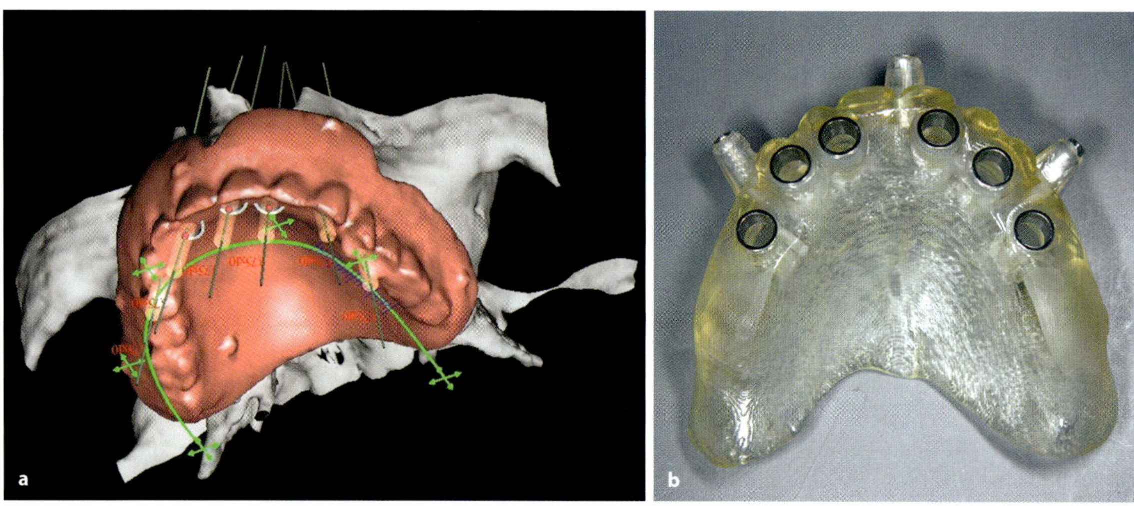

Fig. 128 a, b. Implant insertions with CAD-CAM drilling templates. The CT-based planning of implant position forms the basis for fabricating the drilling template. The template is attached to the jaw with transgingival pins. A specially designed instrument set permits accurate predrilling of the implant beds based on virtual planning (NobelGuide, Nobel Biocare)

intraoperative navigation does not have a significant role to play in standard implantology.

Zygomatic implants are another matter. These oversized dental implants are anchored in the zygoma through an intraoral approach. They represent an alternative – actually a second-line method – to treatment with traditional dental implants. Their indications include the prosthetic rehabilitation of malignant tumor resections when they may be expected to improve the patient's quality of life, especially if life expectancy is limited. They can also be used to treat maxillary defects in cases where bone augmentation is

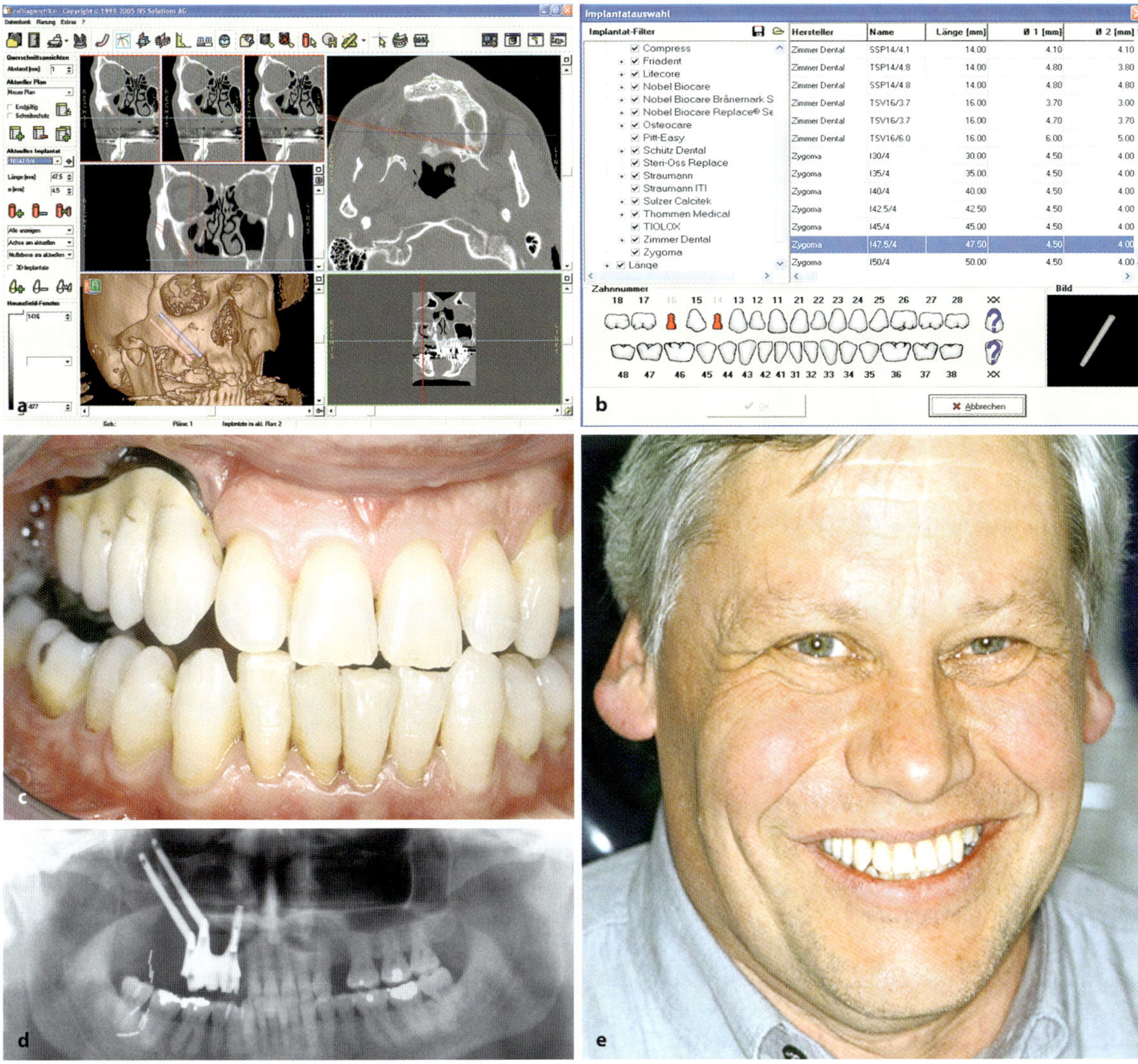

Fig. 129. Navigation-assisted insertion of zygomatic implants. The insertion of two zygomatic implants into the right zygoma was simulated for the prosthetic reconstruction of a maxillary resection (**a**). The selection of implants is based on CAD data supplied by the manufacturer (**b**). The maxillary registration splint is used for navigation-assisted drilling. **c–e** Postoperative clinical and radiographic results

not possible or is unlikely to be successful due to previous failed augmentations. Preoperative planning and intraoperative navigation during the insertion of these implants increase the safety margin for preserving vital structures (orbit, skull base) and help to ensure prosthetically correct positioning, especially during the unilateral placement of two implants. As noted earlier, the implants can be inserted immediately after a tumor resection, but it is far more common for zygomatic implants to be inserted secondarily (Fig. 129). Preoperative planning permits the virtual insertion of implants based on the specifications of the implant

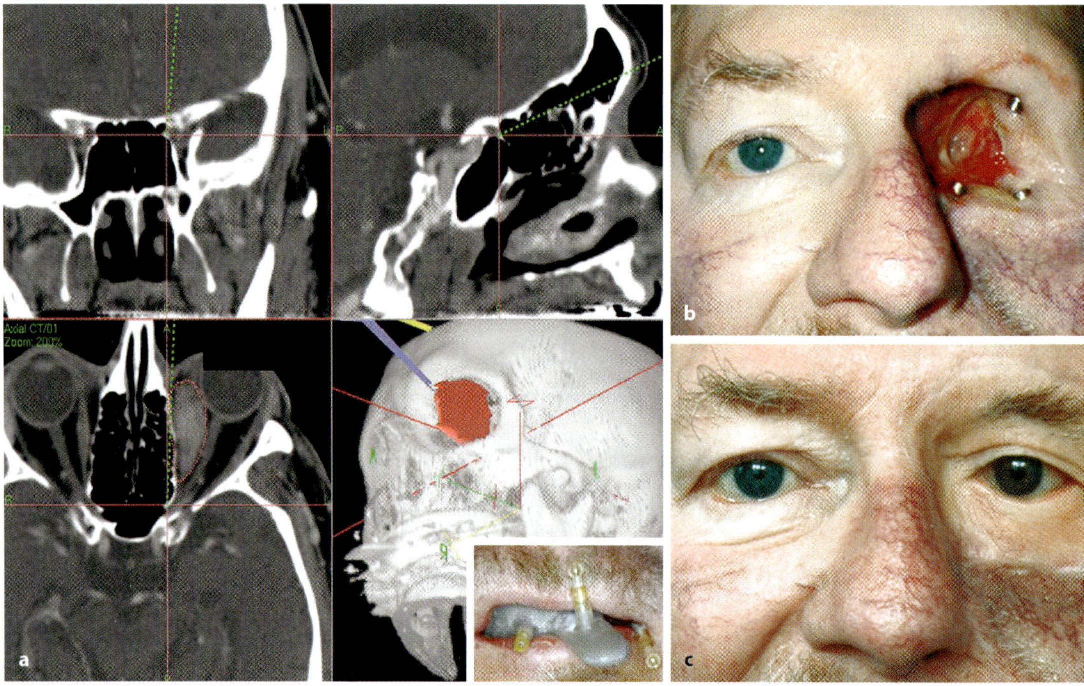

Fig. 130. Navigation-assisted resection of a left orbital tumor (intraoperative navigation, a) and secondary rehabilitation with an implant-anchored ocular prosthesis (b, c). Implant insertion was done with navigational guidance using the same registration splint

manufacturer, just as with standard implants. Visualization of the angled abutments permits optimum prosthetic alignment of the implants in the data set. At operation, the drilling is guided by intraoperative navigation using calibrated handpieces so that the presurgical planning can be transferred to the patient as accurately as possible (Schramm et al. 2000b).

In patients who have undergone orbital exenteration, the CT data sets acquired for the tumor resection can also be used for the simulation and intraoperative insertion of an epithesis for attaching an ocular prosthesis (Fig. 130). This can achieve an implant position that is optimum for the available periorbital bone stock. The same method can be used in the insertion of implants for attaching an auricular prosthesis (Fig. 131).

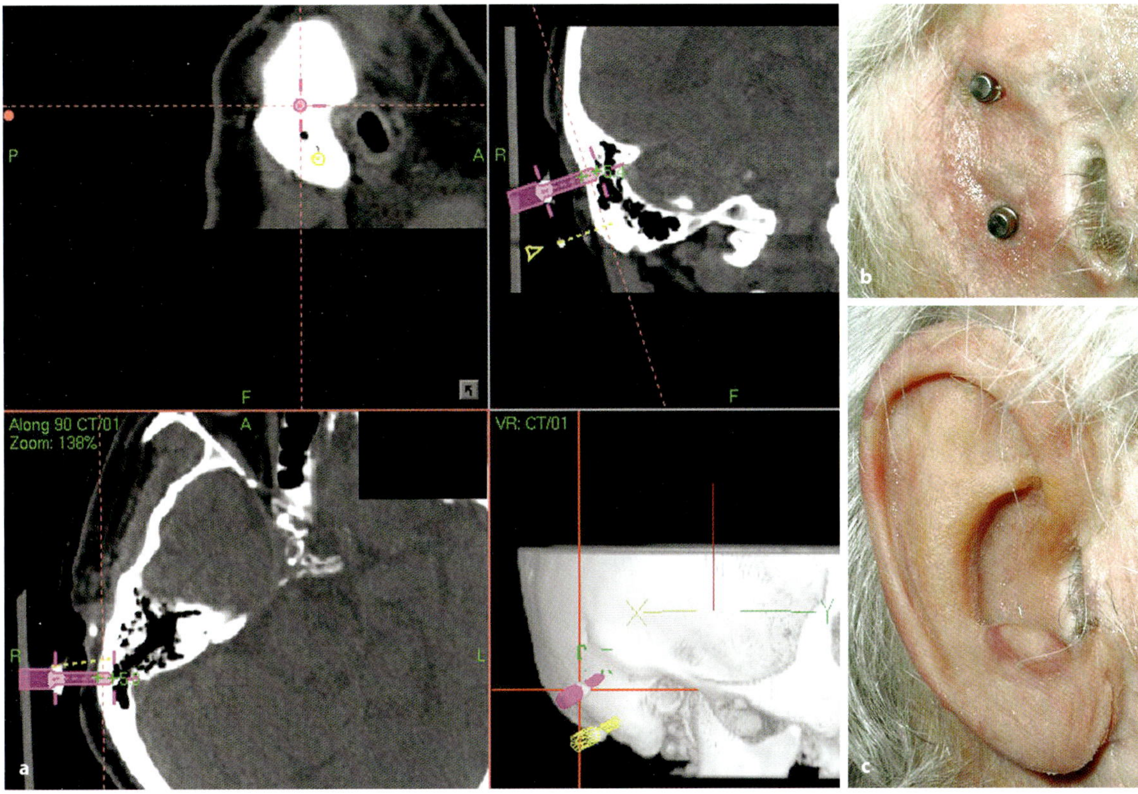

Fig. 131. Navigation-assisted insertion of implants for the attachment of an auricular prosthesis (a). b, c Postoperative clinical appearance with and without the prosthesis in place

References

Abbashi HR (1997): Virtuelle Realität in der Medizin: Stand, Trends, Entwicklung orthopädischer Modelle. Fakultät für theoretische Medizin der Universität Heidelberg, Dissertation

Alp MS, Dujovny M, Misra M, Charbel FT, Ausman JI (1998) Head registration techniques for image-guided surgery. Neurol Res 20:31–37

Altobelli DE, Kikinis R, Mulliken JB, Cline H, Lorensen W, Jolesz F (1993) Computer-assisted three-dimensional planning in craniofacial surgery. Plast Reconstr Surg 92:576–585

Amdur RJ, Gladstone D, Leopold KA, Harris RD (1999) Prostate seed implant quality assessment using MR and CT image fusion. Int J Radiat Oncol Biol Phys 43:67–72

Anon JB, Lipman SP, Oppenheim D, Halt RA (1994) Computer-assisted endoscopic sinus surgery. Laryngoscope 104:901–905

Anon JB, Klimek L, Mösges R, Zinreich SJ (1997) Computer-assisted endoscopic sinus surgery. Adv Sinus Nasal Surg 30:389–401

Apuzzo MLJ, Sabshin JK (1983) Computed tomographic guidance stereotaxis in the management of intracranial mass lesions. Neurosurgery 12:277–284

Arginteanu M, Abbott R, Frempong A (1998) ISG Viewing Wand-guided endoscopic catheter placement for treatment of posterior fossa CSF collections. Pediatr Neurosurg 27:319–324

Arun KS (1987) Least-squares fitting of two 3-D point sets. IEEE Trans. On Pattern Analysis and Machine Intelligence 9:698–700

Bale RJ, Vogele M, Freysinger W, Gunkel AR, Martin A, Bumm K, Thumfahrt WF (1997) Minimally invasive head holder to improve the performance of frameless stereotactic surgery. Laryngoscope 107:373–377

Barnett GH (1996) Surgical management of convexity and falcine meningeomas using interactive image-guided surgery sytems. Neurosurg Clin N Am 7:279–284

Barnett GH, Kormos DW, Steiner CP, Weisenberger J (1993) Intraoperative localization using an armless, frameless stereotactic wand. J Neurosurg 78:510–514

Berry J, O'Malley BW Jr, Humphries S, Staecker H (2003) Making image guidance work: understanding control of accuracy. Ann Otol Rhinol Laryngol 112:689–692

Bettega G, Dessenne V, Raphael B, Cinquin P (1996) Computer-assisted mandibular condyle positioning in orthognatic surgery. Int J Oral Maxillofac Surg 54:553–558

Bill JS, Reuther JF, Dittmann W, Meier JL, Pistner H, Wittenberg G (1995) Stereolithography in oral and maxillofacial operation planning. Int J Oral Maxillofac Surg 24:98–103

Boesecke R, Bruckner T, Ende G (1990) Landmark based correlation of medical images. Phys Med Biol 35:121–126

Bohner P, Holler C, Hassfeld S (1997) Operation planning in craniomaxillofacial surgery. Comput Aided Surg 5:153–161

Brinker T, Aarango G, Kaminski J, Samii A, Thorns U, Vorkapic P, Samii M (1998) An experimental approach to image guided skull base surgery employing a microscope-based neuronavigation system. Acta Neurochir (Wien) 140:883–889

Brix F, Hebbinghaus D, Meyer W (1985) Procedures and equipment for model building in relation to orthopedic and traumatologic surgery planning. Röntgenpraxis 38:290–292

Brown RA (1979) A computerized tomography-computer graphics approach to stereotaxic localisation. J Neurosurg 50:715–720

Bucholz RD, Ho HW, Rubin JP (1993) Variables affecting the accuracy of stereotactic localization using computerized tomography. J Neurosurg 79:667–673

Buchholz RD, Smith KR, Baumann C, McDumont L, Schulz D (1994) Intraoperative localization with an optical digitizer. Stereotact Funct Neurosurg 63:100

Carini S, Caöcagno E, Tortori-Donato P, Andreussi L (1992) A new model for non-invasive, reproducible fixation of a stereotaxic frame using an orthodontic resin plate. Acta Neurochir 118:159–161

Carls FR, Schuhknecht B, Sailer HF (1994) Value of three-dimensional computed tomography in craniomaxillofacial surgery. J Craniomaxillofac Surg 5:282–288

Carney AS, Patel N, Baldwin DL, Coakham HB, Sandeman DR (1996) Intra-operative image guidance in otolaryngology: the use of the ISG Viewing Wand. J Laryngol Otol 110:322–327

Carrau RL, Snyderman CH, Curtin HB, Weissman JL (1994) Computer-assisted frontal sinusotomy. Otolaryngol Head Neck Surg 727–732

Carrau RL, Snyderman CH, Curtin HD, Janeckia IP, Stechison M, Weissman JL (1996) Computer-assisted intraoperative navigation during skull base surgery. Am J Otolaryngol 79:95–101

Casler JD, Doolittle AM, Mair EA (2005) Endoscopic surgery of the anterior skull base. Laryngoscope 115:16–24

Caversaccio M, Ladrach K, Hausler R, Stucki M, Bachler R, Schroth G, Nolte LP (1997) Konzept eines rahmenlosen bildinteraktiven Navigationssystems für die Schädelbasis-, Nasen-, Nasennebenhöhlenchirurgie. Oto Rhino Laryngol Nova 7:121–126

Caversaccio M, Ladrach K, Bachler R, Schroth G, Nolte LP, Hausler R (1998) Computer-assisted surgical navigation with a dynamic mobile framework for the nasal fossae, sinuses and base of the skull. Ann Otolaryngol Chir Cervicofac 115:253–258

Caversaccio M, Nuyens M, Bachler R, Ladrach K, Schroth G, Nolte L, Hausler R (1999) Surgery of the skull base and paranasal sinuses assisted by a computerized navigation system without external orientation support. Acta Otorrinolaringol Esp 50:392–397

Caversaccio M, Nolte LP, Hausler R (2002) Present state and future perspectives of computer aided surgery in the field of ENT and skull base. Acta Otorhinolaryngol Belg 56:51–59

Chabrerie A, Ozlen F, Nakajima S, Leventon ME, Atsumi H, Grimson E, Keeve E, Helmers S, Riviello J Jr, Holmes G, Duffy F, Jolesz F, Kikinis R, McBlack P (1998) 3D reconstruction and surgical navigation in pediatric epilepsy surgery. Pediatr Neurosurg 27:304–310

Chapuis J, Langlotz F, Bläuer M, Halleramnn W, Schramm A, Caversaccio M (2005) A novel approach for computer-aided corrective jaw surgery. In: Computer Aided Surgery Around the Head, 3rd International Symposium Proceedings, Fortschritt-Berichte VDI 17(258):7–8

Cohen DS, Lustgarten JH, Miller E, Khandji AG, Goodman RR (1995) Effects of coregistration of MR to CT images on MR stereotactic accuracy. J Neurosurg 82:772–779

Colchester AC, Zhao J, Holton-Tainter KS, Henri CJ, Maitland N, Roberts PT, Harris CG, Evans RJ (1996) Development and preliminary evaluation of VISLAN, a surgical planning and guidance system using intra-operative video imaging. Med Image Anal 1:73–90

Cook WH, Walker JH, Barr MI (1951) A cytological study of transneuronal atrophy in the rat and the rabbit. J Comp Neurol 94:267–292

Cutting C (1992) Discussion on a stereotactic system for guiding complex craniofacial reconstruction. Plast Reconstr Surg 89:346–348

Davidson M (1938) The indirect traumatic optic atrophies. Am J Ophthalmol 21:7–21

De Greef S, Claes P, Mollemans W, Vandermeulen D, Suetens P, Willems G (2005) Computer-assisted facial reconstruction: recent developments and trends. Rev Belge Med Dent 60:237–249

Desgeorges M, Derosier C, Hor F, Cordoliani YS, Tarina M, Soultrait F De, Bernard C, Khadiri M, Debono B (1997) Réseaux d'imageurs simulation chirurgicale, neurochirurgie guideé par ordinateur. J Neuroradiol 24:108–115

Dittmar C (1873) Über die Lage des sogenannten Gefässzentrums der Medulla oblongata. Ber Saechs Ges Wiss Leipzig (math. Phys) 25:449–469

Dorward NL, Alberti O, Dijkstra A, Buurman J, Kitchen ND, Thomas DG (1997) Clinical introduction of an adjustable rigid instrument holder for frameless stereotactic interventions. Comput Aided Surg 5:180–185

Drake JM, Joy M, Goldenberg A, Kreindler D (1991) Computer- and robot-assisted resection of thalamic astrocytomas in children. Neurosurgery 79:27–33

Dyer PV, Patel N, Pell GM, Cummins B, Sandeman DR (1995) The ISG Viewing Wand: an application to atlanto-axial cervical surgery using the LeFort-I maxillary osteotomy. Br J Oral Maxillofac Surg 33:370–374

Ecke U, Maurer J, Boor S, Khan M, Mann WJ (2003) Common errors of intraoperative navigation in lateral skull base surgery. HNO 51:386–393

Edinger DH (1999) Intraoperative Computernavigation in der Implantologie. Phillip J 3:121–127

Eggers G, Muhling J, Marmulla R (2005) Template-based registration for image-guided maxillofacial surgery. J Oral Maxillofac Surg 63:1330–1336

Ellis E, Tan Y (2003) Assessment of internal orbital reconstructions for pure blowout fractures: cranial bone grafts versus titanium mesh. J Oral Maxillofac Surg 61:442–453

Engelhardt A (2000) Konzept eines navigationsgestützten Therapiesystems für die Mund-, Kiefer- und Gesichtschirurgie. Fakultät für Medizin der Universität Heidelberg, Dissertation

Eufinger H, Weihe S, Rasche C, Wehmöller M, Schramm A, Wittkampf ARM (2001) The use of individual surgical templates in CAS. In: Lemke HU, Vannier MW, Inamura K, Farman AG, Doi K (eds) CARS 2001. Elsevier, New York, pp 117–121

Ewers R, Schicho K, Undt G, Wanschitz F, Truppe M, Seemann R, Wagner A (2005) Basic research and 12 years of clinical experience in computer-assisted navigation technology: a review. Int J Oral Maxillofac Surg 34:1–8

Fleiner B, Hoffmeister B, Kreusch T, Lambrecht K, Lambrecht T (1994) Dreidimensionale Operationsplanung am Modell - eine kritische Bestandsaufnahme. In: Schuchardt K, Schwenzer N (eds) Fortschritte der Kiefer- und Gesichtschirurgie - Ein Jahrbuch, vol XXXIX: Rekonstruktion des Gesichtsschädels. Thieme, Stuttgart, pp 13–16

Freysinger W, Gunkel AR, Martin A, Bale RJ, Vogele M, Thumfahrt WF (1997a) Advancing ear, nose and throat computer-assisted surgery with the armbased ISG Viewing Wand: the stereotactic suction tube. Laryngoscope 67:690–693

Freysinger W, Gunkel AR, Thumfahrt WF (1997b) Image-guided endoscopic ENT surgery. Eur Arch Otorhinolaryngol 254:343–346

Fried MP, Kleefield J, Gopal H, Reardon E, Ho BT, Kuhn FA (1997) Image-guided endoscopic surgery: results of accuracy and performance in a multicenter clinical study using an electromagnetic tracking system. Laryngoscope 43: 594–601

Garston JB (1970) Two cases of optic canal injury. In: Bleeker, Lyle (eds) Fractures of the Orbit. Williams and Wilkins, Baltimore, pp 165–166

Gellrich NC (1999) Controversies and current status of therapy of optic nerve damage in craniofacial traumatology and surgery. Mund Kiefer Gesichtschir 3:176–194

Gellrich NC, Schramm A (2002) Clinical application of computer-assisted reconstruction in complex posttraumatic deformities. In: Ward Booth P, Eppley B, Schmelzeisen R (eds) Maxillofacial Trauma and Esthetic Facial Reconstruction. Elsevier, London, pp 137–153

Gellrich NC, Schramm A, Hammer B, Schmelzeisen R (1999a) The value of computer aided planning and intraoperative navigation in orbital reconstruction. Int J Oral Maxillofac Surg 28:52–53

Gellrich NC, Schramm A, Gutwald R, Schön R, Husstedt H, Schmelzeisen R (1999b) Computer assisted planning and surgery in orbital reconstruction. In: Lemke HU, Inamura K, Vannier MW, Farman AG (eds) CARS 1999. Elsevier, New York. p 1042

Gellrich NC, Schramm A, Schimming R, Gutwald R, Schön R, Schmelzeisen R (2001) Recent advances in reconstruction of major craniofacial deformities: combination of computer-assisted reoperative planning with navigation, distraction and individual implants. Int J Oral Maxillofac Surg 30:65

Gellrich NC, Schramm A, Hammer B, Rojas S, Cufi D, Lagrèze W, Schmelzeisen R (2002a) Computer-assisted secondary reconstruction of unilateral posttraumatic orbital deformities. Plast Reconstr Surg 110:1417–1429

Gellrich NC, Schramm A, Gutwald R, Schmelzeisen R (2002b) Virtuelle Modelloperation und computer-assistierte Orbitarekonstruktion: neue Möglichkeiten in der rekonstruktiven Gesichtschirurgie. In: Wörn H, Mühling J, Vahl C, Meinzer HP (eds) Rechner- und sensorgestützte Chirurgie. Köllen, Bonn, pp 251–257

Gellrich NC, Schramm A, Schipper J, Maier W, Schön R, Schmelzeisen R (2002c) Die computer-gestützte Rekonstruktion der Orbita und des Mittelgesichtes nach ablativer Tumorchirurgie durch 3D-Mesh: Neue Wege in der Primärversorgung von Tumorpatienten. In: Walter GF, Brandis A (eds) Erkrankungen der Schädelbasis.

Giller C, Purdy P (1990) A technique for computer-guided stereotaxis without preoperative head fixation. Comput Med Imaging Graph 14:231–235

Gillespie JE, Isherwood I (1986) Three-dimensional anatomical images from computed tomographic scans. Br J Radiol 59:289–292

Girod S, Keeve E, Girod B (1995) Advances in interactive craniofacial surgery planning by 3D simulation and visualization. Int J Oral Maxillofac Surg 37:120–125

Gladilin E, Zachow S, Deuflhard P, Hege HC (2004) Anatomy- and physics-based facial animation for craniofacial surgery simulations. Med Biol Eng Comput 42:167–170

Goerss S, Kelly PJ, Kall B, Alker GJ (1982) A computed tomographic stereotactic adaptation system. Neurosurgery 54:375–379

Goldware S, Sylvester R, Baker L (1980) Delayed post traumatic optic neuropathy with recovery after unroofing of optic canal. Neuro-ophthalmol 1:77–78

Golfinos JG, Fitzpatrick BC, Smith LR, Spetzler RF (1995) Clinical use of a frameless stereotactic arm: results of 325 cases. J Neurosurg 83:197–205

Grunert P, Darabi K, Espinosa J, Filippi R (2002) Computer-aided navigation in neurosurgery. Neurosurg Rev 26:73–99

Gunkel AR, Freysinger W, Thumfart WF, Pototschnig C (1995) Complete sphenoethmoidectomy and computer-assisted surgery. Acta Otorhinolaryngol Belg 49:257–261

Gunkel AR, Freysinger W, Martin A, Völklein C, Bale RJ, Vogele M, Thumfahrt WF (1997a) 3D image-guided endonasal surgery with a microdebrider. Laryngoscope 107:834–838

Gunkel AR, Freysinger W, Thumfahrt WF, Truppe MJ, Gaber O, Künzler KH, Platzer W, Tiefenbrunner F (1997b) Otorhinolaryngologic computer-assisted biopsies of the iceman. Arch Otolaryngol 123:253–256

Gunkel AR, Freysinger W, Thumfahrt WF (1997c) Computer-assisted surgery in the frontal and maxillary sinus. Laryngoscope 107:631–633

Guthrie BL, Adler JR (1992) Computer-assisted preoperative planning, interactive surgery and frameless stereotaxy. Clin Neurosurg 38:112–131

Haegen TW, Keefe MA, Keefe KS (2005) Use of image-guided systems in the reconstruction of the periorbital region. Arch Facial Plast Surg 7:266–271

Hammer B, Kunz C, Schramm A, deRoche R, Prein J (1999) Repair of complex orbital fractures: technical problems, state-of-the-art, solutions and future perspectives. Ann Acad Med Singapore 28:687–691

Hassfeld S (2000) Rechnerunterstützte Planung und intraoperative Instrumenten-navigation in der Mund-, Kiefer- und Gesichtschirurgie. Eine experimentelle und klinische Studie. In: Habilitationsschriften der Zahn-, Mund- und Kieferheilkunde. Quintessenz, Berlin

Hassfeld S, Mühling J (2001) Computer assisted oral and maxillofacial surgery: a review and an assessment of technology. Int J Oral Maxillofac Surg 30:2–13

Hassfeld S, Mühling J, Zöller J (1994) Planung und Durchführung von Mittelgesichtsverlagerungen mit Hilfe eines 3D-Navigationsgerätes. Mund Kiefer Gesichtschir 18:259–263

Hassfeld S, Mühling J, Zöller J (1995a) Intraoperative navigation in oral and maxillofacial surgery. Int J Oral Maxillofac Surg 24:111–119

Hassfeld S, Zöller J, Wirtz CR, Albert FK, Knauth M, Mühling J (1995b) Computergestützte Chirurgie an der Schädelbasis. Mund Kiefer Gesichtschir 19:216–220

Hassfeld S, Raczkowski J, Bohner P, Hofele C, Holler C, Mühling J, Rembold U (1997) Robotik in der Mund-Kiefer-Gesichtschirurgie. Mund Kiefer Gesichtschir 1:316–323

Hassfeld S, Zöller J, Albert FK, Wirtz CR, Knauth M, Mühling J (1998a) Preoperative planning and intraoperative navigation in skull base surgery. J Craniomaxillofac Surg 26:220–225

Hassfeld S, Mühling J, Zöller J (1998b) Possibilities and developments of intraoperative image-guided surgery in craniofacial surgery. Mund Kiefer Gesichtschir 2:20–24

Hassfeld S, Brief J, Krempien R, Raczkowsky J, Münchenberg J, Giess H, Meinzer HP, Mende U, Wörn H, Mühling J (2000) Computerunterstützte Mund-, Kiefer- und Gesichtschirurgie. Radiologe 40:218–226

Hauser B, Westermann B, Reinhardt H, Probst R (1996) Computerunterstützte Chirurgie der Nasennebenhöhlen mit einem optoelektronischen Ortungssystem. Laryngorhinootologie 75:199–207

Hauser R, Westermann B, Probst R (1997) Noninvasive tracking of patient's head movements during computer-assisted intranasal microscopic surgery. Laryngoscope 107:491–499

Hayashi N, Kurimoto M, Hirashima Y, Ikeda H, Shibata T, Tomita T, Endo S (2001) Efficacy of navigation in skull base surgery using composite computer graphics of magnetic resonance and computed tomography images. Neurol Med Chir (Tokyo) 41:335–339

Heermann R, Schwab B, Issing PR, Haupt C, Hempel C, Lenarz T (2001) Image-guided surgery of the anterior skull base. Acta Otolaryngol 121:973–978

Heiland M, Habermann CR, Schmelzle R (2004) Indications and limitations of intraoperative navigation in maxillofacial surgery. J Oral Maxillofac Surg 62:1059–1063

Heilbrunn MP, McDonald P, Wiker C, Köhler S, Peters W (1992) Stereotactic localization and guidance using a machine vision technique. Stereotact Funct Neurosurg 58:94–98

Hemmy DC, David DJ, Herman GT (1983) Three-dimensional reconstruction of craniofacial deformity using computed tomography. Neurosurgery 13:534–541

Henderson JM, Smith KR, Bucholz RD (1994) An accurate and ergonomic method of registration for image-guided neurosurgery. Comput Med Imaging Graph 18:273–277

Hilbert M, Marmulla R, Strutz J (1998a) Vergleichende Genauigkeitsmessung zwischen einem mechanischen (Viewing Wand) und einem lasergeleiteten mikroskopischen Positionierungssystem (MKM) mit Hilfe eines geometrischen Meßobjekts. HNO 46:44–49

Hilbert M, Müller W, Strutz J (1998b) Entwicklung eines Operationssimulators für Eingriffe an den Nasennebenhöhlen. Laryngorhinootologie 77:153–156

Hill DL, Hawkes DJ, Hussain Z, Green SE, Ruff CF, Robinson GP (1993) Accurate combination of CT and MR data of the head: validation and applications in surgical and therapy planning. Comput Med Imaging Graph 17:357–363

Hill DL, Hawkes DJ, Gleeson MJ, Cox TC, Strong AJ, Wong WL, Ruff CF, Kitchen ND, Thomas DG, Sofat A (1994) Accurate frameless registration of MR and CT images of the head: applications in planning surgery and radiation therapy. Radiology 191:447–454

Hoffmann J, Westendorff C, Troitzsch D, Ernemann U, Reinert S (2004) Image-guided navigation for the control interstitial laser therapy of vascular malformations in the head and neck region. Biomed Tech (Berl) 49:199–201

Hoffmann J, Westendorff C, Leitner C, Bartz D, Reinert S (2005a) Validation of 3D-laser surface registration for image-guided cranio-maxillofacial surgery. J Craniomaxillofac Surg 33:13–18

Hoffmann J, Westendorff C, Schneider M, Reinert S (2005b) Accuracy assessment of image-guided implant surgery: an experimental study. Int J Oral Maxillofac Implants 20:382–386

Hoffmann J, Westendorff C, Gomez-Roman G, Reinert S (2005c) Accuracy of navigation-guided socket drilling before implant installation compared to the conventional free-hand method in a synthetic edentulous lower jaw model. Clin Oral Implants Res 16:609–614

Hohlweg-Majert B, Schon R, Schmelzeisen R, Gellrich NC, Schramm A (2005) Navigational maxillofacial surgery using virtual models. World J Surg 29:1530–1538

Hohoff A, Meier N, Stamm T, Ehmer U, Joos U (2002) Optimizing presurgical orthodontic planning by means of the transverse coordinate simulation system (TCSS). J Craniomaxillofac Surg 30:75–86

Holck DE, Boyd EM Jr, Ng J, Mauffray RO (1999) Benefits of stereolithography in orbital reconstruction. Ophthalmology 106:1214–1218

Horsley V, Clarke RH (1908) The structure and function of the cerebellum examined by a new method. Brain 31:45–124

Horstmann GA, Reinhardt HF (1994a) Micro-stereometry: a frameless computerized navigating system for open microsurgery. Comput Med Imaging Graph 229–233

Horstmann GA, Reinhardt HF (1994b) Ranging accuracy test of the sonic microstereometric system. Neurosurgery 745–755

Howard MA 3rd, Dobbs MB, Simonson TM, LaVelle WE, Granner MA (1995) A noninvasive, reattachable skull fiducial marker system. Technical note. J Neurosurg 83:372–376

Husstedt HW, Heermann R, Becker H (1999) Contribution of low-dose CT-scan protocols to the total positioning error in computer-assisted surgery. Comput Aided Surg 4:275–280

Hwang PH, Maccabee M, Lindgren JA (2002) Headset-related sensory and motor neuropathies in image-guided sinus surgery. Arch Otolaryngol Head Neck Surg 128:589–591

Iseki H, Kawamura H, Tanikawa T, Kawabatake H, Taira T, Takakura K, Dohi T, Hata N (1994) An image-guided stereotactic system for neurosurgical operations. Stereotact Funct Neurosurg 63:130–138

Kajiwara K, Nishizaki T, Ohmoto Y, Nomura S, Suzuki M (2003) Image-guided transsphenoidal surgery for pituitary lesions using Mehrkoordinaten Manipulator (MKM) navigation system. Minim Invasive Neurosurg 46:78–81

Kalfas IH, Kormos DW, Murphy MA, McKenzie RL, Barnett GH, Bell GR, Steiner CP, Trimble MB, Weisenberger JP (1995) Application of frameless stereotaxy to pedicle screw fixation of the spine. J Neurosurg 83:641–647

Kato A, Yoshimine T, Hayakawa T, Tomita Y, Ikeda T, Mitomo M, Harada K, Mogami H (1991) A frameless, armless navigational system for computer-assisted neurosurgery. J Neurosurg 74:845–849

Kavanagh KT (1994) Applications of image-directed robotics in otolaryngologic surgery. Laryngoscope 104:283–293

Kelly PJ (1986) Computer assisted stereotaxis. Neurology 36:535–541

Kikinis R, Gleason, PL, Moriarty TM, Moore MR, Alexander E, Stieg P, Matsumae M, Lorensen WE, Cline HE, Blach PM, Jolesz FA (1996) Computer-assisted interactive three-dimensional planning for neurosurgical procedures. Neurosurgery 38:640–649

Klimek L, Mösges R (1998) Computer-assistierte Chirurgie (CAS) in der HNO-Heilkunde. Laryngorhinootologie 77: 275–282

Klimek L, Mösges R, Lamprecht J, Korves B (1992a) Identifikation und Entfernung orbitaler Fremdkörper mit dem CAS (Computer-Assisted-Surgery) System. Laryngorhinootologie 71:221–223

Klimek L, Klein HM, Mösges R, Schmelzer B, Schneider W, Voy ED (1992b) Methoden zur Simulation operativer Eingriffe in der Kopf-Halschirurgie. HNO 40:446–452

Klimek L, Kainz J, Reul J, Mösges R (1993a) Vermeidung vaskulärer Komplikationen bei der endonasalen Nasennebenhöhlenchirurgie. HNO 41:582–586

Klimek L, Wenzel M, Mösges R (1993b) Computer-assisted orbital surgery. Ophthalmic Surg 24:411–417

Klimek L, Laborde G, Mösges R, Wenzel M (1993c) Ein neues Verfahren zur Entfernung von Fremdkörpern im Kopfbereich. Unfallchirurg 96:213–216

Klimek L, Mösges R, Laborde G, Korves B (1995) Computer-assisted image-guided surgery in pediatric skull-base procedures. Pediatr Surg 1673–1676

Koele W, Stammberger H, Lackner A, Reittner P (2002) Image guided surgery of paranasal sinuses and anterior skull base: five years experience with the InstaTrak-System. Acta Otorhinolaryngol Belg 56:51–59

Koivukangas J, Louhisalmi Y, Alalkuijala J, Oikarinen J (1993) Ultrasound-controlled neuronavigator guided brainsurgery. J Neurosurg 79:36–42

Komori T, Takato T, Akagawa T (1994) Use of a laser-hardened 3D-replica for simulated surgery. Int J Oral Maxillofac Surg 52:516–521

Kondziolka D, Lunsford LD (1996) Intraoperative navigation during resection of brain metastases. Neurosurg Clin N Am 7:267–277

Krückels G, Korves B, Klimek L, Mösges R (1996) Endoscopic surgery of the rhinobasis with a computer-assisted localizer. Surg Endosc 10:453–456

Kurzeja A, Wenzel M, Korves B, Mösges R (1994) Dekompression des Nervus opticus nach Frakturen des Riechschädels mit Hilfe von CAS (Computer Assisted Surgery). Laryngorhinootologie 73:274–276

Laborde G, Gilsbach J, Harders A, Klimek L, Mösges R, Krybus W (1992) Computer assisted localizer for planning of surgery and intra-operative orientation. Acta Neurochir (Wien) 119:166–170

Laborde G, Klimek L, Harders A, Gilsbach J (1993) Frameless stereotactic drainage of intracranial abscesses. Surg Neurol 40:16–21

Lambrecht JT, Brix F (1990) Individual skull model fabrication for craniofacial surgery. Cleft Palate J:382–387

Lattanzi JP, Fein DA, McNeeley SW, Shaer AH, Movsas B, Hanks GE (1997) Computed tomography-magnetic resonance image fusion: a clinical evaluation of an innovative approach for improved tumor localization in primary central nervous system lesions. Radiat Oncol Investig 5:195–205

League D (1995) Interactive, image-guided, stereotactic neurosurgery systems. AORN J 61:360–370

Leemüller R, Bendl R, Schlegel W (1996) Image-guided therapy planning for interventional stereotactic therapy of brain tumors. Radiologe 36:737–743

Lehnhardt E (1973) Die Dekompression des Nervus opticus bei Fraktur der Rhinobasis. HNO 21:158–160

Lehnhardt E, Schultz-Coulon HG (1975) Indication and prognosis of the transethmoidal decompression of the optical nerve in posttraumatic amaurosis. Arch Otorhinolaryngol 209:303–313

Leksell L, Jernberg B (1980) Stereotaxis and tomography. Acta Neurochir 52:1–7

Levin DN, Pelizzari CA, Chen GT, Chen CT, Cooper MD (1988) Retrospective geometric correlation of MR, CT and PET images. Radiology 169:817–823

Linder A, Rasse M, Wolf HP, Millesi W, Englmeier R, Friede I (1995) Indikationen und Anwendung stereolithographischer Schädelrekonstruktionen in der Mund-Kiefer-Gesichtschirurgie. Radiologe 35:578–582

Linney AD, Grindrod SR, Arridge SR, Moss JP (1989) Three-dimensional visualization of computerized tomography and laser scan data for the simulation of maxillo-facial surgery. Med Inform (Lond) 14:109–121

Maciunas RJ, Galloway RL, Fitzpatrick JM, Mandava VR, Edwards CA, Allen GS (1992a) A universal system for interactive image-directed neurosurgery. Stereotact Funct Neurosurg 58:108–113

Maciunas RJ, Galloway RL Jr, Latimer L, Cobb C, Zacharias E, Moore A, Madava VR (1992b) An independent application accuracy evaluation of stereotactic frame systems. Stereotact Funct Neurosurg 58:103–107

Maciunas RJ, Berger MS, Copeland B, Mayberg MR, Selker R, Allen GS (1996) A technique for interactive image-guided neurosurgical intervention in primary brain tumors. Neurosurg Clin N Am 7:245–266

Maes F, Collignon A, Vandermeulen D, Marchal G, Suetens P (1997) Multimodality image registration by maximization of mutual information. IEEE Trans Med Imaging 16: 187–198

Majdani O, Leinung M, Lenarz T, Heermann R (2003) Navigation-supported surgery in the head and neck region. Laryngorhinootologie 82:632–644

Mann W, Klimek L (1998) Indications for computer-assisted surgery in otorhinolaryngology. Comput Aided Surg 3: 202–204

Manwaring KH, Manwaring ML, Moss SD (1994) Magnetic field guided endoscopic dissection through a burr hole may avoid more invasive craniotomies. Acta Neurochir Suppl (Wien) 61:34–39

Marmulla R, Niederdellmann H (1998) Computer-assisted bone segment navigation. J Craniomaxillofac Surg 26:347–359

Marmulla R, Niederdellmann H (1999) Surgical planning of computer-assisted repositioning osteotomies. Plast Reconstr Surg 104:938–944

Marmulla R, Wagener H, Hilbert M, Niederdellmann H (1997a) Precision of computer-assisted systems in profile reconstructive interventions on the face. Mund Kiefer Gesichtschir 11:65–67

Marmulla R, Hilbert M, Niederdellmann H (1997b) Inherent precision of mechanical, infrared and laser-guided navigation systems for computer-assisted surgery. J Craniomaxillofacial Surg 25:192–197

Marmulla R, Hilbert M, Niederdellmann H (1998) Intraoperative Präzision mechanischer, elektromagnetischer, infrarot- und lasergeführter Navigationssysteme in der computergestützten Chirurgie. Mund Kiefer Gesichtschir 2: 145–148

Marmulla R, Hassfeld S, Luth T, Muhling J (2003) Laser-scan-based navigation in cranio-maxillofacial surgery. J Craniomaxillofac Surg 31:267–277

Marmulla R, Luth T, Muhling J, Hassfeld S (2004) Markerless laser registration in image-guided oral and maxillofacial surgery. J Oral Maxillofac Surg 62:845–851

Marmulla R, Eggers G, Muhling J (2005) Laser surface registration for lateral skull base surgery. Minim Invasive Neurosurg 48:181–185

Marsh J, Vannier M (1985) Comprehensive Care of Craniofacial Deformities. Mosby, St. Louis

McDermott MW, Gutin PH (1996) Image-guided surgery for skull base neoplasms using the ISG viewing wand. Neurosurg Clin N Am 7:285–295

Metson R, Glicklich RE, Cosenza M (1998) A comparison of image guidance systems for sinus surgery. Laryngoscope 108:1164–1170

Meyer U, Wiesmann HP, Runte C, Fillies T, Meier N, Lueth T, Joos U (2003) Evaluation of accuracy of insertion of dental implants and prosthetic treatment by computer-aided navigation in minipigs. Br J Oral Maxillofac Surg 41:102–108

Mommaerts MY, Jans G, Vander Sloten J, Staels PF, Van der Perre G, Gobin R (2001) On the assets of CAD planning for craniosynostosis surgery. J Craniofac Surg 12:547–554

Momose KJ, Joseph M (1991) Emergency decompression of the optic nerve in patients who lose vision with craniofacial fractures: the role of radiological examination. Neuroradiology 33:15–17

Mongioj V, Brusa A, Loi G, Pignoli E, Gramaglia A, Scorsetti M, Bombardieri E, Marchesini R (1999) Accuracy evaluation of fusion of CT, MR, and SPECT images using commercially available software packages (SRS PLATO and IFS). Int J Radiat Oncol Biol Phys 43:227–234

Mösges R (1993) Computerunterstützte Chirurgie der Schädelbasisregion: Ergänzung, Revolution oder Science-fiction? Eur Arch Otorhinolaryngol Suppl 1:373–383

Mösges R (1998) Computer-Assistierte Chirurgie im Kopf- und Halsbereich. Forum der Medizin-Informatik 4:4–9

Mösges R, Klimek L (1993) Computer-assisted surgery of the paranasal sinuses. J Otolaryngol 22:69–71

Mösges R, Korves B, Ammon J, Kremer B (1991) Computerunterstützte Positionierung für das Nachladeverfahren mit Iridium-192. HNO 39:429–432

Mukherji SK, Rosenman JG, Soltys M Boxwala A, Castillo M, Carrasco V Pizer SM (1996) A new technique for CT/MR fusion for skull base imaging. Skull Base Surg 6:141–146

Nabavi A, Manthei G, Blomer U, Kumpf L, Klinge H, Mehdorn HM (1995) Neuronavigation. Radiologe 35:573–577

Naumann S (2001) Die Präzision der non-invasiven Oberkiefer-Schienenreferenzierung bei der rahmenlosen Stereotaxie mit einem optischen Navigationssystem am Phantommodell. Fakultät für Medizin der Universität Freiburg, Dissertation

Nilius M (2001) Experimentelle Untersuchung zur Genauigkeit einer nicht invasiven, konfektionierten Navigationsschiene zur rahmenlosen Stereotaxie in der computergestützen Mund-, Kiefer- und Gesichtschirurgie. Fakultät für Medizin der Universität Freiburg, Dissertation

Nolte LP, Visarius H, Arm E, Langlotz F, Schwarzenbach O, Zamorano L (1995) Computer-aided fixation of spinal implants. J Image Guided Surg 1:88–93

Olivier A, Germano IM, Cukiert A, Peters T (1994) Frameless stereotaxy for surgery of the epilepsies: preliminary experience. J Neurosurg 81:629–633

Ossoff RH, Reinisch L (1994) Computer-assisted surgical techniques: a vision for the future of otolaryngology-head and neck surgery. J Otolaryngol 23:354–359

Papadopoulos MA, Christou PK, Christou PK, Athanasiou AE, Boettcher P, Zeilhofer HF, Sader R, Papadopulos NA (2002) Three-dimensional craniofacial reconstruction imaging. Oral Surg Oral Med Oral Pathol Oral Radiol Endod 93:382–393

Parsai EI, Ayyangar KM, Dobelbower RR, Siegel JA (1997) Clinical fusion of three-dimensional images using Bremsstrahlung SPECT and CT. J Nucl Med 38:319–324

Patil AA (1982) Computed tomography-oriented stereotactic system. Neurosurgery 370–373

Paul HA, Bargar WL, Mittlestadt B, Musits B, Taylor RH, Kazanzides P, Zuhars J, Williamson B, Hanson W (1992) Development of a surgical robot for cementless total hip arthroplasty. Clin Orthop 285:57–66

Pelizzari CA, Spelbring DR, Weichelbaum RR, Chen CT (1989) Accurate three-dimensional registration of CT, PET, and/or MR images of the brain. J Comput Assist Tomogr 13:20–26

Perry JH, Rosenbaum AE, Lunsford LD, Swinck CA, Zorub DS (1980) Computed tomography-guided stereotactic surgery: conception and development of a new stereotactic methodology. Neurosurgery 376–381

Perry M, Banks P, Richards R, Friedmann EP, Shaw P (1998) The use of computer-generated three-dimensional models in orbital reconstruction. Br J Oral Maxillofac Surg 36:275–284

Peters TM, Munger CJ, Takahashi AM, Evans AC, Olivier A (1994) Integration of stereoscopic DAS and 3D MRI for image-guided neurosurgery. Comput Med Imaging Graph 18:289–299

Petzold R, Zeilhofer HF, Kalender WA (1999) Rapid prototyping technology in medicine: basics and applications. Comput Med Imaging Graph 23:277–284

Ploder O, Wagner A, Enislidis G, Ewers R (1995) Computergestützte intraoperative Visualisierung von dentalen -Implantaten. Radiologe 35:569–572

Postec F, Bossard D, Disant F, Froehlich P (2002) Computer-assisted navigation system in pediatric intranasal surgery. Arch Otolaryngol Head Neck Surg 128:797–800

Raabe A, Krishnan R, Wolff R, Hermann E, Zimmermann M, Seifert V (2002) Laser surface scanning for patient registration in intracranial image-guided surgery. Neurosurgery 50:797–801

Raabe A, Krishnan R, Seifert V (2003) Actual aspects of image-guided surgery. Surg Technol Int 11:314–319

Ramieri G, Spada MC, Biancji SD, Berrone S (2000) Dimensions and volumes of the orbit and orbital fat in posttraumatic enophthalmos. Dentomaxillofac Radiol 29:302–311

Ramsay JH (1979) Optic nerve injury in fracture of the canal. Br J Ophthalmol 63:607–610

Randelzhofer P, de la Barrera JM, Spielberg M, Kurtz C, Strub JR (2001) Three-dimensional navigation in oral implantology: a preliminary investigation. Int J Periodontics Restorative Dent 21:617–626

Raveh J, Vuillemin T (1988) The surgical one-stage management of combined cranio-maxillo-facial and frontobasal fractures. J Craniomaxillofac Surg 16:350–358

Reinhardt HF, Zweifel HJ (1990) Interactive sonar-operated device for stereotactic and open surgery. Stereotact Funct Neurosurg 55:393–397

Reinhardt HF, Horstmann GA, Gratzl O (1991) Mikrochirurgische Entfernung tiefliegender Gefäßmißbildungen mit Hilfe der Sonar-Stereometrie. Ultraschall Med 12:80–84

Reinhardt HF, Horstmann GA, Gratzl O (1993) Sonic stereometry in microsurgical procedures for deep-seated brain tumors and vascular malformations. Neurosurgery 51–57

Reinhardt HF, Trippel M, Westermann B, Horstmann GA, Gratzl O (1996) Computer assisted brain surgery for small lesions in the central sensorimotor region. Acta Neurochir (Wien) 138:200–205

Roberts DW, Strohbehn JW, Hatch JF, Murray W, Kettenberger H (1986) A frameless stereotactic integration of computerized tomographic imaging and the operating microscope. J Neurosurg 65:545–549

Roessler K, Ungersboeck K, Aichholzer M, Dietrich W, Czech T, Heimberger K, Matula C, Koos WT (1998a) Image-guided neurosurgery comparing a pointer device system with a navigating microscope: a retrospective analysis of 208 cases. Minim Invasive Neurosurg 41:53–57

Roessler K, Ungersboeck K, Aichholzer M, Dietrich W, Goerzer H, Matula C, Czech T, Koos WT (1998b) Frameless stereotactic lesion contour-guided surgery using a computer-navigated microscope. Surg Neurol 49:282–289

Rojas S, Schramm A, Gellrich NC (2001) La navegación quirúrgica en el campo de la cirugía craneofacial: una revisión y evaluación de la tecnología y sus aplicaciones prácticas. Cirurgia Plastica 11:131–142

Roth M, Lanza DC, Zinreich J, Yousem D, Scanlan KA, Kennedy DW (1995) Advantages and disadvantages of 3D computed tomography intraoperative localization for functional endoscopic sinus surgery. Laryngoscope 105:1279–1286

Sader R, Zeilhofer H-F, Kliegis U, Deppe H, Horch HH (1997) Über die Genauigkeit von 3D-gestützten Operationsplanungen mit Rapidprototyping-Techniken. Mund Kiefer Gesichtschir 1:61–64

Sandemann DR, Patel N, Chandler C, Coakham HB, Griffith HB (1994) Advances in image-directed neurosurgery: preliminary experience with the ISG viewing wand compared with the Leksell G frame. Br J Neurosurg 8:529–544

Santler G (1998) The Graz hemisphere splint: a new precise, non-invasive method of replacing the dental arch of 3D-models by plaster models. J Craniomaxillofac Surg 26:169–173

Santler G (2000) 3-D COSMOS: a new 3-D model based computerised operation simulation and navigation system. J Craniomaxillofac Surg 28:287–293

Schipper J, Klenzner T, Berlis A, Maier W, Offergeld C, Schramm A, Gellrich NC (2005) Objectivity of therapeutic results following skull base surgery using virtual model analysis. HNO Dec 10 [Epub ahead of print]

Schlöndorff G, Mösges R, Meyer-Ebrecht D, Krybus W, Adams L (1989) CAS: Ein neuartiges Verfahren in der Kopf- und Halschirurgie. HNO 37:187–190

Schmelzeisen R, Schramm A (2002) Computer-assisted reconstruction of the facial skeleton. Arch Facial Plast Surg 5:437

Schmelzeisen R, Schramm A, Schön R (2000) Future perspectives in craniomaxillofacial reconstruction. Asian Dentech Proc 1:7–12
Schmelzeisen R, Gellrich NC, Schramm A, Schön R, Otten JE (2002a) Navigation-guided resection of temporomandibular joint ankylosis promotes safety in skull base surgery. J Oral Maxillofac Surg 60:1275–1283
Schmelzeisen R, Schramm A, Gellrich NC (2002b) Variationen des navigationsgestützten Zugangs zur lateralen Schädelbasis. In: Bootz F, Strauss G (eds) Die Chirurgie der lateralen Schädelbasis. Springer, Berlin Heidelberg New York, pp 128–137
Schramm A (2001) Navigational procedures in orthognathic surgery. J Kor Assoc Oral Maxillofac Surg 27:24–26
Schramm A, Gellrich NC, Schön R, Naumann S, Bühner U, Schmelzeisen R (1999a) Non-invasive referencing in computer assisted surgery. Med Biol Eng Comput 37:644–645
Schramm A, Gellrich NC, Gutwald R, Thoma L, Schmelzeisen R (1999b) Reconstructive computer assisted surgery of deformities by mirroring CT data sets. Comput Biol Med 37:974–975
Schramm A, Gellrich NC, Schön R, Schimming R, Schmelzeisen R (1999c) Advantages of computer assisted surgery in the treatment of cranio-maxillofacial tumors. In: Lemke HU, Inamura K, Vannier MW, Farman AG (eds) CARS 1999. Elsevier, New York, pp 903–907
Schramm A, Gellrich NC, Schipper J, Schön R, Buitrago-Téllez C, Schmelzeisen R (2000a) Sind rechnergeführte Navigationsverfahren bei schädelbasisnahen Eingriffen noch entbehrlich? Journal DGPW 21:32–33
Schramm A, Gellrich NC, Schimming R, Schmelzeisen R (2000b) Rechnergestützte Insertion von Zygomatikumimplantaten (Brånemark-System) nach ablativer Tumorchirurgie. Mund Kiefer Gesichtschir 4:292–295
Schramm A, Gellrich NC, Gutwald R, Schipper J, Bloss HG, Hustedt H, Schmelzeisen R, Otten JE (2000c) Indications for computer assisted treatment of cranio-maxillofacial tumors. Comput Aided Surg 5:343–352
Schramm A, Gellrich NC, Randelzhofer P, Schneider U, Gläser R, Schmelzeisen R (2000d) Use and abuse of navigational surgery in oral implantation. In: Lemke HU, Vannier MW, Inamura K, Farman AG, Doi K (eds). CARS 2000. Elsevier, New York, pp 923–926
Schramm A, Gellrich NC, Swaid S, Gutwald R, Schimming R Schmelzeisen R (2000e) Optic nerve decompression: advances and perspectives. J Craniomaxillofac Surg 28:30
Schramm A, Gellrich NC, Schimming R, Schön R, Gutwald R, Schmelzeisen R (2001a) Computer aided planning and intraoperative navigation in cranio-maxillofacial distraction. Int Poster J Dent Oral Med 3:105
Schramm A, Gellrich NC, Gutwald R, Schön R, Schimming R, Schmelzeisen R (2001b) Primary and secondary orbital reconstruction: indication for computer assisted treatment? Int J Oral Maxillofac Surg 30:92
Schramm A, Gellrich NC, Nilius M, Schön R, Schimming R, Gutwald R, Schmelzeisen R (2001c) Intraoperative accuracy of non-invasive registration in computer assisted craniomaxillofacial surgery. In: Lemke HU, Vannier MW, Inamura K, Farman AG, Doi K (eds). CARS 2001. Elsevier, New York, p 1152
Schramm A, Gellrich NC, Schimming R, Schön R, Gutwald R, Schmelzeisen R (2002a) Non-invasive registration in computer assisted cranio-maxillofacial surgery. In: Wörn H, Mühling J, Vahl C, Meinzer HP (eds) Rechner- und sensorgestützte Chirurgie. Köllen, Bonn, pp 258–269
Schramm A, Gellrich NC, Schön R, Gutwald R, Schmelzeisen R (2002b) Navigational maxillofacial surgery using virtual models. In: Tachibana E, Furukawa T, Mukai Y, Ma H (eds) Proc Intern Symp Modelling Applic, Daegu, Korea. pp 71–76
Schramm A, Schön R, Rücker M, Barth E-L, Zizelmann C, Gellrich N-C (2006) Computer assisted oral and maxillofacial reconstruction. Int J Comp Techn (CIT) 14:71–77
Schwestka-Polly R, Roese D, Kuhnt D, Hille KH (1993) Application of the model-positioning appliance for three-dimensional positioning of the maxilla in cast surgery. Int J Adult Orthodon Orthognath Surg 8(1):25–31
Selesnick SH, Kacker A (1999) Image-guided surgical navigation in otology and neurotology. Am J Otol 20:688–693
Siessegger M, Mischkowski RA, Schneider BT, Krug B, Klesper B, Zöller JE (2001) Image guided surgical navigation for removal of foreign bodies in the head and neck. J Cranio Maxillofac Surg 29:321–325
Sipos EP, Tebo SA, Zinreich SJ, Long DM, Brem H (1996) In vivo accuracy testing and clinical experience with the ISG Viewing Wand. Neurosurgery 39:194–202
Smith KR, Frank KJ, Bucholz RD (1994) The Neurostation: a highly accurate, minimally invasive solution to frameless stereotactic neurosurgery. Comput Med Imaging Graph 18:247–256
Spetzger U, Krombach GA, Reinges MT, Gilsbach JM, Schmidt T (1996) Navigierte Mikroneurochirurgie: Erfahrungen mit dem EasyGuide Neuro. Kontraste 9:2–8
Spiegel EA, Wycis HT, Marks M (1947) Stereotactic apparatus for operations on the human brain. Science 106:349–350
Stutzin JM, Cutting CB, McCarthy JG, Dufresne CR (1988) Radiographical documentation of direct injury of the intracanalicular segment of the optic nerve in the orbital apex syndrome. Ann Plast Surg 20:368–373
Takato T, Harii K, Hirabayashi S, Komuro Y, Yonehara Y, Susami T (1993) Mandibular lengthening by gradual distraction: analysis using accurate skull replicas. Br J Plast Surg 46: 686–693
Takizawa T (1993) Neurosurgical navigation using a noninvasive stereoadapter. Surg Neurol 40:299–305
Takizawa T, Soto S, Sanou A, Murakami Y (1993) Frameless isocentric stereotactic laser beam guide for image-directed microsurgery. Acta Neurochir (Wien) 125:177–180

Thoma L (1998) Computergestützte Planung und Durchführung einer Rekonstruktion im Bereich der Mund-, Kiefer- und Gesichtschirurgie. Fakultät für Mathematik und Informatik, Abt. Informationswissenschaft der Universität Konstanz: Diplomarbeit

Thomas DG, Gill SS, Wilson CB, Darling JL, Parkins CS (1990) Use of relocatable stereotactic frame to integrate positron emission tomography and computed tomography images: application in human malignant brain tumours. Stereotact Funct Neurosurg 54–55:388–392

Thumfahrt WF, Gunkel AR (1997) Neueste Entwicklungen in der intraoperativen 3D-Navigation im Hals-Nasen-Ohrenbereich. Laryngorhinootologie 76:700–703

Thumfahrt WF, Freysinger W, Gunkel AR, Truppe M (1997) 3D image-guided surgery on the example of the 5300-year-old Innsbruck iceman. Arch Otolaryngol 117:131–134

Troitzsch D, Hoffmann J, Dammann F, Bartz D, Reinert S (2003) Registration using three-dimensional laser surface scanning for navigation in oral and craniomaxillofacial surgery. Zentralbl Chir 128:551–556

Tronnier VM, Wirtz CR, Knauth M, Bonsanto MM, Hassfeld S, Albert FK, Kunze S (1996) Intraoperative computer-assisted neuronavigation in functional neurosurgery. Stereotact Funct Neurosurg 66:65–68

Truppe MJ, Freysinger W, Gunkel AR, Thumfart WF (1996) Remote-guided surgical navigation in ENT surgery. Stud Health Techn Inform 29:280–282

Vannier MW, Marsh JL (1996) Three-dimensional imaging, surgical planning, and image-guided therapy. Radiol Clin North Am 34:545–563

Vannier MW, Marsh JL, Warren JO (1984) Three dimensional CT reconstruction images for craniofacial surgical planning and evaluation. Radiology 150:179–184

Vannier MW, Marsh JL, Tsiaras A (1995) Craniofacial surgical planning and evaluation with computers. In: Taylor RH, Lavallee S, Burdea GC, Mösges R (eds) Computer-integrated Surgery: Technology and Clinical Applications. MIT Press, London

Vaughan ED (1996) The maxillofacial surgeon and cranial base surgery. Br J Oral Maxillofac Surg 34:4–17

Vinas FC, Zamorano L, Buciuc R, Li Hang Q, Shamsa F, Jiang Z, Diaz FG (1997) Application accuracy study of a semipermanent fiducial system for frameless stereotaxis. Comput Aided Surg 2:257–263

Vougioukas VI, Hubbe U, van Velthoven V, Freiman TM, Schramm A, Spetzger U (2004) Neuronavigation-assisted cranial reconstruction. Neurosurgery 55:162–167

Vrionis FD, Foley KT, Robertson JH, Shea JJ (1997) Use of cranial surface anatomic fiducials for interactive image-guided navigation in the temporal bone: a cadaveric study. Neurosurgery 40:755–763

Wagner A, Ploder O, Enislidis G, Truppe M, Ewers R (1995) Virtual image guided navigation in tumor surgery: technical innovation. J Craniomaxillofac Surg 23:271–273

Wagner A, Ploder O, Enislidis G, Truppe M, Ewers R (1996) Image-guided surgery. Int J Oral Maxillofac Surg 25:147–151

Wagner A, Rasse M, Millesi W, Ewers R (1997) Virtual reality for orthognathic surgery: the augmented reality environment concept. J Oral Maxillofac Surg 55:456–462

Wagner A, Wanschitz F, Birkfellner W, Zauza K, Klug C, Schicho K, Kainberger F, Czerny C, Bergmann H, Ewers R (2003) Computer-aided placement of endosseous oral implants in patients after ablative tumour surgery: assessment of accuracy. Clin Oral Implants Res 14:340–348

Waldhart E, Röthler G, Norer B, Puelacher W (2000) Versorgung von Mittelgesichtsfrakturen. Mund Kiefer Gesichtschir 4:118–125

Walker DG, Ohaegbulam C, Black PM (2002) Frameless stereotaxy as an alternative to fluoroscopy for transsphenoidal surgery: use of the InstaTrak-3000 and a novel headset. J Clin Neurosci 9:294–297

Walters H, Walters DH (1986) Computerised planning of maxillo-facial osteotomies: the program and its clinical applications. Br J Oral Maxillofac Surg 24:178–189

Wang Z, Wang D, Chen Q, Luo D, Shen J (2002) Modification and application of anterior skull base microsurgery with navigation system. Zhonghua Yi Xue Za Zhi 82:879–882

Watanabe E, Watanabe T, Manaka S, Mayanagi Y, Takakura K (1987) 3D digitizer (Neuronavigator): new equipment for computed tomography-guided stereotactic surgery. Surg Neurol 27:543–547

Watanabe E, Mayanagi Y, Kosugi Y, Manaka S, Takakura K (1991) Open surgery assisted by the Neuronavigator, a stereotactic, articulated, sensitive arm. Neurosurgery 28: 792–799

Watzinger F, Wanschitz F, Wagner A, Enislidis G, Millesi W, Baumann A, Ewers R (1997) Computer-aided navigation in secondary reconstruction of post-traumatic deformities of the zygoma. J Craniomaxillofac Surg 25:198–202

Watzinger F, Wanschitz F, Rasse M, Millesi W, Schopper C, Kremser J, Birkfellner W, Sinko K, Ewers R (1999a) Computer-aided surgery in distraction osteogenesis of the maxilla and mandible. J Oral Maxillofac Surg 28:171–175

Watzinger F, Birkfellner W, Wanschitz F (1999b) Positioning of dental implants using computer-aided navigation and an optical tracking system: case report and presentation of a new method. J Craniomaxillofac Surg 27:77–81

Weihe S, Wehmöller M, Hassfeld S, Schramm A, Raczkowsky J, Gellrich NC, Eufinger H (2002) Der Einsatz von Resektionsschablonen, Navigation und Robotern zur Knochenresektion und einzeitigen Rekonstruktion mittels individueller CAD/CAM-Implantate im Bereich des Hirnschädels. In: Wörn H, Mühling J, Vahl C, Meinzer HP (eds) Rechner- und sensorgestützte Chirurgie. Köllen, Bonn, pp 227–235

Wenzel M, Klimek L, Korves B, Schütz W (1994) Extraktion von orbitalen Fremdkörpern mit Hilfe eines neuartigen Bildverarbeitungssystems. Ophthalmologe 91:31–35

Westendorff C, Hoffmann J, Troitzsch D, Dammann F, Reinert S (2004) Ossifying fibroma of the skull: interactive image-guided minimally invasive localization and resection. J Craniofac Surg 15:854–858

Westermann B, Trippel M, Reinhardt H (1995) Optically-navigable operating microscope for image-guided surgery. Minim Invasive Neurosurg 38:112–116

Westermark A, Zachow S, Eppley BL (2005) Three-dimensional osteotomy planning in maxillofacial surgery including soft tissue prediction. J Craniofac Surg 16:100–104

Wirtz CR, Kunze S (1998) Neuronavigation: Computerassistierte Neurochirurgie. Dt Aerztebl 95:1865–1871

Woods RP, Mazziotta JC, Cherry SR (1993) MRI-PET registration with automated algorithm. J Comput Assist Tomogr 17:536–546

Zamorano L, Kadi AM, Dong A (1992) Computer-assisted neurosurgery: simulation and automation. Stereotact Funct Neurosurg 59:115–122

Zamorano L, Nolte L, Jiang C, Kadi M (1993a) Image-guided neurosurgery: frame-based and frameless approaches. Neurosurg Operative Atlas 3:403–422

Zamorano L, Nolte L, Adi AM, Jiang Z (1993b) Interactive intraoperative localization using an infrared-based system. Neurol Res 15:290–298

Zeilhofer HF, Kliegis U, Sader R, Horch HH (1997) Videomatching als intraoperative Navigationshilfe bei profilverbessernden Operationen. Mund Kiefer Gesichtschir 1: 68–70

Zizelmann C, Gellrich NC, Metzger MC, Schoen R, Schmelzeisen R, Schramm A (2005a) Computer-assisted reconstruction of orbital floor based on cone beam tomography. Br J Oral Maxillofac Surg Aug 8 [Epub ahead of print]

Zizelmann C, Schramm A, Schon R, Ridder GJ, Maier W, Schipper J, Gellrich NC (2005b) Computer assisted methods in reconstructive and function-preserving orbital surgery. New capabilities of computer assisted preoperative surgical planning (CAPP) and computer assisted surgery (CAS). HNO 53:428–4